Nancy Clark's

Sports Nutrition Guidebook

FOURTH EDITION

Nancy Clark, MS, RD, CSSD

Healthworks Fitness Center

Chestnut Hill, MA

Human Kinetics

Library of Congress Cataloging-in-Publication Data

Clark, Nancy, 1951-
  [Sports nutrition guidebook]
  Nancy Clark's sports nutrition guidebook / Nancy Clark. -- 4th ed.
    p. cm.
  Includes bibliographical references and index.
  ISBN-13: 978-0-7360-7415-5 (soft cover)
  ISBN-10: 0-7360-7415-5 (soft cover)
  1. Athletes--Nutrition. I. Title. II. Title: Sports nutrition
guidebook.
  TX361.A8C54 2008
  613.2'024--dc22   2007051946

ISBN-10: 0-7360-7415-5 (print)
ISBN-13: 978-0-7360-7415-5 (print)
ISBN-10: 0-7360-8086-4 (Adobe PDF)
ISBN-13: 978-0-7360-8086-6 (Adobe PDF)
ISBN-10: 0-7360-7877-0 (Mobipocket)
ISBN-13: 978-0-7360-7877-1 (Mobipocket)
ISBN-10: 0-7360-7878-9 (Kindle)
ISBN-13: 978-0-7360-7878-8 (Kindle)

This publication is written and published to provide accurate and authoritative information relevant to the subject matter presented. It is published and sold with the understanding that the author and publisher are not engaged in rendering legal, medical, or other professional services by reason of their authorship or publication of this work. If medical or other expert assistance is required, the services of a competent professional person should be sought.

The Web addresses cited in this text were current as of January 2008, unless otherwise noted.

Developmental Editor: Heather Healy; **Assistant Editor:** Carla Zych; **Copyeditor:** Patricia McDonald; **Proofreader:** Jim Burns; **Indexer:** Nan N. Badgett; **Permission Manager:** Carly Breeding; **Graphic Designer:** Nancy Rasmus; **Graphic Artist:** Kim McFarland; **Cover Designer:** Keith Blomberg; **Photo Office Assistant:** Jason Allen; **Art Manager:** Kelly Hendren; **Associate Art Manager:** Alan L. Wilborn; **Illustrator:** Roberto Sabas; **Printer:** Versa Press

Human Kinetics books are available at special discounts for bulk purchase. Special editions or book excerpts can also be created to specification. For details, contact the Special Sales Manager at Human Kinetics.

Printed in the United States of America   10   9   8   7   6   5   4

The paper in this book is certified under a sustainable forestry program.

Human Kinetics
Web site: www.HumanKinetics.com

United States: Human Kinetics
P.O. Box 5076
Champaign, IL 61825-5076
800-747-4457
e-mail: humank@hkusa.com

Canada: Human Kinetics
475 Devonshire Road, Unit 100
Windsor, ON N8Y 2L5
800-465-7301 (in Canada only)
e-mail: info@hkcanada.com

Europe: Human Kinetics
107 Bradford Road
Stanningley
Leeds LS28 6AT, United Kingdom
+44 (0)113 255 5665
e-mail: hk@hkeurope.com

Australia: Human Kinetics
57A Price Avenue
Lower Mitcham, South Australia 5062
08 8372 0999
e-mail: info@hkaustralia.com

New Zealand: Human Kinetics
Division of Sports Distributors NZ Ltd.
P.O. Box 300 226 Albany
North Shore City, Auckland
0064 9 448 1207
e-mail: info@humankinetics.co.nz

*With appreciation for their patience, understanding,
and love, I dedicate this book to my husband, John,
and my children, John Michael and Mary.
They feed my heart, nourish my soul,
and empower my spirit.*

CONTENTS

PREFACE

"My diet is horrible. I'm so good at exercising—but I am so bad at eating right."

"I'm training hard but not getting the results I want. Something must be wrong with my diet."

"I feel so confused about what to eat. What *is* a well-balanced diet?"

These are just a few of the questions and concerns both casual exercisers and competitive athletes share with me when I'm coaching them to win with good nutrition. More than ever, they feel confused about what and when to eat; how to fuel before, during, and after exercise; how to find their way through the jungle of engineered sports foods; and how to choose the best diet to help them lose fat and build muscle.

There is no doubt in my mind that eating the right foods at the right times significantly improves performance and weight—as well as future health and well-being. I've helped many competitive athletes build bigger muscles, run faster marathons, and compete with higher energy. I've also helped many fitness exercisers train better, lose weight, and achieve dramatic results. Yet, too many active people fail to eat well and are reluctant to do anything about it. They think eating well equates to denying their hunger and depriving themselves of flavorful and fun foods. This is not the case.

Nancy Clark's Sports Nutrition Guidebook, Fourth Edition, clarifies the confusion about how much carbohydrate, protein, and fat you should consume and teaches you how to enjoy a variety of tasty, nutrient-rich foods that can give you the winning edge. You'll learn the latest information about the topics that matter most to active people:

- How to lose undesired body fat and have energy to exercise
- When to eat so you optimize energy, muscle growth and repair, and performance—no more running out of gas during workouts (or the workday, for that matter!)
- The proper balance and best sources of carbohydrate, to fuel your muscles, and protein, to build your muscles, including sample menus and suggestions
- How much dietary fat is OK to eat and how to choose foods with health-protective fats
- How to consume enough protein at meals, even if you are a vegetarian
- How to sneak more fruits and veggies into your daily food plan so you effortlessly enjoy these nutrient-dense sources of vitamins and minerals
- Ways to tame the cookie monster (hint: the cookie monster visits when you get too hungry)

If your goal is to move to the next level of performance and health, the up-to-date information in this book can help you get there. You'll find answers to your questions about the glycemic index, amino acids, energy drinks, commercial sports foods, high fructose corn syrup, muscle cramps, organic foods, hyponatremia, and recovery foods as well as tips on how to apply this information to your sports diet and training program. Whatever you do, don't show up for exercise but neglect to show up for winning meals and sports snacks!

With best wishes for good health, high energy, and success with food,

Nancy Clark, MS, RD, CSSD
Healthworks Fitness Center
1300 Boylston Street
Chestnut Hill, MA 02467
www.nancyclarkrd.com

ACKNOWLEDGMENTS——————

I'd like to acknowledge and express my sincere thanks to my family. Without the love and support of my husband, John; my son, John Michael; and my daughter, Mary; I would lack the purpose, meaning, and balance that brings energy and inspiration to my life.

To my running buddies, Jean Smith and Catherine Farrell, I extend my appreciation for sharing life's marathons with me.

To my clients, who teach me about sports nutrition up close and personal, I extend my gratitude. By entrusting me with their experiences, they help me to help others with similar nutrition concerns. Throughout this book, I have shared their stories, but I have changed their names and occupations to protect their privacy.

I'm appreciative of the numerous recipe contributors as well as my faithful recipe testers: my neighbors, Joan and Rex Hawley; my mother and brother, Janice and Warren Clark; and my immediate family.

And last but not least, I thank the staff at Human Kinetics for their support of this book, from the first edition to this fourth edition. Special thanks to Rainer Martens, Martin Barnard, and Jason Muzinic as well as Heather Healy, Alexis Koontz, Kim McFarland, Sue Outlaw, Nancy Rasmus, and Carla Zych.

PART I

Everyday Eating for Active People

CHAPTER 1 ——————

Building a High-Energy Food Plan

"Nutrition is my missing link. I know I could feel better, have more energy, and have better workouts if I were to eat better. But I get confused about what to eat and overwhelmed by my busy lifestyle. Help!"

—Paul

If you are like Paul and the majority of my clients, you know that food is important for fueling the body and investing in overall health, but you don't quite manage to eat right. Perhaps you sleep through breakfast, work through lunch, skimp on meals, or stuff yourself with not-so-healthful snacks. Students, parents, business people, casual exercisers, and competitive athletes alike repeatedly express their frustrations about trying to eat high-quality diets. The stress and fatigue associated with long work hours, well-intentioned attempts to lose weight, and efforts to schedule exercise can all mean that food becomes more of a source of stress than one of life's pleasures. Given today's grab-and-go culture, eating well can seem harder than ever.

In this chapter, you'll learn how to eat right and fuel your body appropriately all day long, even if you have a stressful lifestyle. Whether you work out at the health club, compete with a varsity team, aspire to be an Olympian, or simply are busy playing with your kids, you can nourish yourself with a diet that supports good health and high energy, even if you are eating on the run.

A key to eating well is preventing yourself from getting too hungry. When people get too hungry, they tend to care less about what they choose to eat and more about rewarding themselves with a treat. To prevent hunger, you need to eat throughout the day in order to offer your body and your brain a steady supply of fuel. This is contrary to the standard pattern of undereating by day only to overeat at night. By preventing hunger, you can curb your physiological desire to eat excessive treats as well as tame your psychological desire to reward yourself with, let's say, a scrumptious chocolate brownie.

In the upcoming chapters, I offer information on how to manage meals—breakfasts, lunches, dinners, and snacks—but in this chapter, I cover the day-to-day basics of how to choose the best foods to build a winning sports diet.

Creating a Winning Eating Plan

As you start to create your healthful eating plan, keep in mind these three concepts:

1. **Eat three kinds of food at meals.** The more different types of foods you eat, the more different types of vitamins, minerals, and other nutrients you consume. Instead of eating a repetitive menu with the same 10 to 15 foods each week, target 35 different types of foods per week. You can do this by eating not just Bran Flakes topped with banana for breakfast, but many different brands of cereal topped with a variety of different fruits; not just a turkey sandwich for lunch, but different types of breads and sandwich fillings; not just spinach in the salad, but lots of different colorful vegetables. Start counting!

2. **Choose foods in their natural state.** For instance, choose oranges rather than orange juice, bananas rather than commercial energy bars, whole-wheat bread rather than white bread, baked potatoes rather than French fries. Foods in their natural state and foods that have been lightly processed have more nutritional value and less sodium, trans fat, and other health-eroding ingredients.

3. **Think moderation.** Enjoy a foundation of healthful foods, but don't deprive yourself of enjoyable foods. Rather than categorize a food as being good or bad for your health, think about moderation, and aim for a diet that offers 85 to 90 percent quality foods and about 10 percent foods with fewer nutritional merits. This way, even soda pop and chips can fit into a nourishing diet, if desired; you just need to balance them with healthier choices during the

rest of the day. You can also compensate for an occasional greasy sausage and biscuit breakfast by selecting a low-fat turkey sandwich for lunch and grilled fish for dinner.

What Shape Is Your Diet?

Whereas a well-rounded diet is the desired shape of good nutrition, many of my clients eat a linear diet: apples, apples, apples; energy bars, energy bars, energy bars; pasta, pasta, pasta. Repetitive eating keeps life simple, minimizes decisions, and simplifies shopping, but it can result in an inadequate diet and chronic fatigue. If your diet looks more like a line than a circle filled two-thirds with fruits, vegetables, and whole grains and one-third with protein- and calcium-rich foods, keep reading. You'll learn how to eat more of the best foods, eat less of the rest, and create a food plan that invests in high energy, good health, top performance, and weight management.

The Food Pyramid

Every five years, the U.S. government updates its nutrition recommendations. In 2005, it also updated the food pyramid. The new pyramid, with no words or hierarchy of foods, has left many athletes confused about how to build a better diet. Here's a brief summary of some of the pyramid's key points:

- Each of the different wedges in the pyramid represents a different food group. The variety of wedges symbolizes the variety of foods that we need to form a balanced diet.
- The larger the wedge, the larger the recommended number of servings from that food group.
- The broad base and narrow top of each wedge symbolize that we should choose portion sizes that vary according to our calorie needs.
- The wedge shape also suggests we should eat a big base of nutrient-dense foods and taper off our intake of processed foods with less nutritional value. (That is, eat more apples, less apple pie; enjoy more carrot sticks, less carrot cake.)
- The stairs symbolize the message of taking small steps to a healthier lifestyle.
- The person running up the stairs symbolizes the importance of daily exercise.

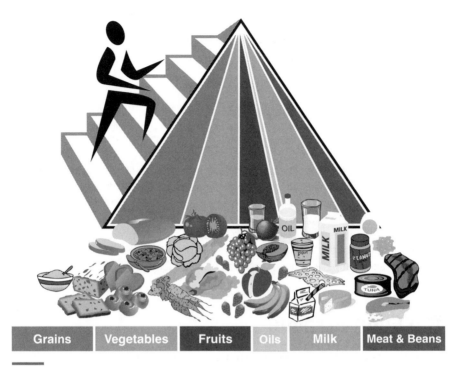

| Grains | Vegetables | Fruits | Oils | Milk | Meat & Beans |

The food pyramid.

From the U.S. Department of Agriculture (USDA). www.MyPyramid.gov

- The person also symbolizes that the pyramid can be personalized. At www.MyPyramid.gov, you can get a personalized online food plan, based on your estimated calorie needs, that defines the amounts of fruits, vegetables, grains, protein, and dairy foods you need for good health.

One key to building a healthy sports diet is to consume a variety of nutrient-dense foods from the five basic food groups (fruits, vegetables, grains, lean protein, and low-fat dairy foods). For more details about each food group, keep reading this chapter.

The food pyramid's guidelines for an 1,800-calorie food plan (a minimal amount for most athletes, including most of those who want to lose body fat) include the following:

- **Fruit:** 1 1/2 cups of fruit or juice per day. This is easy—a refreshing smoothie with a banana, berries, and orange juice will do that job.
- **Vegetables:** 2 1/2 cups (about 400 g) per day with a variety of colors. A big bowlful of salad with tomato, peppers, carrots, and baby spinach fulfills the vegetable requirement, no sweat.

- **Grains:** 6 ounces (175 g) of grain foods, of which at least half are whole grain. (Look for *whole* before the grain name on the ingredient list.) One ounce = one slice bread or 1/2 cup cooked pasta or rice. Eating whole-grain Wheaties at breakfast and a sandwich on rye bread at lunchtime can balance white rice or pasta served at dinner.

- **Dairy:** 3 cups (720 ml) of low-fat or fat-free milk or yogurt. One and a half ounces (60 g) of natural cheese or two ounces of processed cheese equates to 1 cup (240 ml) of milk.

- **Meat and alternatives:** five one-ounce equivalents. One ounce (28 g) of meat is equal to 1 egg, 1 tablespoon of peanut butter, or 1/2 ounce of nuts. This translates into a small portion of a protein at two meals per day.

Don't Just Eat, Eat Better

To help you select a high-quality sports diet—even if you are eating on the run and prefer to cook as little as possible—use the following information to help you not just eat, but eat better.

Whole Grains and Starches

If you eat well, there is a "whole" in your diet—whole grains! Wholesome breads, cereals, and other grain foods are the foundation of an optimal diet, particularly a high-performance sports diet. Grains that are unrefined or only lightly processed are excellent sources of carbohydrate, fiber, and B vitamins. They fuel your muscles, protect against needless muscular fatigue, and reduce problems with constipation if they're fiber rich. And despite popular belief, the carbohydrate in grains is not fattening; excess calories are fattening. Excess calories often come from the various forms of fat (butter, mayonnaise, gravy) that accompany rolls, sandwich bread, rice, and other types of carbohydrate. If weight is an issue, I recommend that you limit the fat but enjoy fiber-rich breads, cereals, and other whole grains. These foods help curb hunger and assist with weight management. Wholesome forms of carbohydrate should be the foundation of both a weight-reduction program and a sports diet.

Grains account for about 25 percent of the calories consumed in the United States, but unfortunately for our health, most of the grains we eat are refined—white bread, white rice, products made with white flour. The refining process strips grains of their bran and germ, thereby removing fiber, antioxidants, minerals, and other health-protective compounds. People who habitually eat diets based on refined grains tend to have a higher incidence of chronic diseases, such as adult-onset diabetes and heart disease. People who habitually eat whole grains enjoy a 20 to 40 percent lower risk of heart disease and stroke (Flight and Clifton 2006).

When selecting grains, try to choose ones that have been only lightly processed, if processed at all. For example, brown rice, whole-wheat bread, and stoned-wheat crackers offer more B vitamins, potassium, and fiber than do refined white rice, white bread, and white crackers. Other whole grains include rye crackers, Triscuits (preferably the low-fat variety), popcorn, corn tortillas, whole-wheat pita bread, bulgur, and barley.

How Much Is Enough?

To get adequate carbohydrate to fully fuel your muscles, you need to consume carbohydrate as the foundation of each meal. You can do this by eating at least 200 to 300 calories of grain foods per meal—one bowl of cereal, two slices of bread, 1 cup of rice. This is not much for hungry exercisers who require 600 to 900 calories per meal. Most active people commonly need to eat (and should eat) double or even triple the standard servings listed on the label of a cereal or pasta box.

Top Choices

If refined white grains (white flour, bread, rice, pasta) dominate your grain choices, here are some tips to boost your intake of whole grains, which offer more health value yet are tasty and readily available. Note that *wheat* on a label may not mean *whole wheat*, and a dark color might be just from food coloring, so be sure to look for the word *whole*. And whatever you do, don't try to stay away from grains, thinking they are fattening. That is not the case.

Put a "Whole" in Your Diet

Whole grains offer hundreds of phytochemicals that play key roles in reducing the risk of heart disease, diabetes, and cancer. For a food to be called a *whole grain*, one of the following should be listed first in the ingredient list on the food label:

Amaranth	Triticale
Brown rice	Whole-grain barley
Buckwheat bulgur (cracked wheat)	Whole-grain corn
Millet	Whole oats or oatmeal
Popcorn	Whole rye
Quinoa	Whole wheat
Sorghum	Wild rice

Whole-grain cereals. Wheaties, Cheerios, Total, Kashi, and Shredded Wheat are examples of whole-grain cereals. Look for the words *whole grain* on the cereal box or in the list of ingredients.

Oatmeal. When cooked into a tasty hot cereal or eaten raw as in muesli, oatmeal makes a wonderful breakfast that helps lower cholesterol and protect against heart disease. Some people even keep microwaveable packets of instant oatmeal in their desk drawers for cozy afternoon snacks. Oatmeal (instant and regular) is a whole-grain food with slow-to-digest carbohydrate that offers sustained energy and is perfect for a preexercise snack.

Bagels and muffins. Bagels (pumpernickel, rye, whole wheat) and low-fat muffins (bran, corn, oatmeal) are more healthful than doughnuts, buttered toast, croissants, pastries, or muffins made with white flour. Add a tub of yogurt plus a small container of orange juice and you have a meal on the run that's easily available from a convenience store or cafeteria, if not from home.

Whole-grain and dark breads. When it comes to choosing bread products, remember that whole-grain breads tend to have more nutritional value than do white breads. At the supermarket, select the hearty brands that have whole wheat, rye, or oatmeal listed as the first ingredient. Keep wholesome breads in the freezer so that you'll have a fresh supply on hand for toast, sandwiches, or a snack. When at the sandwich shop, request the turkey with tomato on dark rye.

Stoned-wheat and whole-grain crackers. These low-fat munchies are a perfect high-carbohydrate snack for your sports diet. Be sure to choose wholesome brands of crackers with low fat content, not the ones that leave you with greasy fingers. Look for Ak-Mak, Dr. Kracker, Finn Crisp, Kavli, RyKrisp, Triscuit Thin Crisps, Wasa, and Whole Foods 365 Baked Woven Wheats (among others).

Popcorn. Whether popped in air or in a little canola oil, popcorn is a fun way to boost your whole-grain intake. The trick is to avoid smothering it in butter or salt. How about sprinkling it with Mexican or Italian seasonings or a seasoned popcorn spray?

Vegetables

Like fruits, vegetables contribute important carbohydrate to the foundation of your sports diet. Vegetables are what I call nature's vitamin pills because they are excellent sources of vitamin C, beta-carotene (the plant form of vitamin A), potassium, magnesium, and many other vitamins, minerals, and health-protective substances. In general, vegetables offer a little more nutritional value than fruits. Hence, if you don't eat much fruit, you can compensate by eating more veggies. You'll get similar vitamins and minerals, if not more.

How Much Is Enough?

The recommended intake is at least 2 1/2 cups of vegetables per day (preferably more). Many busy people rarely eat that much in a week. If you are vegetable challenged, the trick is to eat large portions when you do eat vegetables—a big pile rather than a standard serving—and that can equate to 2 1/2 cups in one sitting. Then, to really invest in your health, try to do that twice a day, such as eating a big colorful salad with lunch and a bunch of broccoli with dinner. The food industry is working hard to make eating vegetables as easy as opening a bag of leafy greens, baby carrots, or peeled and cubed butternut squash.

Top Choices

Any vegetable is good for you. Of course, vegetables fresh from the garden are best, but they are often impossible to obtain. Frozen vegetables are a good second choice; freezing destroys little nutritional value. Canned vegetables are also a good choice; rinsing them with plain water can reduce their higher sodium levels. Because canned vegetables are processed quickly, they retain many of their nutrients. Overcooking is a prime nutrient destroyer, so cook fresh or frozen vegetables only until they are tender-crisp, preferably in the microwave oven, steamer, or wok. Heat canned vegetables just until warm; there's no need to boil them.

Dark, colorful vegetables usually have more nutritional value than paler ones. If you are struggling to improve your diet, boost your intake of colorful broccoli, spinach, peppers, tomatoes, carrots, and winter squash. They are more nutrient dense than pale lettuces, cucumbers, zucchini, mushrooms, and celery. (In no way are these pale vegetables bad for you; the colorful ones just offer more vitamins and minerals.) Here's the scoop on a few of the top vegetable choices.

Broccoli, spinach, and peppers (green, red, or yellow). These low-fat, potassium-rich vegetables are loaded with vitamin C and the health-protective carotenes that are the precursors of vitamin A. One medium stalk (one cup) of steamed broccoli offers you a full day's worth of vitamin C, as does half a large pepper. I enjoy munching on a pepper instead of an apple for a snack; it offers more vitamins and potassium and fewer calories. What a nutrition bargain!

Tomatoes and tomato sauce. In salads or on pasta or pizza, tomato products are another easy way to boost your veggie intake. They are good sources of potassium, fiber, and vitamin C (one medium-size tomato provides half the vitamin C you need each day); carotenes; and lycopene, a phytochemical that might protect against certain cancers. Tomato juice and vegetable juice are additional suggestions for fast-laners who lack the time or interest to cook. They can enjoyably drink their veggies! Commercial tomato products tend to be high in sodium, however, so people with high blood pressure should limit their intake or choose the low-sodium brands. Some "salty sweaters," however, welcome tomato or V8 juice after a hard workout; the sodium helps replace the sodium lost in sweat (see chapter 8).

Cruciferous vegetables (members of the cabbage family). Cabbage, broccoli, cauliflower, brussels sprouts, collards, kale, kohlrabi, turnip, and mustard greens may protect against cancer. Do your health a favor by focusing on these choices. You can't go wrong eating piles of these.

If you are eating too few vegetables, be sure the ones you eat are among the best. The information in table 1.1 can help guide your choices, as can the information in the salad section in chapter 4.

Table 1.1   Comparing Vegetables

Vegetable	Amount	Calories	A (IU*)	C (mg)	Potassium (mg)
Asparagus	8 spears cooked	35	980	30	260
Beets	1/2 cup boiled	35	30	5	260
Broccoli	1 cup cooked	50	3,500	75	330
Brussels sprouts	8 medium cooked	60	1,100	100	500
Cabbage, green	1 cup cooked	30	200	35	145
Carrot	1 medium raw	30	20,250	10	230
Cauliflower	1 cup cooked	30	20	55	180
Celery	1 7-in. stalk	5	55	5	115
Corn	1/2 cup frozen	65	180	5	120
Cucumber	1/3 medium	15	220	5	150
Green beans	1 cup cooked	45	180	15	370
Kale	1 cup cooked	40	9,600	55	300
Lettuce, iceberg	7 leaves	15	455	5	160
Lettuce, romaine	2 cups shredded	15	2,900	30	320
Mushrooms	1 cup pieces raw	20	0	2	260
Onion	1/2 cup chopped	30	0	5	125
Peas, green	1/2 cup cooked	60	530	10	135
Pepper, green	1 cup diced	30	630	90	180
Potato, baked	1 large with skin	220	0	50	1,700
Spinach	1 cup cooked	40	14,750	20	840
Squash, summer	1 cup cooked	35	520	10	345
Squash, winter	1 cup baked	80	7,200	20	890
Sweet potato	1 medium baked	120	25,000	30	400
Tomato	1 small raw	25	770	25	275
Recommended intake:	Men		>3,000	>90	>4,700
	Women		>2,310	>75	>4,700

*International units
Created from data in J. Pennington, 1998, *Bowes & Church's food values of portions commonly used*, 17th ed. (Philadelphia, PA: Lippincott, Williams & Wilkins).

Fruits

Fruits add to the strong foundation of carbohydrate needed for your sports diet. Fruits are rich not only in carbohydrate but also in fiber, potassium, and many vitamins, especially vitamin C. The nutrients in fruits improve healing; aid in recovery after exercise; and reduce the risk of cancer, high blood pressure, and constipation.

How Much Is Enough?

The food pyramid recommends at least 1 1/2 cups of fruit or juice per day—this translates into only one or two standard pieces of fruit. The Centers for Disease Control and Prevention (CDC) encourages consuming even more to help prevent many of the diseases of aging. If you have trouble getting even a little fruit into your daily menus, I recommend scheduling it into your breakfast routine. An 8-ounce (240 ml) glass of orange juice and a medium banana on your cereal will cover your minimum fruit requirement for the entire day. Strive to consume more fruit at other eating occasions throughout the day by having dried fruit instead of an energy bar for a preexercise snack, or drink a fruit smoothie for a postexercise recovery shake. Any fruit is better than no fruit!

Top Choices

If you have trouble including fruit in your diet because it spoils before you get around to eating it or because it is not readily available, the following tips will help you balance your fruit intake better. Make these foods a top priority in your good nutrition game plan.

Citrus fruits and juices. Whether it's the whole fruit or fresh, frozen, or canned juice, citrus fruits such as oranges, grapefruits, clementines, and tangerines surpass many other fruits or juices in vitamin C and potassium content.

If the hassle of peeling an orange or a grapefruit is a deterrent for you, just drink its juice. The whole fruit has slightly more nutritional value, but given the option of a quick glass of juice or nothing, juice does the job. Just 8 ounces (240 ml) of orange juice provides more than the daily reference intake of 75 milligrams of vitamin C; all the potassium you may have lost in an hour-long workout; and folic acid, a B vitamin needed for building protein and red blood cells. Choose the OJ with added calcium to give your bone health a boost.

To boost your juice intake, stock up on cans of frozen juice concentrate, buy juice boxes for lunch or snacks, and look for cans or bottles of juice in vending machines. Better yet, stock whole oranges in your refrigerator and pack them in your gym bag.

Bananas. This low-fat, high-potassium fruit is perfect for busy people, and it even comes prewrapped. Bananas are excellent for replacing potassium lost in sweat. The potassium protects against high blood pressure. To boost your banana intake, add sliced banana to cereal, pack a banana in your lunch bag for a satisfying dessert, or keep them on hand for a quick and easy energy-boosting snack. My all-time favorite combination is banana with peanut butter, stoned-wheat crackers, and a glass of low-fat milk—a well-balanced meal or snack that includes four kinds of foods (fruit, nuts, grain, dairy), with a nice foundation of carbohydrate (banana, crackers) and protein (peanut butter, milk) as the accompaniment.

To prevent bananas from becoming overripe, store them in the refrigerator. The skin may turn black from the cold, but the fruit itself will be fine. Another trick is to keep (peeled) banana chunks in the freezer. These frozen nuggets taste just like banana ice cream but have far fewer calories; they also blend nicely with milk to make creamy smoothies. (See the recipe for fruit smoothies on page 398.)

Without a doubt, bananas are among the most popular sports snacks. I once saw a cyclist with two bananas safely taped to his helmet, ready to grab when he needed an energy boost.

Cantaloupe, kiwi, strawberries, and other berries. These nutrient-dense fruits are also good sources of vitamin C and potassium. Many of my clients keep berries and chunks of melon in the freezer, ready and waiting to be made into a smoothie for breakfast or a pre- or postworkout refresher.

Dried fruits. Convenient and portable, dried fruits are rich in potassium and carbohydrate. They travel well; keep baggies of dried fruit and nuts (as in a trail mix) in your gym bag instead of yet another energy bar.

If you are eating too little fruit, be sure that the fruit you eat is nutritionally the best. The information in table 1.2 can help guide your choices.

Is Organic Better?

Many of my clients wonder if they should spend their food budgets on organic fruits and vegetables. Are organic foods better, safer, and more nutritious? The simple answer is they can be better for the small farmers and are possibly better for the environment, but they are not significantly better in terms of nutritional value. It's debatable whether they are significantly safer. Here's a closer look at the story as we know it to date.

To start, *organic* refers to the way farmers grow and process fruits, vegetables, grains, meat, poultry, eggs, and dairy products. Only foods that are grown and processed according to USDA organic standards can be labeled *organic*. (Note: The food-label terms *natural*, *hormone free*, and *free range* do not necessarily mean *organic*.) Organic farmers do not use chemical fertilizers, insecticides, or weed killers on crops.

Table 1.2   Comparing Fruits

Fruit	Amount	Calories	A (IU)	C (mg)	Potassium (mg)
Apple	1 medium	80	75	10	160
Apple juice	1 cup	115	0	2	300
Apricots	10 halves dried	85	2,550	1	480
Banana	1 medium	105	90	10	450
Blueberries	1 cup raw	80	145	20	260
Cantaloupe	1 cup pieces	55	5,160	70	495
Cherries	10 sweet	50	145	5	150
Cranberry juice	1 cup	140	10	90	55
Dates	5 dried	115	20	–	270
Figs	1 medium raw	35	70	1	115
Grapefruit	1/2 medium pink	40	155	45	170
Grapefruit juice	1 cup white	95	25	95	400
Grapes	1 cup	60	90	5	175
Honeydew melon	1 cup cubes	60	70	40	460
Kiwi	1 medium	45	135	75	250
Orange, navel	1 medium	60	240	75	230
Orange juice	1 cup fresh	110	500	125	500
Peach	1 medium	35	465	5	170
Pineapple	1 cup raw	75	35	25	175
Pineapple juice	1 cup	140	13	25	335
Prunes	5 dried	100	830	2	310
Raisins	1/3 cup	150	5	2	375
Strawberries	1 cup raw	45	40	85	245
Watermelon	1 cup	50	585	15	185
Recommended intake:	Men		>3,000	>90	>4,700
	Women		>2,310	>75	>4,700

Created from data in J. Pennington, 1998, *Bowes & Church's food values of portions commonly used*, 17th ed. (Philadelphia, PA: Lippincott, Williams & Wilkins).

Nor do they use growth hormones, antibiotics, and medications to enhance animal growth and prevent disease.

Organic fruits and vegetables can cost about 30 percent more than standard produce, if not more. Are they worth the extra cost? In terms of taste, some athletes claim organic foods taste better. Taste is subjective and may relate to the fact that freshly grown foods have more flavor. In terms of nutrition, some research suggests that organic foods may have slightly more minerals and antioxidants than do conventionally grown counterparts, but the differences are insignificant (Winter and Davis 2006). You could adjust for the difference by eating a larger portion.

One important reason to buy organic—preferably locally grown organic—is to help sustain the earth and replenish its resources. Buying

The Nutrition Rainbow

Strive to eat a variety of colors of fruits and vegetables. Each color offers different kinds of the health-protective phytochemicals that are linked to reducing the risk of cancer and heart disease.

Color	Fruits	Vegetables
Red	Strawberries, watermelon	Red peppers, tomatoes*
Green	Kiwi, grapes, honeydew melon	Peas, beans, spinach, broccoli
Blue or purple	Blueberries, grapes, prunes	Eggplant, beets
Orange	Mango, peaches, cantaloupe	Carrots, sweet potato, pumpkin
Yellow	Pineapple, star fruit	Summer squash, corn
White	Banana, pears	Garlic, onions

*Technically, tomatoes are a fruit.

The following tips can help you enjoy a more colorful diet:

Breakfast

Wake up with a big swig of orange juice.

Add banana or berries to cold cereal.

Cook hot cereal with raisins and dried fruits.

Whip together a smoothie with berries, juice, banana, and yogurt.

Lunch

Include a handful of baby carrots.

Munch on a red pepper, as you would an apple.

Put dried cranberries or canned mandarin oranges in your salad.

Choose vegetable or tomato soup.

Snacks

Keep dried apricots and pineapple in your desk drawer.

Sip on V8 juice.

Bring a week's supply of fruit (five apples, five oranges) to work with you on Monday.

Dinner

Enjoy an extra-large portion of broccoli (fresh or frozen).

Buy precut fresh winter squash that is ready to cook.

Smother pasta with extra tomato sauce.

Order pizza with extra peppers or broccoli.

Choose Chinese stir-fry with extra veggies.

locally grown foods supports the small farmers and helps them earn a better living from their farmland. Otherwise, farmers can easily be tempted to sell their land for house lots or industrial parks—and there goes more beautiful open green space.

Yet, if you buy organic foods from a large grocery store chain, you should think about the whole picture. Because organic fruits, for example, are in big demand, they may need to be transported for thousands of miles, let's say from California to Massachusetts. This transportation process consumes fuel, pollutes the air, and hinders the establishment of a better environment. Does this really fit the ideal vision of *organic*? The compromise is to buy any kind of locally grown produce whenever possible.

A second potential reason to choose organic relates to reducing the pesticide content in your body and the potential risk of cancer and birth defects. The Environmental Protection Agency has established standards that require a 100- to 1,000-fold margin of safety for pesticide residues. They have set limits based on scientific data that indicate a pesticide will not cause "unreasonable risk to human health." According to Richard Bonanno, PhD, agricultural expert at University of Massachusetts-Amherst and a farmer himself, 65 to 75 percent of conventionally grown produce has no detectible pesticides. (When used properly and applied at the right times, pesticides degrade and become inert.) Results of testing vegetables from farms in Massachusetts showed no pesticide residues in 100 percent of the samples. Bonanno reports that only 0.5 percent of conventionally grown foods (but 3 to 4 percent of imported foods) are above EPA standards. A 2005 survey of 13,621 food samples revealed pesticide residue exceeding the tolerance was 0.2 percent (USDA Pesticide Data). Yet, watchdog groups (www.foodnews.org) remind us that small amounts of pesticides can accumulate in the body. This may be of particular concern during vulnerable periods of growth, such as early childhood.

Clearly, whether or not to buy organic foods becomes a matter of personal values. Bonanno sees "organic," in part, as a marketing ploy; organic foods are portrayed as being safer and better. He argues that we do not have a two-tier food system in the United States—with wealthier people who can afford to buy organic foods being the recipients of safer foods.

So what's a hungry but poor athlete to do?

- Eat a variety of foods to minimize exposure to a specific pesticide residue.
- Carefully wash and rinse fruits and vegetables under running water; this can remove 99 percent of any pesticide residue (depending on the food and the pesticide).
- Peel foods such as apples, potatoes, carrots, and pears (but then, you also peel off important nutrients).

- Remove the tops and outer portions of celery, lettuce, and cabbage.
- Buy organic versions of the foods you eat most often, such as organic apples if you are a five-a-day apple eater.
- Sometimes (if not all the time), buy organic versions of the fruits and veggies that are known to have the highest pesticide residue, even after having been washed. According to the Environmental Working Group (2006), the "dirty dozen" includes the following fruits and vegetables: apples, cherries, imported grapes, nectarines, peaches, pears, strawberries, red raspberries, potatoes, bell peppers, celery, and spinach.
- Save money by choosing conventionally grown versions of the "clean dozen" (with little or no pesticide residue): banana, kiwi, pineapple, mango, papaya (note that foods such as papaya, mango, and banana have their own protective shell, so this reduces pesticide exposure on the flesh of the fruit), asparagus, avocado, broccoli, cauliflower, onion, sweet corn, and green peas.

When all is said and done, whether or not to make the extra shopping trip and pay the higher price is an individual decision. Yes, buying locally grown organic foods can help save the small farms, but whether or not organic foods are better, safer, and more nutritious is debatable.

Low-Fat Dairy Products

Dairy foods such as low-fat milk, yogurt, and cheese are not only quick and easy sources of protein but are also rich in vitamin D (if fortified) and calcium, a mineral that is particularly important, not only for growing children and teens but also for women and men of all ages. A diet rich in calcium and vitamin D helps maintain strong bones, reduces the risk of osteoporosis, protects against high blood pressure, and may help prevent weight gain (Caan et al. 2007). Vitamin D may be helpful in preventing and treating diseases other than cancer, such as fibromyalgia, diabetes mellitus, multiple sclerosis, and rheumatoid arthritis (Lappe et al. 2007).

Dairy products are not the only natural sources of calcium, but they tend to be the most concentrated and convenient sources for those who eat on the run. If you prefer to limit your consumption of dairy products because you are lactose intolerant or are biased against dairy, you may have difficulty consuming the recommended intake of calcium from natural foods. For example, to absorb the same amount of calcium that you would obtain from one glass of milk, you'd need to consume either 3 cups of broccoli, 8 cups of spinach, 2 1/2 cups of white beans, 6 cups of pinto beans, 6 cups of sesame seeds, or 30 cups of unfortified soy milk.

Calcium-fortified foods, such as calcium-enriched soy milk, orange juice, or breakfast cereals such as Total, can help you reach your calcium goals. Table 1.3 lists a few of the more common calcium sources and the amount of the source that provides a serving of calcium (300 mg). The table also provides the amount of vitamin D supplied by these common sources.

Fat-free or low-fat milk (cow's or soy) and other foods rich in calcium and vitamin D should be an important part of your diet throughout your lifetime. Because your bones are alive, they need calcium and vitamin D daily. Children and teens need calcium for growth. Adults also need calcium to maintain strong bones. Although you may stop growing by age 20, you don't reach peak bone density until age 30 to 35. The amount of calcium stored in your bones at that age is a critical factor in your susceptibility to fractures as you grow older. After age 35, bones start to thin as a normal part of aging. A calcium-rich diet, in combination with resistance exercise and strong muscles, can slow this process.

Many of my clients tell me, "I don't drink milk, but I do take a calcium supplement." I remind them that calcium supplements are incomplete

Table 1.3   Calcium Equivalents

Calcium-rich food	Amount*	Vitamin D (IU)
Dairy		
Milk (fortified)	1 cup (240 ml)	100
Milk powder	1/3 cup dry (75 ml)	100
Yogurt	1 cup	100
Cheese, cheddar	1.5 oz (45 g)	5-15
Cottage cheese	2 cups	—
Frozen yogurt	1 1/2 cups	—
Pizza, cheese	2 slices	—
Protein		
Soy milk, enriched	1 cup (240 ml)	40-120
Tofu	5 oz (150 g)	—
Salmon, canned with bones	4 oz (125 g)	700
Sardines, canned with bones	3 oz (90 g)	230-400
Almonds	3/4 cup (170 g)	—
Vegetables		
Broccoli, cooked	3 cups (500 g)	—
Collard or turnip greens, cooked	1 cup (200 g)	—
Kale or mustard greens, cooked	1 1/2 cups (200 g)	—
Bok choy	2 cups (340 g)	—
Calcium-fortified foods		
Total cereal	1 cup (30 g)	40
Orange juice, calcium & D enriched	1 cup (240 ml)	100

*The amount represents 1 serving of calcium (300 mg).

substitutes for calcium-rich dairy products. Low-fat milk and yogurt offer a full spectrum of important vitamins, minerals, and protein; a calcium supplement offers only calcium (and maybe vitamin D). Milk, for example, is rich in not only calcium and vitamin D but also potassium and phosphorous—nutrients that work in combination to help your body use calcium effectively. Milk is also one of the best sources of riboflavin, a vitamin that helps convert the food you eat into energy. Active people, who generate more energy than their sedentary counterparts, need more riboflavin. If you don't eat dairy products, your riboflavin intake is likely to be poor.

Granted, taking a calcium supplement is better than consuming no calcium. But I highly recommend a nutrition consultation with a registered dietitian to ensure appropriate calcium intake from your daily food choices. This nutrition professional can help you optimize your diet so that you get the right balance of all the nutrients you need for good health and optimal sports performance. (See the Dietitian section in appendix A for information on finding a registered dietitian in your area.)

How Much Is Enough?

As you can see in table 1.4, calcium needs vary according to age, with growing teens needing four servings and most adults three servings. This may seem like a lot if you are not a milk drinker, but even weight-conscious athletes can easily consume the recommended daily minimum of three servings of low-fat dairy foods for only 300 calories. Try to get at least half, if not all, of your calcium requirements from food.

Table 1.4 Calcium Requirements

Age	Calcium target (mg)	Number of servings
Children		
1-3 years	500	2
4-8 years	800	3
Teenagers		
9-18 years	1,300	4
Women		
19-50 years	1,000	3
>50 years (menopausal)	1,200-1,500	4-5
Amenorrheic athletes	1,200-1,500	4-5
Pregnant or breastfeeding	1,000-1,500	3-5
Men		
19-50 years	1,000	3
>50 years	1,200	4

Some people have trouble digesting milk because they lack an enzyme (lactase) that digests milk sugar (lactose). These lactose-intolerant people can often tolerate yogurt, hard cheeses, or even small amounts of milk taken with a meal. They can also drink soy milk or Lactaid milk, a lactose-free brand available at supermarkets. All too often, my lactose-intolerant clients neglect the fact that their bodies still need calcium from alternative calcium sources.

Boosting Your Calcium Intake

Here are some tips to help you boost your calcium intake to build and maintain strong bones:

- For breakfast, enjoy cereal with 1 cup of low-fat or skim milk (or soy milk).
- With crunchy cereal, such as granola, use yogurt in place of milk.
- With hot cereal, cook the cereal in milk, or mix in 1/3 cup of powdered milk.
- When grabbing a quick meal, choose pizza with low-fat mozzarella cheese or sandwiches with low-fat cheese.
- Choose a postworkout chocolate milk chug for an excellent recovery food.
- Boost the calcium in salads by adding low-fat grated cheese, cottage cheese, or tofu cubes.
- In a blender, mix soft tofu or plain yogurt with salad seasonings for a calcium-rich dressing. Read the labels on the tofu containers, and choose the brands processed with calcium sulfate; otherwise, the tofu will be calcium poor.
- Drink a glass of low-fat, skim, or soy milk with lunch, snacks, or dinner.
- Add extra milk (instead of cream) to coffee, and enjoy lattes.
- Take powdered milk to the office to replace coffee whiteners.
- Drink milk-based hot cocoa in place of coffee.
- Make shakes and smoothies using milk as the base.
- Snack on fruit-flavored yogurt rather than ice cream.
- Enjoy pudding made with low-fat milk for a tasty low-fat calcium treat.
- Eat canned salmon or sardines with bones for an easy lunch option; serve with crackers.
- Add tofu to Oriental soups or stir-fried meals.

Top Choices

To consume the amount of calcium you need to build and maintain strong bones (1,000 to 1,500 mg per day), you should plan to include a calcium-rich food in each meal.

Milk, low-fat or nonfat, fortified with vitamin D. Low-fat or skim milk is an excellent source of calcium. It has most of the fat removed but retains all the calcium and protein. A glass of whole milk (3.5 percent fat) has the same amount of fat as two pats of butter, but skim milk (0 percent fat) has almost no fat. Calcium-fortified soy milk is also a fine alternative.

Yogurt, low-fat or nonfat. Plain yogurt is one of the richest food sources of calcium. Note that frozen yogurt product (and ice cream for that matter) is only a fair source of calcium. I consider both types of treats sugar-based foods that contain a little milk, not milk-based foods. One cup of soft-serve frozen yogurt equals 1/3 a cup of milk in terms of calcium but comes with twice as many calories.

Low-fat cheese. Because many brands of fat-free cheese tend to be unpalatable, I suggest that you enjoy small portions of the low-fat options. They are usually tasty and add both calcium and protein to sandwiches, pasta, chili, and other vegetarian meals.

Dark green veggies. Broccoli, bok choy (a vegetable common in Chinese cookery), kale, and collards are among the best vegetable sources of calcium. Spinach, Swiss chard, and beet greens also contain calcium, but your body can absorb very little of it because these veggies have a type of fiber that binds the calcium and hinders absorption.

Protein-Rich Foods

Protein from animal sources (meats, seafood, eggs, and poultry) and plant sources (beans, nuts, and legumes) is also important in your daily diet, but you should eat protein as the accompaniment to the carbohydrate found in fruits, vegetables, and grains. If one-quarter to one-third of your plate at two of your daily meals is covered with a protein-rich food, you can get the right amount of the amino acids you need to build and repair muscles. By choosing darker meats with iron and zinc, you reduce the risk of iron-deficiency anemia.

How Much Is Enough?

Athletes tend to eat either too much or too little protein, depending on their health consciousness, accuracy of nutrition education, or lifestyle. Some athletes fill up on too much meat. Others proclaim themselves vegetarian, yet they sometimes neglect to replace the beef with beans and are, in fact, only non-meat-eaters—and often protein deficient, at that.

Although slabs of steak and huge hamburgers have no place in any athlete's diet—or anyone's diet—adequate amounts of protein are important for building muscles and repairing tissues. (Excess protein isn't stored as bulging muscles.) The purpose of this section is to highlight quick and easy protein choices. See chapter 7 for sport-specific protein needs.

For most people, including athletes, a daily total of about 5 to 7 ounces (150 to 200 g) of protein-rich food plus the protein you get in two to three servings of milk, yogurt, or cheese (which you consume for calcium) offers adequate protein. Five ounces for a day is much less than the portions most Americans eat in one meal: 10-ounce steaks, 6-ounce chicken breasts, slabs of roast beef. Many athletes polish off their required protein by lunchtime and continue to eat one to two times more than they need.

Other people, however, miss out on adequate protein when they eat only veggies in a salad for lunch or stir-fried for dinner. Dieters, for example, who dine exclusively on salads and vegetables commonly neglect their protein needs.

Top Choices

All types of protein-rich foods contain valuable amino acids. See table 1.5 for a comparison of some popular protein-rich foods. The following choices can enhance your sports diet.

Chicken and turkey. Poultry generally has less saturated fat than red meats, so it tends to be a more heart-healthful choice. Just be sure to buy skinless chicken or discard the fatty skin before cooking. Cooked until crispy, poultry skin can be a big temptation.

Fish. Fresh, frozen, or canned fish provides not only a lot of protein but also the omega-3 fat that protects your health. The recommended target is 12 ounces (350 g), or two to three servings, of canned or fresh fish per week. The best choices are the oilier varieties that live in cold ocean waters, such as salmon, mackerel, albacore tuna, sardines, bluefish, and herring, but any fish is better than no fish. Chapter 2 offers more fish information.

Lean beef. A lean roast-beef sandwich made with two thick slices of whole-grain bread for carbohydrate is an excellent choice for protein as well as iron (prevents anemia), zinc (needed for muscle growth and repair), and B vitamins (help produce energy). Top round (such as you'd buy at a deli), eye of round, and round tip are among the leanest cuts of beef. A lean roast-beef sandwich is preferable in terms of heart health and nutritional value to a grilled-cheese sandwich, chicken salad sandwich, or hamburger because of these nutrients and the lower fat content.

Peanut butter. Although peanut butter by the jarful can be a dangerous diet breaker, a few tablespoons on whole-grain bread, crackers, a bagel,

Table 1.5 Comparing Protein Content of Commonly Eaten Foods

Food sources	Protein (g)
Animal protein	
Egg white, 1	3
Beef, roast, 4 oz (120 g) cooked	30
Chicken breast, 4 oz (125 g) cooked*	30
Tuna, 1 can (6 oz)	30-40
Plant protein	
Nuts, 1 oz (1/4 cup or 30 g)	6
Soy milk, 1 cup (240 ml)	7
Lentils, 1/2 cup (100 g)	7
Hummus, 1/2 cup (125 g)	8
Peanut butter, 2 tbsp	9
Tofu, 4 oz (125 g)	11
Boca burger, 2.5 oz (70 g)	13
Dairy products	
Cheese, American, 1 slice (2/3 oz)	6
Milk, 1 cup (240 ml)	6-7
Yogurt, 6 oz (175 g) tub	6-7
Cheese, cheddar, 1 oz (30 g)	7
Milk powder, 1/3 cup (75 g)	8
Cottage cheese, 1/2 cup (113)	15
Breads, cereals, grains	
Bread, 1 slice	2
Cold cereal, 1 oz (30 g)	2
Rice, 1/3 cup dry (65 g) or 1 cup cooked	4
Oatmeal, 1/2 cup dry (40 g) or 1 cup cooked	5
Pasta, 2 oz (60 g) dry or cooked	8
Starchy vegetables**	
Peas, 1/2 cup cooked	2
Carrots, 1/2 cup cooked	2
Corn, 1/2 cup cooked	2
Beets, 1/2 cup cooked	2
Winter squash, 1/2 cup	2
Potato, 1 small	2

*4 oz (125 g) cooked (approx. size of deck of cards) = 5-6 oz (150-175 g) raw.

**Whereas starchy vegetables contribute a little protein, most watery vegetables (and fruits) offer negligible amounts of protein. They may contribute a total of 5 to 10 g of protein per day, depending on how much you eat.

or a banana for a satisfying snack or a quick meal offer protein, vitamins, and fiber. A source of plant protein, peanut butter is cholesterol free and a good source of health-protective polyunsaturated fat. People who eat at least two servings of peanut butter (or peanuts) per week tend to have a lower risk of heart disease (Kris-Etherton et al. 2001). The all-natural brands have a tiny bit less "bad" trans fat, but the difference is very small. So enjoy this childhood favorite!

Canned beans. Vegetarian refried beans (tucked into a tortilla sprinkled with salsa and shredded low-fat cheese and then heated in the microwave oven), hummus (as a dip with baby carrots), and canned garbanzo or kidney beans (added to a salad) are three easy ways to boost your intake of plant protein, which is also an excellent sources of carbohydrate. If you tend to avoid beans because they make you flatulent, try eating them with Beano, a product available at many health-food stores and pharmacies that takes the gas out of vegetarian diets.

Tofu. Tofu is an easy addition to a meatless diet because you don't have to cook it. It has a mild flavor, so you can easily add it to salads, chili, spaghetti sauce, stir-fry dishes, and casseroles. Look for tofu in the vegetable section of your grocery store. Buy "firm" tofu for slicing or cutting into cubes, "soft" or "silken" tofu for blending into smoothies or dips.

Even those who don't cook can easily incorporate adequate protein into a day's diet. Simply buy lean roasted beef, rotisserie chicken, and turkey breast at the deli counter, or open a can or foil pouch of tuna, salmon, or chicken.

Fat and Oils

A food plan need not be fat free to be healthful. Fat may be nutrient poor, but it adds flavor and enjoyment to your diet. Hungry athletes will have a far easier time consuming the calories they need when the food is tasty and enjoyable. And despite popular belief, a little fat does not negate all the positive aspects of your overall healthful sports diet, although too much saturated and trans fat can be harmful to your health.

In particular, you want to limit your intake of "hard" fat, such as beef lard and butter; use more "soft" fat, such as olive and canola oils; and stay away from partially hydrogenated trans fat, which, until recently, had been prevalent in many commercially prepared foods such as crackers, cakes, cookies, chips, pastries, and the chocolate covering on energy bars. Trans fat is created in an industrial process that adds hydrogen to mono- and polyunsaturated fats. This converts them into a partially hydrogenated oil (the term on the food label).

The American Heart Association recommends avoiding trans fat because it raises the bad LDL cholesterol and lowers the good HDL cholesterol.

Try to consume less than 1 percent of your calories from trans fat; that's only 18 calories—2 grams of fat—if you eat 1,800 calories; a large order of French fries might have 6 grams of trans fat. With new laws that require trans fat to be identified on labels, food companies have scrambled to find trans-fat-free alternatives that offer the same light and flaky pastries and crunchy chips—a tall order!

How Much Is Enough?

About 20 to 35 percent of the calories in your diet can appropriately come from fat. According to the food pyramid, about 5 teaspoons of fat per day are appropriate for an 1,800-calorie food plan. Some people eat way too much fat—buttery, cheese-filled omelets for breakfast; burgers and fries for lunch; and fried chicken for dinner. If you tend to choose high-fat foods at each meal, strive to correct the imbalance by choosing lower-fat foods for at least two of your three meals. If you fill up on fatty snacks (chips, cookies, ice cream), try eating larger portions of wholesome foods at meals in order to curb your appetite for artery-clogging snacks.

Top Choices

The following forms of fat are a positive addition to your sports diet because they are health enhancing.

Olive oil. This monounsaturated fat is associated with low risk of heart disease and cancer. Use it for salads, sauteing, and keeping pasta from sticking together. If you use olive oil for its health-giving properties, buy the unrefined extra-virgin olive oil (despite its higher cost). Extra-virgin olive oil offers more phenolic compounds—powerful antioxidants that can reduce inflammation (Fitó et al. 2007).

Peanut butter (and other nut butters). All-natural brands are best because they are less processed, but even Skippy, Jif, and other commercial peanut butters offer predominantly health-protective fat.

Walnuts, almonds, and other nuts. Thought to be protective against heart disease, nuts (and nut oils, such as walnut oil) are a fine addition to salads, cooked vegetables, and even pasta meals.

Flaxseed (ground) and flax oil. Flax contains an omega-3 fat that the body converts into small amounts of the health-protective EPA and DHA contained in fish. Sprinkle ground flaxseed on cold cereal, blend it into shakes, and add it to pancake batter.

Sugars and Sweets

Even a well-balanced diet can include some sugar and sweets; the key is moderation. The plan is to first fill up on healthful foods, and then, if desired, enjoy a little fun food for a small treat. That is, there is little wrong with enjoying a bit of chocolate after a lunchtime sandwich. But there is a lot wrong with eating chocolates for lunch. Given that 10 percent of your calories can appropriately come from sugar, the following foods are some of the better ways to spend those calories.

Molasses. Confirming the rule that the darker the food is, the more nutrients it has, molasses is among the darkest of sugars, and it has the most nutrients. Molasses is a fair source of potassium, calcium, and iron—if you eat several tablespoons. For a change of taste, add a tablespoon to milk for taffy milk, mix some in yogurt, or spread it on a peanut butter sandwich.

Berry jams. Because of the seeds in raspberry, strawberry, and blackberry jams, these sweet spreads have a little fiber that somewhat boosts their healthfulness. Preferable to strained jellies, the jams offer slightly more fruit value, but you still have to count them as primarily sugar.

Building a Strong Sports Diet

Now that you have read this chapter, you know which foods are the best choices. The trick is to assemble the best foods into wholesome meals and snacks. I recommend that you try to choose from at least three out of five food groups at each meal. The following chart shows how this might work.

Food group	Meal 1	Meal 2	Meal 3
1. Grain	Oatmeal	Whole-wheat wrap	Pizza crust
2. Fruit	Raisins	Apple	Green peppers
3. Vegetable		Lettuce, tomato	Tomato sauce
4. Dairy	Low-fat milk	Low-fat yogurt	Cheese
5. Protein	Almonds	Turkey	

Foods made from a combination of ingredients can create a well-balanced meal in one dish. For example, vegetable pizza topped with peppers, onions, and mushrooms is far from junk food. It offers calcium-rich dairy food (from the low-fat mozzarella); vegetables rich in potassium, beta-carotene, and vitamin C (from the tomato sauce and vegetable toppings); and carbohydrate-rich grain foods in the (preferably whole-wheat) crust. A dinner of thick-crust pizza with a foundation of carbohydrate better fits the pyramid plan than does a fried-chicken dinner that is mostly greasy protein.

Eating well need not be a major task. You simply need to do the following:

- Eat a variety of wholesome foods to consume a bigger variety of health-protective nutrients. Choose more of the best foods and less of the rest.
- Fuel your body on a regular schedule, eating every two to four hours rather than having one or two big meals per day.
- Eat when you are hungry, and then stop when you are content. When eating at restaurants, be cautious of "value meals" that emphasize large portions. They lead to overeating and poor health.
- Take mealtimes seriously. The following chapters offer additional tips to help you choose a sports diet that will invest in good health and high energy for sports, exercise, and a nourishing life.

Balancing Act

How can I tell if I am choosing a well-balanced diet? You can consume the recommended intake of the vitamins, minerals, amino acids (the building blocks of protein), and other nutrients you need for good health within 1,200 to 1,500 calories if you wisely select from a variety of wholesome foods. Because many active people consume 2,000 to 5,000 calories (depending on their age, level of activity, body size, and gender), they have the chance to consume abundant amounts of vitamins and other nutrients. Dieters, on the other hand, tend to take in fewer calories, so they need to carefully select nutrient-dense foods— foods that offer the most nutritional value for the least amount of calories—to reduce the risk of consuming a nutrient-deficient diet.

To determine if your daily food intake is balanced and adequate, you can track your diet on the Internet using any number of Web sites. See appendix A for a list of sites, or simply search the Web for "nutrient analysis programs."

CHAPTER 2

Eating to Stay Healthy for the Long Run

Few people fully appreciate the power of food in the prevention and treatment of the so-called diseases of aging, which are, in reality, diseases of inactivity and poor nutrition. In this day and age where people are taking all sorts of medications to lower cholesterol, blood sugar, and blood pressure and to deal with other health concerns, we forget that, just as the wrong foods can be powerfully bad for your health, the right foods can be powerfully health protective. By eating wisely, you are investing in your good health and top performance; alternatively, you can eat poorly and end up with your poor health controlling you and your life.

No single medicine is as powerful as a healthful diet. Luckily, the wholesome foods you need to protect your health are the same foods that should be part of your sports diet. By routinely choosing the best sports foods, you'll be better able to enjoy lifelong health and high energy.

Confusion abounds about foods that are "good" or "bad" for your health. My clients repeatedly ask me, "What foods should I avoid?" My standard answer is that the only "bad" foods are foods that are moldy or poisonous (or foods you are allergic to); all other foods, in moderation, can be balanced into a healthful food plan.

Although there is no such thing as a bad food, there is a bad diet. Repeatedly eating meals and snacks of junk foods filled with saturated fat and refined sugars can, indeed, contribute to obesity, heart disease, cancer, hypertension, diabetes, kidney failure, and other diseases associated with excessive eating. As I outline in chapter 1, choosing a nutrition game plan based on wholesome grains, fruits, vegetables, nuts, lean protein, and low-fat dairy foods—in addition to leading an active lifestyle—clearly invests in optimal health and sports performance. The purpose of this chapter is to help you make the best food choices for lifelong well-being.

Diet and Heart Health

Heart disease is the number one killer of both men and women in America. Women tend to think cancer is the number one killer, but that is not the case. Heart disease and stroke account for 38 percent of deaths among women (Mosca et al. 2007), whereas cancer accounts for about 22 percent. Two ways to reduce your risk of heart disease are being physically fit and eating wisely. Yet, active people often believe they are exempt from the food rules about heart-healthy eating; they assume that being physically fit protects them from heart disease. Wrong! A friend of mine, a seemingly healthy 48-year-old marathoner, died suddenly of a massive heart attack. He'd run 2 hours 10 minutes, stopped his watch, and was later found dead in the running path. Everyone was shocked.

Unfortunately, even the most health-conscious people can find themselves confused by the constant updates and changes to heart-health information. This leaves us wondering what the real answers are to questions such as the following: Is beef bad? What about eggs? Should I use butter or margarine? The answers vary from person to person because we each have a unique genetic makeup. It won't be long before dietary recommendations will be based on genetic tests. But for today, here are suggestions for optimizing your diet, based on the latest nutrition studies.

Know Your Numbers

Cholesterol is a waxy substance that accumulates in the walls of the blood vessels throughout the body, especially those in the heart, and contributes to hardening of the arteries. This buildup limits blood flow to the heart muscle and contributes to heart attacks. You consume cholesterol when you eat animal foods; cholesterol is a part of animal cells. Your body also makes cholesterol. Foods with saturated fat (butter, lard) and partially hydrogenated or trans fat can increase the level of cholesterol in the blood, thereby increasing the risk of cardiovascular (*cardio* = heart; *vascular* = blood vessel) disease. Table 2.1 provides the amounts of cholesterol and fat found in common foods.

Because genetics play a large role in heart and blood vessel health, you may have a blood cholesterol level that puts you at a high risk for

Table 2.1   Fat and Cholesterol in Common Foods

Food product	Amount	Fat (g)	Cholesterol (mg)
Milk			
Nonfat	1 cup (240 ml)	0	5
2% fat	1 cup (240 ml)	5	20
Whole	1 cup (240 ml)	8	35
Cheese			
Cheddar	1 oz (30 g)	10	30
Mozzarella, part skim	1 oz (30 g)	5	15
Cottage cheese, 1% fat	1/2 cup (115 g)	1	5
Ice cream			
Expensive brands			
16% fat	1/2 cup (125 g)	12-18	40-50
Less-expensive brands			
10% fat	1/2 cup (125 g)	5-10	30-35
Low fat	1/2 cup (125 g)	3-5	10-20
Meats and fish (cooked)			
Pork, roast loin	4 oz (125 g)	8	85
Beef, 90% lean hamburger	4 oz (125 g)	18	95
Ham, canned lean	4 oz (125 g)	6	50
Chicken, roast breast	4 oz (125 g)	2	95
Tuna, canned white	4 oz (125 g)	3	45
McDonald's Big Mac	1	29	75
McDonald's Filet-o-Fish	1	18	35

Nutrient data from food labels, McDonald's Corporation (www.mcdonalds.com) and J. Pennington, 1998, *Bowes & Church's Food Values of Portions Commonly Used*, 17th ed. (Philadelphia: Lippincott).

developing cardiovascular disease even if you eat a healthy diet. One 28-year-old triathlete was dismayed when he discovered his cholesterol was very high. He likely inherited this trait from his father and grandfather, both of whom had heart attacks in their 50s.

By knowing your cholesterol level, you can assess your risk of developing heart disease. Make an appointment with your doctor to get your blood tested for these health indicators:

- Total cholesterol. Your body contains different types of cholesterol, including HDL and LDL. The sum of the types of cholesterol is called your total cholesterol. The desired level is less than 200 milligrams of total cholesterol per deciliter of blood.

- HDL cholesterol. High-density lipoprotein cholesterol is the "good stuff" that carries the bad cholesterol out of the arteries. The desired level is more than 60 milligrams HDL per deciliter to protect against heart disease.

- LDL cholesterol. Low-density lipoprotein cholesterol is the "bad stuff" that clogs arteries. A level greater than 160 milligrams per deciliter is associated with a higher risk of heart disease. The optimal LDL level is less than 100 milligrams per deciliter.

- Ratio of total cholesterol to HDL. At least 25 percent of your total blood cholesterol should be HDL. Because exercise tends to boost HDL, active people often have a higher percentage of this good cholesterol. Their total cholesterol may be higher than that of a sedentary person, but as long as 25 percent of it is HDL, these individuals have a lower risk of heart problems. The higher the HDL percentage, the better.

After you know your blood cholesterol level, you'll be better able to determine how strict you need to be with your diet. For example, if your level is far less than 200 milligrams and your 97-year-old parents are still alive and thriving, you can be less obsessive about your eating habits than can your buddy whose cholesterol is a risky 250 milligrams and whose father died suddenly of a heart attack at age 54.

Another possible blood test for people with a family history of heart disease but no obvious risk factors is a test that checks levels of artery-clogging particles called apolipoproteins and determines the ratio of apoB to apoA-1. A third possible test is for CRP, or C-reactive protein, a measure of inflammation. Arteries weakened by inflammation are also associated with a higher risk of heart disease. Although none of these tests will predict with certainty whether or not you will have a heart attack, they can offer a suggestion of where you stand when it comes to heart disease.

Eat for Heart Health

By tweaking your daily food intake to include heart-healthy choices, you can make several small changes that accumulate to make a big difference in the long run. The American Heart Association (AHA) recommends a variety of diet and lifestyle choices to reduce your risk for cardiovascular disease (Lichtenstein et al. 2006)*. You should review your physical activity and calorie intake to ensure they are in balance. Doing so will help you reach or maintain a healthy weight. You should also strive to consume a diet that is rich in vegetables, fruits, and whole-grain, high-fiber foods. The guidelines also recommend consuming 8 ounces (250 g) of oily fish per week.

Another part of achieving a healthy diet is to limit your intake of saturated fats, trans fats, and cholesterol. Saturated fats should account for no more than 7 percent of your total calories, and trans fat for no more than 1 percent of your total calories. Limit your cholesterol intake to less than 300 mg per day. You can achieve these goals by choosing lean meats or vegetable alternatives; by selecting fat-free (skim), 1%-fat, and low-fat dairy products; and by minimizing your comsumption of partially hydrogenated fats.

Other choices that can reduce your risk of heart disease include controlling your weight by limiting your intake of beverages and foods with added sugars, choosing and preparing foods with little or no salt, and consuming alcohol in moderation (if at all). And when you dine away from home you can make reasonably healthful choices by following AHA's recommendations for eating out.

This book provides you with detailed information you can use to follow the AHA's guidelines successfully.

*Adapted from A.H. Lichtenstein et al., 2006, "Diet and lifestyle recommendations revision 2006: A scientific statement from the American Heart Association Nutrition Committee," *Circulation* 114(1): 82-96.

Lean Beef and Heart Health

Athletes commonly shun beef, believing it to be an artery clogger. Although that is true for greasy burgers and sausages, small portions of lean beef aren't so bad after all. In fact, lean beef is an excellent source of iron, zinc, and other nutrients athletes need. Despite popular belief, beef is not exceptionally high in cholesterol; it has a cholesterol value similar to that in chicken and fish. Additionally, we now know that cholesterol, which was once thought to contribute to heart disease, is less of a culprit than saturated fat. However, beef tends to have more saturated fat than chicken or fish, so that's why it still has a bad name among health watchers. Saturated fat is hard at room temperature. For example, the hard fat on uncooked steak is different from chicken fat, which is softer and less saturated.

The AHA recommends that we consume less than 7 percent of our calories from saturated fat; the average intake in the United States is about 11 percent. The Web site www.americanheart.org/facethefats has a fat calculator that helps you determine how much of each type of fat can fit into your daily food plan. If you are on an 1,800-calorie reducing diet, 7 percent is just about the amount of saturated fat you'd consume in a McDonald's Quarter Pounder with Cheese. If you are very active and require 3,000 calories per day, 7 percent of calories from saturated fat equates to the amount in two double cheeseburgers.

But not all beef is fatty. In the past decade, the healthfulness of beef and other meats has improved because farmers have learned how to raise leaner animals and because butchers are trimming more of the fat from the meat in stores. You can easily fit beef (and pork and lamb) into a heart-healthy sports diet if you select lean cuts, such as eye of round, rump roast, sirloin tip, flank steak, top round, and tenderloin, and eat smaller portions, limiting yourself to a piece of lean protein about the size of the palm of your hand. You can more easily consume lean beef when you are preparing meals at home than when you are in a restaurant that prides itself on juicy, tender (read as "loaded with saturated fat") beef.

Fish and Heart Health

If good health is your wish, get hooked on fish. Research indicates that fish may guard against not only heart disease but also hypertension, cancer, arthritis, asthma, and who knows what else. The omega-3 fatty acids, the special polyunsaturated fat found in fish oil, block many harmful biochemical reactions that can cause blood to clot (predisposing you to heart attack and stroke) and the heart to beat irregularly (as occurs during a heart attack). Some researchers believe that fish oils can prevent heart disease from beginning rather than merely having a beneficial effect after the onset of the disease.

A comparison of the rates of death from heart disease of men in a fishing village and the rates of death of men in a farming village suggests a 4 times lower incidence of heart disease among the men in the fishing village. They ate 10 times more fish than the farmers and had much higher blood levels of the health-protective omega-3 fat (Torres et al. 2000). A study of almost 85,000 U.S. nurses suggests that women who ate fish two to four times a week had a 31 percent lower risk of heart disease compared with those who rarely ate fish (Hu et al. 2002).

The American Heart Association recommends eating about 8 oz (250 g) of oily fish per week (that's one large or two small fish servings) to help reduce your risk of heart disease. Eating fish for dinner not only contributes fish oil to your diet but also displaces meat-based meals high in saturated fat. Table 2.2 can help guide your fish choices so you select the fish highest in omega-3 fat. Just be sure that your fish is prepared in low-fat ways, not fried or broiled in butter. If you shy away from cooking fish, simply take advantage of precooked tuna (mixed with low-fat mayonnaise), salmon, and sardines in cans or foil pouches.

Be careful about eating too much fish, however. Unfortunately, the fish highest in omega-3 fatty acids also deliver a dose of methylmercury from industrial pollution of the oceans. Long-term consumption of mercury can contribute to neurological and cardiovascular problems in

Table 2.2   Fish Highest in Omega-3 Fatty Acids

Fish, 6 oz cooked (8 oz raw); 175 g cooked (250 g raw)	Grams of omega-3 fat (EPA and DHA)**
Salmon, Atlantic, farmed	2.0-3.6
Sardines, in sardine oil, 3 oz (90 g)	2.0-3.4
Salmon, Atlantic, wild	1.8-3.1
Swordfish*	0.7-3.1
Salmon, coho, farmed	3.0
Trout, rainbow, farmed	2.0
Trout, rainbow, wild	1.7
Salmon, coho, wild	1.4
Sardines, in vegetable oil, 3 oz (90 g)	1.0
Halibut	0.8
Tuna, albacore white, canned, 3 oz (90 g)*	0.7
Tuna, fresh*	0.5
Pollock	0.4
Lobster, 3 oz (90 g)	0.1-0.4
Shrimp, 3 oz (90 g)	0.3
Alternative sources	
Smart Balance Omega Plus spread, 1/2 tbsp	0.08
Orange juice, omega-3 fortified, 8 oz (240 ml)	0.05
Egg, 1 omega-3 rich	0.05-0.11
Silk Plus Omega-3 DHA soy milk, 8 oz (240 ml)	0.03

*Highest in mercury; limit to 6 oz (175 g) per week.
**EPA and DHA are two types of omega-3 fat.
Data from the American Heart Association and food labels.

adults, as well as cause significant damage to the developing brains of infants and children. If you are into sport fishing, eating sushi, or having tuna every day for lunch—and enjoy high-mercury fish several times a week—take heed. The mercury can accumulate in your body and create health problems (numbness and tingling in hands and feet, fatigue, muscle pain).

Yet, the FDA advises pregnant women that they can and should safely enjoy up to 12 ounces (340 g) of fish a week because fish oil is important for normal brain development. The 12 ounces includes a large safety margin, but pregnant women should avoid shark, swordfish, king mackerel, and tile fish and limit their intake of albacore tuna to not more than one 6-ounce can per week. These fish are long-lived and large; they accumulate mercury in their tissues over time by eating a lot of smaller mercury-containing fish. The safest fish are shrimp, salmon, pollock, catfish, and canned light tuna. For a list of fish oil and mercury in commonly consumed seafood, visit the American Heart Association's Web site and do a search for "fish." To calculate your potential mercury intake, go to www.gotmercury.org.

If you are not a fish fan, and if you have heart disease, the American Heart Association suggests fish oil capsules as an alternative: 850 to 1,000 milligrams EPA plus DHA; 2,000 to 4,000 milligrams if you have high triglycerides (Kris-Etherton, Harris, and Appel 2002; Mosca et al. 2007). But be aware: Fish oil supplements contain only a small amount of omega-3s compared with a fish dinner, so you may need to take several capsules to get the equivalent of one 4-ounce (120 g) serving of salmon. For more information about fish oil supplements, visit the Web site of the National Institutes of Health Office of Dietary Supplements (www. ods.od.nih.gov).

An alternative way to ingest omega-3 fat is from plant sources, such as flaxseed oil, walnuts, tofu, soy nuts, canola oil, and olive oil. Plant sources offer a less potent type of omega-3s, but any omega-3 is better than none. You can also buy foods fortified with omega-3s, such as some brands of orange juice, margarine, yogurt, and eggs.

Soy Foods and Heart Health

At one time, soy was believed to lower the bad LDL cholesterol and increase the good HDL cholesterol. This shift would offer protection against heart disease. The current research suggests that soy—and substances in soy called isoflavones—do not protect against heart disease. Yet, soy products can still be beneficial because of their high content of polyunsaturated fat, fiber, vitamins, and minerals (Sacks et al. 2006). Soy foods are also low in saturated fat, so when you choose soy foods for dinner, you forgo prime rib and other artery-clogging choices.

Eggs and Heart Health

Eggs have gotten a bad rap when it comes to healthy eating. Medical experts have told us that eating eggs is bad because a single egg has 210 milligrams of cholesterol. This just about hits the American Heart Association's recommended limit of 300 milligrams per day. But more recent studies suggest that egg cholesterol may have little effect on many people's blood cholesterol levels, especially in combination with an overall low-saturated-fat diet (Katz et al. 2005; Kritchevsky and Kritchevsky 2000). In fact, an estimated 85 percent of Americans can eat a high-cholesterol diet with no elevation of blood cholesterol. Among 49 healthy men and women who ate two eggs daily for six weeks, blood cholesterol levels remained stable (Katz et al. 2005).

To date, it is unclear whether the cholesterol you eat affects the cholesterol in your blood, because most of the blood's cholesterol is made in the liver. We do know that dietary fat affects the way the body disposes of cholesterol. In particular, saturated fat (such as butter and beef fat) appears to inhibit the body's ability to get rid of the bad form of cholesterol (low-density lipoprotein, or LDL) that clogs arteries. We also know that some people respond more readily than others to a low-cholesterol diet, and dietary recommendations need to be individualized.

So, when it comes to eggs, you should limit your intake if you have a high blood cholesterol level and a family history of heart disease. The American Heart Association recommends a limit of three eggs per week, including those used in cooking. Otherwise, if you have low blood cholesterol and no family history of heart disease, this highly nutritious protein source can likely be eaten without concern as a part of your balanced nutrition plan.

For dieters who want to lose weight to help reduce their risk of heart disease, eggs may even be a positive addition to their diets. Eating two eggs with two slices of toast and some jam for breakfast has been shown to be more satiating than eating the same number of calories in the form of a bagel with cream cheese and a little yogurt. The egg breakfast maintained satiety, so the subjects felt less hungry and ate about 250 fewer calories the rest of the day (Vander Wal et al. 2005).

When choosing eggs, you may want to buy brands such as Eggland's Best, which contain health-protective omega-3 fatty acids (110 mg per egg). These "designer eggs" are produced from chickens given a special vegetarian feed that includes canola oil, which improves the fat content of the egg yolk. They also contain more vitamin E than other eggs and are preferable to standard eggs for a heart-healthier diet.

Oatmeal for Heart Health

The type of fiber (soluble fiber) found in oats as well as in barley, lentils, split peas, and beans protects against heart disease. Find ways to include more of these foods in your diet. For example, trade a meat sandwich for a hummus wrap or some hearty lentil soup and some whole-grain bread.

Research suggests that eating a bowlful of oatmeal (1 1/2 cups cooked) each day can help people attain lower cholesterol levels, especially when eaten as part of a low-fat diet, and especially when the person has elevated cholesterol levels to begin with (Expert Panel 2001). In a six-week study of healthy adults who ate oatmeal for breakfast, cholesterol dropped 10 points (Katz et al. 2005). Of course, a low-fat diet is as important as eating the oatmeal; that is, you cannot eat oatmeal for breakfast, have a cheesesteak sub for lunch and pepperoni pizza for dinner, and expect your blood cholesterol to drop!

If you don't have time to cook oatmeal at home, enjoy one or two packets of instant oatmeal for a midmorning or afternoon snack. Or do what I do—simply add raw oats (either instant or old fashioned) to your cold cereal. Wheaties and raw oats is my favorite way to get two whole grains in one tasty bowl.

Cooking Oils for Heart Health

When it comes to selecting heart-healthy fat for cooking, the rule of thumb is "the softer the better." That is, soft (liquid) vegetable oils have a higher percentage of unsaturated fat compared with harder (solid) fat such as margarines and butter. Olive oil and canola oil are the two preferred types of fat to include in a heart-healthy diet. These oils are rich in monounsaturated fat and are considered better choices than safflower, corn, sunflower, and other polyunsaturated vegetable oils. Use olive and canola oils with salads, pesto, and pasta and when sautéing. Just be sure to use only moderate amounts if you want to lose body fat. Their calories, although preferable to the calories from butter or lard, still count and add up quickly.

Cooking with olive and canola oil is far more healthful than using butter, stick margarine, bacon grease, lard, salt pork, and animal fat, which are all solid at room temperature. If you use a significant amount of margarine, you may want to use Take Control, a margarine with sterols, a substance that interferes with the absorption of dietary cholesterol. Two tablespoons a day (to equate to 2 grams of plant sterol per day) can contribute to lower LDL (bad) cholesterol by 10 percent or more.

Nuts and Peanut Butter for Heart Health

Although many people try to stay away from nuts and peanut butter because they fear them as being fattening, research with more than 260,000 people indicates that eating one serving of nuts or peanut butter five times a week can reduce the risk of heart disease by 50 percent (Kris-Etherton et al. 2001). Research also indicates that eating nuts can reduce the risk of type 2 diabetes by about 25 percent (Jiang et al. 2002). Nuts are rich in monounsaturated fat (as well as folate, niacin, thiamin, magnesium, fiber, and other health-protective nutrients). Adding walnuts to oatmeal, peanut butter to a bagel, sliced almonds in a salad, and mixed nuts to dried fruit for trail mix are just a few simple ways to include these health-protective foods in your daily diet—to say nothing of enjoying a good old peanut butter sandwich for lunch.

The trick with nuts and peanut butter is to keep the portion within your calorie budget. For 170 calories, you can enjoy an ounce (30 g) of nuts: about 22 almonds, 28 peanuts, 20 pecans, 45 pistachios, 10 walnuts, or 1/4 cup sunflower seeds. The good news is that nuts are very satisfying, and an ounce (or less) will curb your hunger for a while. Dieters can lose weight and keep it off when they include nuts, peanut butter, and other types of healthful fat as a part of their daily diets (McManus et al. 2001).

FITTING FAT INTO YOUR DIET   Both a sports diet and a heart-healthy diet limit fat to 20 to 35 percent of calorie intake. The American Heart Association advises eating more of the good plant and fish oils and less of the saturated animal fat. It also recommends cutting back on partially hydrogenated vegetable oils (trans fat), coconut oils, and palm oils, three highly saturated vegetable oils commonly used in processed foods.

By rationing your intake of fried foods and foods obviously high in fat (butter, margarine, mayonnaise, salad dressing, ice cream, cookies, chips), you'll end up with a diet that's about 25 percent fat. You really don't need to calculate and count grams of fat. But if you are an avid label reader, like many of my clients, you may want to more precisely know your fat budget. I advise most athletes to aim for a diet that contains 25 percent fat to allow space for plenty of carbohydrate to fuel their muscles.

If you have a very high cholesterol level, your physician may recommend a diet that is 20 percent fat. This restriction is for people clinically endangered by heart disease, not for healthy people who already have low cholesterol levels. I talk often to food fanatics with low cholesterol who try to eliminate all fat from their diets. They burden themselves with needless restrictions; a low-fat diet need not be a no-fat diet. Some fat is important for absorbing vitamins A, D, E, and K; fueling your muscles; and satisfying your appetite.

Your weight in kilograms (1 kilogram is 2.2 pounds) is a rough estimation of the number of grams of fat you can healthfully include in your diet. For a more precise calculation, follow these three steps:

1. Estimate how many calories you need per day (see chapter 15 for instructions).

2. Multiply your total daily calories by 25 percent to determine the number of fat calories you can appropriately eat.

3. Divide your allotted fat calories by 9 to determine the number of grams of fat in your daily fat budget (1 gram of fat is 9 calories).

Hence, if you are an active woman who eats about 2,000 calories per day, 500 of them could appropriately come from fat, and you could consume about 56 grams of fat per day:

$$0.25 \times 2{,}000 \text{ total cal} = 500 \text{ cal fat}$$
$$500 \text{ cal fat} \div 9 \text{ cal/g} = 56 \text{ g fat}$$

HOW MUCH FAT IS OKAY? The following table can help you determine your target fat intake. If you are underweight or very active, you may want more calories from (healthful) fat to help boost your total calorie intake. Plan to eat more heart-healthy fat, such as peanut butter, nuts, and olive or canola oils. Read food labels to learn the fat content of the foods you commonly eat (see appendix A for other dietary analysis tools).

Calorie needs per day	20% fat (g)	25% fat (g)	30% fat (g)
1,500	30	40	50
1,800	40	50	60
2,000	45	55	65
2,400	55	65	80
2,600	60	70	85

Supplements for Heart Health

Questions arise about the role of vitamin supplements to enhance heart health. Living healthfully could be so much easier if we could just take a pill that could compensate for both suboptimal eating and suboptimal genetics. Unfortunately, the vitamin and antioxidant studies that looked for reduction in heart disease saw few benefits—and even potential harm—from taking high doses of beta-carotene, selenium, and vitamin E. The same goes for folate and other B vitamins; research results have been disappointing. Hence, the AHA highly encourages you to get your vitamins and antioxidants from fruits, vegetables, whole grains, and vegetable oils. The right foods can be powerfully health promoting! See chapter 11 for more information about vitamin supplements.

Diet and Cancer

In the United States, cancer follows heart disease as the most frequent cause of death. Cancer isn't one disease; it is many. Each has its own high-risk groups, its own incidence and cure rates, and its own causes. Diet is a factor in an estimated 35 percent of cancer cases, and a healthier diet may cut your risk more than you may think.

Despite the gloomy news that two out of every five of us will get cancer, the encouraging news is that dietary changes can prevent perhaps one-third of cancer deaths. For example, people who eat at least five servings a day of fruits and vegetables have a 40 percent lower risk for certain cancers (lung, colon, stomach, esophagus, and mouth) compared with people who eat two or fewer servings of fruits and vegetables. A fruit-filled, high-fiber, cancer-protective diet is also a top-performance sports diet. Indulge in good health for high energy.

Protective Nutrients

One key to the role of diet in preventing cancer may lie in an antioxidative capacity, or a nutrient's ability to deactivate harmful chemicals in the body known as free radicals. Free radicals are formed daily through normal body processes. Environmental pollutants such as cigarette smoke, automobile exhaust, radiation, and herbicides also generate free radical precursors. These unstable compounds can attack, infiltrate, and injure vital cell structures. Fortunately, our bodies have natural control systems that deactivate and minimize free radical reactions within the cells. These natural control systems involve many vitamins and minerals, including these:

- **Carotenoids.** These precursors of vitamin A are found in plants and then converted into vitamin A in the body. Beta-carotene, as well as the more than 40 other carotenoids found in orange and green fruits and vegetables, helps prevent the formation of free radicals. Some of the best sources include carrots, spinach, sweet potatoes, kale, apricots, and cantaloupe. (If you eat too many carotene-rich vegetables and fruits, your skin might turn yellow. If it does, simply cut back.)

- **Vitamin C.** This vitamin guards against harmful reactions within the cells. The best sources include kiwi, citrus fruits, broccoli, green and red peppers, and strawberries. The body's tissues become saturated with vitamin C at about 200 milligrams a day, an amount easily attainable by eating the recommended four cups of fruits and vegetables.

- **Vitamin E.** Vitamin E protects the cell walls from free radical damage. Be sure to include some foods rich in vitamin E when balancing your daily calorie budget, but consume them carefully because they are calorie dense. The best sources are vegetable oils (and foods made with them, such as salad dressings), almonds, peanuts, sunflower and sesame seeds, wheat germ, and whole grains (see table 2.3). The recommended dietary allowance (RDA) for vitamin E is 15 milligrams.

Table 2.3   Vitamin E in Foods

Food	Portion	Vitamin E (mg)
Sunflower seeds	1/4 cup (30 g)	28
Almonds	1/4 cup (30 g)	14
Oil, safflower	1 tbsp	6
Wheat germ	1/4 cup (30 g)	5
Peanuts	1/4 cup (30 g)	4
Oil, canola	1 tbsp	3
Oil, olive	1 tbsp	2
Spinach, cooked	1 cup (44 g)	2

Data from J. Pennington, 1998, *Bowes & Church's Food Values of Portions Commonly Used*, 17th ed. (Philadelphia: Lippincott).

- **Selenium.** Selenium protects the cell walls from free radical damage and enhances the immune system's response with increased resistance to cancer growth. The best sources of selenium include seafood such as tuna fish, meats, eggs, milk, whole grains, and garlic. Supplements are not recommended because of the danger of toxicity with long-term supplementation over 200 micrograms.

Other cancer protectors include foods rich in fiber. Although population studies suggest that people who eat a lot of fiber from grains, fruits, and vegetables have a lower risk of cancer, scientists are unclear if the fiber is the protective nutrient. In addition to the known vitamins and minerals in grains, fresh fruits, and vegetables, these fiber-rich foods contain hundreds, perhaps thousands, of other lesser-known substances called phytochemicals that may protect our health. That's why you want to put more energy into eating a varied diet than wondering which fiber supplement to choose.

For more information about diet and cancer prevention, see the 2007 Diet and Cancer Report by the World Cancer Research Fund and the American Institute for Cancer Research (see Cancer in appendix A). A few of the key points of the report include eating mostly foods of plant origin, enjoying at least 14 ounces of vegetables and fruits every day, limiting intake of red meat to 18 ounces per week, avoiding processed meats (like hot dogs, bologna, and pepperoni), limiting alcohol intake, and aiming to meet nutritional needs through diet alone. The report does not recommend dietary supplements for cancer prevention.

Although researchers at one time hoped that high intakes of antioxidants from pills would reduce the incidence of some types of cancer, the current evidence is disappointing. Apart from the possibility that vitamin

E and selenium may reduce the risk of prostate cancer (and eye problems such as macular degeneration), several large studies have shown few health benefits from supplemental antioxidants. The studies that drove the hope that antioxidants would protect against cancer came from people who ate lots of fruits and vegetables (and had higher blood levels of antioxidants). Most health professionals today emphasize the importance of obtaining these nutrients from food, not from supplements. Scientists have yet to pinpoint which of the thousands of substances in fruits and vegetables are protective.

So, be sure to eat lots of broccoli, carrots, sweet potatoes, and other colorful vegetables and remember that no amount of supplementation will compensate for a fast-food diet low in fruits and vegetables and a stress-filled, health-eroding lifestyle.

Cancer Prevention

Eating a low-fat diet may be a second dietary key to reducing cancer risk, particularly if it leads to reducing excess body fat. Population studies suggest that people who eat low-fat diets have a lower incidence of cancer. The National Research Council recommends that we eat less than 30 percent of our total calories as fat, eat more fruits and vegetables rich in beta-carotene and vitamin C (review tables 1.1 and 1.2), and eat more whole grains. Voila—a high-carbohydrate sports diet! Fatty fish can also be included among cancer-protective foods. The omega-3 fatty acids may slow tumor growth.

Cancer (and other health problems) can be affected by not only your diet but also your lifestyle. Relaxation, peace of mind, a positive outlook on life, a contented spirit, absence of envy, love of mankind, and faith are powerful health-promoting factors without which optimal health cannot be achieved. This holistic approach to cancer prevention and health protection includes nourishing yourself with pleasant, well-balanced, low-fat meals; enjoying exercise as part of your daily routine; and taking time to smell the roses.

Diet and High Blood Pressure

High blood pressure, or hypertension, is a major risk factor for heart disease and the chief risk factor for stroke. Hypertension affects approximately 25 to 30 percent of Americans. By having your blood pressure measured, you can determine if it is in a healthy range. The normal pressure is 120 over 80, and a measure that exceeds 140 over 90 is considered high. Blood pressure tends to increase with age.

What Causes Hypertension?

Risk factors that can predispose people to hypertension include obesity, smoking, high stress, poor kidney function, and poor diet. Most regular exercisers are not obese, do not smoke, and eat a healthier-than-average diet, thus eliminating several risk factors. Many active people, in fact, have low blood pressure. But you cannot change additional predisposing factors—such as your genetics, age, and race—that can sometimes cause high blood pressure in spite of all your good health habits. You also cannot overlook the fact that blood pressure increases as we age; as many as 70 percent of people over age 65 have high blood pressure. In a study of people 30 to 54 years of age with borderline high blood pressure, those who reduced their sodium intake for 10 to 15 years experienced 25 percent fewer heart attacks and other cardiovascular events compared with those who consumed their standard sodium-rich meals (Cook et al. 2007).

If you have high blood pressure, you may believe that salt causes the problem and that reducing salt intake will lower your high blood pressure, but that's not always true. Only 10 percent of high blood pressure cases in the United States have a known cause. In the remaining 90 percent, no one cause can be identified. Health professionals debate whether the broad recommendation to reduce sodium intake is necessary. Yet, in Finland, because of a consistent salt education campaign, the Finns reduced their salt intake by about one-third over 30 years. This was associated with a large decrease in blood pressure and a dramatic 75 to 80 percent decline in deaths from heart disease and stroke in Finnish people younger than 65 years of age (Karppanen and Mervaala 2006). Reducing your daily sodium intake to reduce your risk of cardiovascular disease seems a wise investment for the long run.

Athletes and Salt

Salt is a compound of 40 percent sodium and 60 percent chloride. The sodium helps maintain proper fluid balance between the water in and around your body's cells; thus, you do need some sodium—about 1,000 milligrams per day. Many Americans, however, routinely consume up to seven times that amount.

The 2005 *Dietary Guidelines for Americans* recommend consuming less than 2,300 milligrams of sodium per day (a teaspoon of salt is about 2,300 mg). You lose sodium when you perspire heavily, and some athletes lose more than others. Most active people, though, can get adequate sodium from the amounts that naturally occur in foods. If you will be exercising moderately hard for more than four to six hours in the heat, you should purposefully consume salt. You should also consume salt if you exercise intensely for shorter periods. For example, the sodium in the sweat of professional football players varied widely from about 1,500 to 11,000 milligrams during two-hour summer practices (Greene et al. 2007). See chapters 8 and 10 for information on replacing sodium lost in sweat.

The daily value for sodium seems low for sweaty athletes. Consuming a low-sodium diet may be less of a priority if you routinely train hard and sweat heavily, have normal or low blood pressure, and have no family history of hypertension. If you have low sweat losses, however, reducing your daily sodium intake is likely a wise health investment.

Reducing Your Salt Intake

Food type	Average sodium content	Comments
Cereal (cold)	250 mg/oz (/30 g)	Read food label; varies by brand
Baked goods	250 mg/serving	Once a day, if at all
Cheese (low fat)	200 mg/oz (/30 g)	Moderate amounts; 1-2 oz/day
Breads	150 mg/slice	Read food label; varies by brand
Milk, yogurt (low fat)	125 mg/8 oz (/240 ml or g)	Read food label
Meat, fish, poultry	80 mg/4 oz (/115 g)	Unprocessed, unsalted
Eggs	60 mg/egg	Unprocessed, unsalted
Butter, margarine	50 mg/pat	Unsalted butter is an option
Vegetables	10 mg/serving	Fresh and frozen; if canned, rinse well
Fruit, juice	5 mg/serving	Naturally low in sodium

If you want a diet that is conducive to low blood pressure, your best bet is to buy foods in their natural state, such as raw unsalted peanuts, fresh (not canned) vegetables, and so on. Plan to eat lots of fresh fruits, vegetables, low-fat dairy products, and lean protein. Here is how foods compare in terms of sodium content:

Commercially prepared foods are the biggest contributor to sodium in the diet, so eating more unprocessed foods is the simplest way to lower your salt intake. (Fast-food eaters commonly consume more than 5,000 mg of sodium per day.) If you are overweight, try to lose a little weight to lower your blood pressure. Eating less of the following foods will also lower your sodium intake and may contribute to a greater reduction in blood pressure:

- Commercially prepared foods such as frozen dinners, canned soups, and instant meals unless they are labeled *low sodium*. Processed foods account for 75 percent of the sodium in the American diet.

Hungry athletes who eat a lot of convenience foods can easily consume a lot of sodium. Here's how: 1 cup of Ragu spaghetti sauce contains 1,140 milligrams of sodium; 1 cup of Rice-A-Roni contains 1,030 milligrams; a can of Campbell's chicken noodle soup contains 2,225 milligrams; and a 15-ounce (425 g) can of Beefaroni contains 1,980 milligrams.

- Table salt. Remove the saltshaker from the table. Omit or reduce salt from cooking and baking. You can often leave it out without affecting the outcome. If you must add salt, add it right before serving, not during cooking, to keep it on the food's surface so it tastes saltier.
- Obviously salty foods such as salted crackers, chips, pretzels, popcorn, salted nuts, olives, and pickles. Buy low-sodium versions, if they're available.
- Smoked and cured meats and fish such as ham, bacon, sausage, corned beef, hot dogs, bologna, salami, pepperoni, lox, and pickled herring. Choose low-sodium versions if you like these foods.
- Cheeses, in particular processed and low-fat cheeses, some of which may be higher in sodium than the regular form.
- Seasonings and condiments such as ketchup, mustard, relish, Worcestershire sauce, soy sauce, steak sauce, MSG, and garlic salt.
- Baking soda, seltzers, and antacids. Also, some laxatives may be high in sodium.

To add flavor to your foods, experiment with herbs and spices. When you try a new seasoning, cautiously add a small amount. Some tried-and-true combinations include the following:

- Beef—dry mustard, pepper, marjoram, red wine, or sherry
- Chicken—parsley, thyme, sage, tarragon, curry, white wine, or vermouth
- Fish—bay leaf, cayenne pepper, dill, curry, onions, garlic
- Eggs—oregano, curry, chives, pepper, tomatoes, pinch of sugar

The DASH Diet

To clarify the connection between blood pressure and diet, the National Institutes of Health funded a large study of dietary approaches to stop hypertension (DASH). The DASH diet requires twice the average daily servings of fruits, vegetables, and dairy foods; one-third the usual intake of beef, pork, and ham; one-half the typical use of fat, oils, and salad dressings; and one-quarter the ordinary number of snacks and sweets

(Blackburn 2001). When more than 400 people followed the DASH diet for three months, their blood pressure dropped. The researchers concluded that a diet rich in calcium, potassium, magnesium, and fiber contributes to lower blood pressure. When people simultaneously reduce sodium intake, their blood pressure drops even more. Those consuming 1,500 milligrams of sodium a day experience a greater drop in blood pressure than those who eat 3,300 milligrams (the typical American intake). For more details about the DASH diet, see the hypertension section in appendix A.

The DASH study points out that blood pressure is affected by more than just sodium intake. The same fruits, vegetables, whole grains, and low-fat dairy products and meats that optimize your sports diet can also optimize your health. Eating a potassium-rich diet seems to guard against hypertension. Potassium helps make arteries stronger and better able to withstand the blood vessel damage that can occur with aging. Calcium may offset the effect of too much sodium in the diet. Refer to tables 1.1 and 1.2 (pages 11 and 14) for the potassium content of some popular fruits and vegetables and table 1.3 (page 19) for a list of calcium-rich foods.

Increasing Your Potassium Intake

If sodium is the bad guy that contributes to high blood pressure, then potassium is the good guy that helps lower blood pressure. Potassium is found in most whole foods: fruits, vegetables, whole-grain breads and cereals, lentils, beans, nuts, and protein foods. Refined or highly processed foods, sweets, and oily foods (e.g., salad dressing, butter) are poor sources of potassium. You can increase your potassium intake by eating the following kinds of foods:

- Whole-wheat, oatmeal, and dark breads instead of white bread and flour products.
- More salads and raw or steamed veggies cooked in only a small amount of water, because the potassium leaches into the water. Steaming removes only 3 to 6 percent of the potassium, as compared with 10 to 15 percent with boiling. Microwaving is best for optimal potassium retention.
- Potatoes more often than rice, noodles, or pasta.
- Natural fruit juices instead of fruit-flavored beverages or soft drinks.

The suggested daily intake for potassium is 4,700 milligrams a day for the average person. The typical American diet contains 4,000 to 7,000 milligrams of potassium. A small amount of potassium is lost in sweat; one pound of sweat loss may contain 85 to 105 milligrams.

Diet and Diabetes

With the current epidemic of obesity that is plaguing the United States, a concurrent epidemic of diabetes is tagging alongside, not only in adults but also among children, who have grown accustomed to eating supersized fast foods and spending too much time in front of TV and computer screens instead of playing outside and moving their bodies. Although one type of diabetes, insulin-dependent diabetes, is the result of the body's inability to produce adequate insulin to carry blood sugar into the cells, a second and more common type of diabetes, type 2 diabetes, commonly occurs in people who are overweight and underfit. These people need to lose weight, exercise more, and eat better-quality foods (or take medications). If not, the resulting high levels of blood glucose increase their risk of heart attacks, strokes, kidney disease, blindness, and amputation of limbs.

Many people think eating lots of sugar causes diabetes. Wrong. Being overweight and underfit are the bigger culprits. In a study of 3,200 people (average age in the 50s) who were overweight and had elevated blood glucose, both when fasting and after eating meals (a risk factor for diabetes), some of the subjects were given medicine (metformin) to lower their blood glucose. Others were instructed to exercise at least 150 minutes per week (five times a week for 30 minutes) and to lose weight (about 7 percent of their body weight, or about 11 pounds for a 160-pound person). And some were told to make no changes (these people made up the control group).

The subjects who became more active and lost a little bit of weight dramatically reduced their risk of developing diabetes—by 58 percent. In contrast, the group that took medicine experienced a 31 percent drop during the almost three-year study. The bottom line: Food and exercise are better than medicine! By getting active and staying active throughout your life, you'll greatly reduce your risk of developing adult-onset diabetes (as well as other diseases of aging) (Knowler et al. 2002). The best cure for diabetes is prevention. For more in-depth information about diabetes, see the resources in appendix A.

Diet and Bone Health

Osteoporosis, or thinning of the bones with aging, results in hunched backs and brittle bones that break easily. Particularly among older post-menopausal women, osteoporosis is a serious health problem. In a survey of more than 200,000 healthy women 50 years or older, 40 percent had osteopenia (reduced bone mass, the early stage of osteoporosis) and

7 percent had osteoporosis—and they didn't even know it. The women diagnosed with osteoporosis were four times more likely to fracture a bone within the next 12 months; those with osteopenia were almost two times more likely (Siris et al. 2001). Osteoporosis is also a major concern for men older than 70, so men need to take care of their bones in their earlier years as well.

Younger female athletes who have stopped having regular menstrual periods are also at risk for low bone density that can develop into osteoporosis. Both amenorrheic and postmenopausal women lack adequate estrogen, a hormone that contributes to menstruation and helps maintain bone density. The low bone density of a 29-year-old woman, a former amenorrheic runner, has left her living in pain and doubting if her bones will be able to withstand the weight of a pregnancy.

The good news is that osteoporosis is a preventable condition. It is not an inevitable result of old age. You can reduce your risk of developing osteoporosis with these life-long, good-health habits:

- **Calcium-rich diet.** A lifelong calcium-rich diet will help you build strong bones as well as maintain bone density by reducing the rate of calcium loss thereafter. To ensure the best protection, aim to consume 1,000 to 1,300 milligrams of calcium per day. You should also consume 400 to 800 international units of vitamin D per day, which will help your body absorb the calcium you consume. If you are a parent, be sure your 11- to 14-year-old kids consume more milk than soda pop. Calcium is most important in the three years surrounding puberty and up to about age 30.

  In chapter 1, I talk about how to include in your daily diet the calcium necessary for lifelong fitness. Unfortunately, the typical 25- to 40-year-old woman consumes only half the recommended intake of 1,000 milligrams. This may be one reason why about 25 percent of women over 65 years have osteoporosis (of whom 12 percent may die from medical complications). These women might have reduced their risk by consuming more calcium-rich foods throughout their lifetimes.

  If you think taking calcium pills is the simple alternative to drinking milk, think again. Women who get their calcium from food sources tend to have stronger bones than those who rely on supplements (Napoli et al. 2007).

- **Regular exercise.** Participate in a regular exercise program that includes weight-bearing aerobic and muscle-building exercises. (If you are a swimmer or cyclist, you may want to cross-train with some jogging, jumping rope, or other weight-bearing exercise to enhance bone strength.) Accompany these bone-strengthening exercises with adequate calcium and vitamin D.

- **Normal hormones.** Women with estrogen deficiency have lower bone mineral density despite high calcium intake and participation in a weight-bearing exercise program. (That's one reason why amenorrheic female athletes are at high risk for stress fractures.) Athletes with amenorrhea commonly take the birth control pill, believing it will protect their bones, but research suggests this may be ineffective (Weaver et al. 2001). The better bet for athletes with amenorrhea is to eat enough to support regular menses (Nattiv 2007).

- **Low sodium intake.** Because too much salt interferes with the retention of calcium (Sellmeyer, Schloetter, and Sebastian 2002), your best bet is to moderate your salt intake, especially if you have a genetic predisposition to osteoporosis.

Unfortunately, too many women follow too few of these guidelines. I once counseled a very thin 24-year-old amenorrheic aerobics instructor who had the bones of a 60-year-old. She rarely drank milk (believing it to be a fattening fluid), ate a restrictive diet low in calories and protein, and was always trying to be thinner despite her obvious leanness.

Boosting Your Calcium Consumption

An excellent way to boost your calcium intake is with yogurt. That's because yogurt offers not only more calcium cup for cup than milk (400 versus 300 mg) but also contains probiotics—health-protective bacteria that boost your immune system and enhance digestion. When buying yogurt, look for "live and active cultures" on the label. Yogurt is especially healthful if you have had antibiotic treatment. Antibiotics kill both the good bacteria that live in your gut and the bad bacteria that cause health problems; yogurt helps replenish the good ones. The bacteria also digest most of the lactose (milk sugar) in yogurt, so many people who are lactose intolerant can enjoy yogurt as a milk alternative.

Because flavored yogurts can have a high sugar content—above and beyond the 12 grams of naturally occurring milk sugar in 8 ounces (240 ml) of milk—your best bet is to choose plain yogurt and add a teaspoon of honey or jam, or add plain yogurt to flavored yogurt. You'll come out way ahead in terms of sugar content. Remember, frozen yogurt has no active cultures but a high sugar content and marginal nutritional value. Don't fool yourself!

For athletes, yogurt is an easy-to-digest carbohydrate–protein combination that is a smart choice before and after exercise. A study of fatigued athletes suggests that those who regularly consumed yogurt had better immune function (Clancy et al. 2006). How about a postexercise fruit and yogurt smoothie?

Little did she know that her diet was contributing to the amenorrhea and that she was putting herself at risk of developing stress fractures, an early sign of poor bone health. She thought that exercise would keep her bones strong because she'd heard that exercise helps maintain bone density. Exercise does help, but calcium, estrogen, and adequate calories are simultaneously essential.

Her doctor advised her to regain her menstrual period to protect her bone health. Because lack of menstruation is associated with inadequate nutrition, I recommended that she boost her calorie intake by consuming more protein- and calcium-rich low-fat milk and yogurt. After two months of dietary improvements, she regained her menstrual period—a good step toward lifelong health. See chapter 16 for more information about amenorrhea and appendix A for more about osteoporosis.

Fiber for Good Health

Fiber is one of the components that make "good carbohydrate"—found in foods such as whole grains, legumes, fruits, vegetables—good. Fiber is the part of plant cells that humans can't digest. Food processing—such as milling whole wheat into white flour and peeling skins—removes the fiber. So, to reach the target intake of at least 25 grams of fiber per day, try to eat foods in their natural state.

Having heard claims that fiber lowers blood cholesterol, promotes regular bowel movements, and improves blood sugar control, sports-active people are seeking out high-fiber, carbohydrate-rich foods, or the "good carbohydrate" that should be the foundation of a sports diet. Although it's difficult to tease out which of these benefits are related to fiber and which to the other healthful components of fruits, vegetables, whole grains, beans, legumes, and nuts, you won't go wrong adding roughage to your diet.

Until recently, fiber was thought to reduce the risk of colon cancer. Disappointing results from recent studies fail to show a protective benefit of fiber (Rock 2007). Yet, fiber's positive association with lowering the risk of heart disease, helping to control diabetes, aiding with weight control, and preventing and treating constipation offer more than enough reasons to stack your diet with fiber-rich foods.

Types of Fiber

You should try to eat a variety of fiber-rich foods on a daily basis because different foods offer different types of fiber with different health benefits. You should consume both of the two main types of fiber:

- **Insoluble fiber.** This type of fiber gives plants their structure. It does not dissolve in water. Common sources are wheat bran, vegetables, and whole grains. Insoluble fiber absorbs water, increases fecal bulk, and makes the stools easier to pass.

- **Soluble fiber.** This type of fiber forms a gel in water. It is found in oatmeal, barley, and kidney beans (as well as in pectin and guar gums, two fibers often added to foods and listed among the ingredients). Soluble fiber lowers blood cholesterol, particularly in people with elevated cholesterol. Soluble fiber can also help stabilize blood glucose levels, making fiber-rich snacks a wise pre-exercise choice (assuming they settle comfortably and don't make you "gas propelled"). Some sustaining preexercise snacks include oatmeal as well as beans and legumes, such as lentil soup, refried beans, and hummus, as tolerated.

You can increase your fiber intake to the U.S. dietary guidelines' recommended 28 grams per 2,000 calories by taking the following actions:

- Enjoy fruits and vegetables at as many meals and snacks as possible.
- Choose a high-fiber cereal (with at least 5 grams of fiber per serving), or mix high- and low-fiber cereals. Top the cereal with berries and other fruits.
- Buy 100 percent whole-grain breads, cereals, and crackers.
- Opt for brown rice, quinoa, wheat berries, and other whole grains.
- Add wheat germ, ground flaxseed, nuts, or sesame seeds to yogurt, cereals, and baked goods.
- Eat more beans—in chili, sprinkled on salads, mixed with rice, made into hummus, and added to soups.
- Snack on popcorn (homemade, using canola oil) or dried fruits and nuts.
- Read food labels. Unexpected foods, such as some brands of orange juice and yogurt, have added fiber.

The information in table 2.4 can help you choose the foods richest in fiber.

Fiber Myths

Despite popular belief, fiber does not hasten the time it takes for food to pass through your system. It may increase fecal weight and the number

Table 2.4   Fiber in Foods

Cereal	Fiber (g)	Grain	Fiber (g)
Fiber One	14	Bulgur, 1 cup	8
All-Bran Extra Fiber, 1/2 cup	13	Brown rice, 1 cup	4
All-Bran, 1/2 cup	10	Triscuits, 7	4
Kashi Go Lean, 1 cup	8	Popcorn, 3 cups	3
Raisin Bran, 1 cup	7	Multigrain bread, 1 slice	2
Cheerios, 1 cup	3	Spaghetti, 1 cup	2
Oatmeal, 1 packet instant	3	White rice, 1 cup	1
Vegetables	**Fiber (g)**	**Fruits**	**Fiber (g)**
Brussels sprouts, 1 cup	6	Pear, 1 medium	4
Spinach, 1 cup	5	Apple, 1 medium	4
Potato, 1 large with skin	5	Prunes, 5 dried	3
Peas, 1/2 cup	4	Orange, 1 medium	3
Carrot, 1 medium	2	Banana, 1 medium	3
Corn, 1/2 cup	2	Kiwi, 1 medium	3
Lettuce, 1 cup	1	Raisins, 1/4 cup	2
Legumes	**Fiber (g)**	**Nuts and seeds**	**Fiber (g)**
Lentils, boiled, 1/2 cup	8	Flaxseed, 1 tbsp	3
Chickpeas, canned, 1/2 cup	5	Almonds, 1 oz (~22)	3
Kidney beans, canned, 1/2 cup	5	Peanut butter, 2 tbsp	2
Soy nuts, 1/4 cup	3	Cashews, 1 oz (~18)	1

Data from food labels and J. Pennington, 2004, *Bowes & Church's Food Values of Portions Commonly Used*, 18th ed. (Philadelphia: Lippincott Williams & Wilkins).

of trips to the bathroom, but it usually does not increase transit time. Transit time varies for each person, but it normally averages between two and four days. This varies according to stress, exercise, and diet. Your best bet as an active person is to determine the right combination of fiber-rich foods that promotes regular bowel movements for your body. You may need to restrict your fiber intake if exercise itself becomes a powerful bowel stimulant.

To Your Good Health

Whether you want to reduce your risk of cancer, heart disease, high blood pressure, or diabetes, health professionals agree that your best bet is a diet rich in fruits, vegetables, whole grains, and low-fat dairy; moderate in lean protein (which is low in saturated fat); and reduced in sodium (fewer processed foods). So please, think twice before you dig your grave with your knife and fork. Keep in mind these basic messages:

- Enjoy adequate, but not excessive, portions of lean meats (see chapter 7).

- Plan one or two fruits or vegetables into every meal. Breakfast can easily include orange juice and a banana; lunch a handful of baby carrots and an apple; dinner a double portion of mixed vegetables.

- Boost your intake of "good fat" (within your calorie budget) by choosing olive and canola oils for cooking and margarines made with olive or canola oil for spreads. Enjoy more nuts and nut butters.

Fruits and Veggies Matter

No matter what your health concerns—preventing cancer, heart disease, diabetes, obesity, high blood pressure, whatever—the bottom-line message from every health organization (including the American Heart Association; the American Cancer Society; the National Heart, Lung and Blood Institute; and the USDA) is to eat more fruits and vegetables. Yet, more than 90 percent of Americans fail to consume the recommended amount.

Ideally, you should include a hefty portion of fruit or veggies in every meal and snack. Here are some tips to help you boost your intake of these carbohydrate-rich foods that not only fuel your muscles but also protect your good health:

- Whip together a fruit smoothie for breakfast: orange juice, banana, frozen berries.
- To your egg (white) omelet, add diced peppers, tomato, mushrooms.
- Add blueberries or sliced banana to pancakes; top with applesauce.
- No fresh fruit for your cereal? Use canned peaches, raisins, or frozen berries.
- Put leftover dinner veggies into your lunchtime salad or soup.
- Keep within easy reach grab-and-go snacks, such as small boxes of raisins, trail mix with dried fruit, frozen 100 percent fruit juice bars, cherry tomatoes, baby carrots, and celery sticks.
- Add shredded carrots to casseroles, chili, lasagna, meatloaf, or soup.

For additional tips and recipes using fruits and vegetables, see the recipes in part IV and the Recipes section in appendix A.

By combining the best food choices from the food guide pyramid with a regular exercise program, you can invest in your future well-being. Although genetics do play a strong role in heart disease, cancer, hypertension, and osteoporosis, you can help put the odds in your favor by eating wisely. As Hippocrates said, "Let food be thy medicine."

CHAPTER 3

Breakfast: The Key to a Successful Sports Diet

Just as your car works better when it has fuel in its tank, your body works better when you give it adequate morning fuel. Yet, many people push their bodies through a busy day with an empty fuel tank. The result is low energy, cravings for sugary foods, a high intake of sweets and treats, and often undesired weight gain. There's no doubt in my mind: Breakfast is the most important meal of the day. Eat up!

Don't Skip Breakfast

Of all the nutrition mistakes you might make, skipping breakfast is the biggest. Raiya, an early-morning exerciser at her local YMCA, learned this the hard way: She collapsed from low blood sugar after one of her morning workouts. She managed to struggle through the hour-long stationary cycling class but felt very light-headed and dizzy, and she ended up in a heap on the floor, surrounded by the other frightened exercisers. She had blacked out because she had no fuel to feed her brain.

Raiya's story is a dramatic example of how skipping breakfast can hinder your workouts as well as leave you drained for the rest of the day. In comparison, a high-energy breakfast sets the stage for a high-energy day. Nevertheless, many active people come up with familiar excuses for skipping the morning meal:

"I'm not hungry in the morning."

"I don't have time."

"I don't like breakfast foods."

"I'm on a diet."

"If I eat breakfast, I feel hungrier all day."

Excuses, excuses. If you skip breakfast, you're likely to concentrate less effectively in the late morning, work or study less efficiently, feel irritable and short tempered, or fall short of energy for your afternoon workout. If you are a breakfast-skipping parent, your kids are more likely to skip breakfast, too, and the result is more snacking, irregular eating patterns, and a poorer-quality diet—all of which can influence their (and your) energy and weight (Affenito 2007). For every flimsy excuse to skip breakfast, there's an even better reason to eat it. Keep reading!

No Morning Appetite?

If you are not hungry for breakfast, you probably ate too many calories the night before. I often counsel people who eat a huge dinner at 9:00 p.m., mindlessly munch through a bag of chips while watching TV at night, or devour a bedtime bowl of ice cream as their reward for having survived a busy day. These snacks can certainly curb a morning appetite. Unfortunately for your health, when evening snacks replace a wholesome breakfast, you can end up with an inadequate sports diet.

Mark, a 35-year-old computer programmer and runner, wasn't hungry for breakfast for another reason: His morning workout killed his appetite. However, by 10:00 a.m. his appetite came to life again. He'd try to hold off until lunchtime, but he raided the candy machine three out of five workdays. I recommended that Mark keep some breakfast foods at work—energy bars, trail mix, packets of instant oatmeal. These nonperishable foods would be ready and waiting for a hassle-free yet nourishing meal.

For morning exercisers, a wholesome breakfast that combines carbohydrate with a little protein—cereal with milk, granola with yogurt, toast with peanut butter—promptly replaces the depleted glycogen stores and helps refuel and heal the muscles so they'll be refreshed for the next training session. The sooner you eat, the more quickly you'll recover. For more information on refueling after exercise, see chapter 10.

A recovery breakfast is particularly important if you do two workouts per day. I often talk with triathletes who say they're not yet hungry for breakfast after the first workout, which might be a morning run. They then skimp at lunchtime, afraid that a substantial meal might interfere with their afternoon workout. They end up dragging themselves through a poor training session. In this situation, I recommend having breakfast, lunch, or brunch around 10:00 or 11:00. The food will be adequately digested in time to fuel the muscles that afternoon. Refreshing liquids throughout the morning, such as juice, chocolate milk, and smoothies, can help refuel you as well as quench your thirst. You'll discover that you have more energy and a better second workout.

You Do Have Time for Breakfast

"I just don't have time to eat breakfast. I get up at 5:30, go to the rink, skate for an hour, then dash to school by 7:45." Obviously, this ice hockey player's morning schedule didn't allow him to relax and enjoy a leisurely meal. However, Nick still needed the energy to tackle his high school classes.

I reminded Nick that breakfast doesn't have to be a sit-down, cooked meal. It can be a substantial snack after hockey practice while riding to school. I advised him to plan and prepare a breakfast-to-go the night before. If he could make time to train for hockey, he could make time to eat right for training.

Nick discovered that his "duffle-bag breakfast" was indeed worth the effort. Two peanut butter and banana sandwiches and a bottle of juice satisfied his ravenous appetite and improved his ability to concentrate at school. No longer did he sit in class counting the minutes until lunch and listening to his stomach grumble. Rather, he was able to concentrate on his class work and even improve his grades.

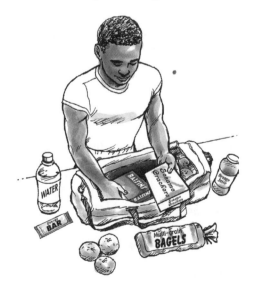

Maria, a nurse who was training for her first marathon, had the same excuse of no time for breakfast. She'd rise at 6:00 and be at the hospital by 6:45; she didn't want to eat breakfast at that early hour, claiming her stomach was not awake. However, by her break time at 10:00 she'd be grumpy, unable to focus on her work, and ravenously looking for the doughnuts or cookies that were in the nurses' station, begging to be eaten.

I recommended that Maria eat something nutritious between 7:00 and 9:00 to curb the overwhelming 10:00 a.m. hunger that interfered with her ability to concentrate and be pleasant to her patients. Maria made the effort to do one of the following every day:

- Bring a sandwich to work to eat within four hours of waking.
- Buy a bagel, yogurt, and orange juice at the coffee shop.
- Take an earlier break and enjoy a hot breakfast at the cafeteria.
- Keep emergency food in her desk drawer: granola bars, crackers, peanuts, and dried fruits.

She soon became a breakfast advocate, feeling so much better when well fueled rather than half starved.

If you lack creative quick-fix breakfast ideas, the following food choices can help you make a fast break to becoming a regular breakfast eater:

- Yogurt. Keep your refrigerator well stocked; add cereal for crunch.
- Banana. Eat an extra-large one, chased by a large glass of milk.
- Blender drink. Whip together juice, fruit, and yogurt or dried milk (or protein powder).
- Raisins and peanuts. Prepacked in small plastic bags, these are ready to get tucked in your pocket.
- Whole-wheat bagel. Spread it with peanut butter, then wash it down with a large glass of milk.
- Graham crackers. These are a crunchy favorite with a latte made with low-fat milk.
- Pita bread. Stuff it with low-fat cheese, cottage cheese, hummus, sliced turkey, or other handy fillings.

Breakfast for Dieters

Everyone who wants to lose weight knows diets start at breakfast, right? Wrong! Skipping breakfast to save calories is an unsuccessful approach to weight loss. Research confirms that dieters who skip breakfast tend to gain weight over time (Neumark-Sztainer et al. 2006). If you are tempted to save calories by skimping on breakfast, remember that you don't gain weight by eating this meal. You do gain weight if you skip breakfast, get too hungry, and then overindulge at night. If you are going to skip any meal, skip dinner rather than breakfast. Your goal should be to fuel by day and eat a little less at night.

A survey of almost 3,000 dieters who have lost more than 30 pounds (14 kg) and have kept it off for at least a year reports that 78 percent of the dieters ate breakfast every day, and 88 percent ate breakfast five or more days a week. Only 4 percent reported never eating breakfast. The breakfast eaters also reported being slightly more active during the day. This study suggests that breakfast is indeed an important part of a successful weight loss program (Wyatt et al. 2002). Another study of breakfast and weight control suggests that dieters who ate breakfast were less likely to snack impulsively later in the day and ate an overall lower-fat diet (Schlundt et al. 1992). You can't go wrong with eating breakfast!

Time and again I advise dieters to fuel during the day and eat less at night. Time and again they look at me with fear in their eyes. As Pat, an at-home mom who wanted to lose some weight, explained, "If I eat breakfast, I get hungrier and seem to eat more the whole day." Her breakfast was only half of a dry bagel, enough to get the digestive juices flowing, but not enough to satisfy her appetite. When she ate a substantial 500-calorie breakfast, she felt fine and didn't overindulge later in the afternoon. Although she initially couldn't believe that the following 500-calorie breakfasts would help her lose weight, she discovered they did:

Breakfast on the run	Calories
Bagel, medium large	300
Vanilla yogurt	200
Total	**500**
Nontraditional breakfast	
2 slices of cheese pizza	500
Total	**500**
Desk-drawer breakfast	
Instant oatmeal, 2 packets	250
Raisins, 1 small box (1.5 oz)	130
Powdered milk, 1/2 cup	120
Total	**500**

If you are watching your weight and for some reason overeat at breakfast, let's say at a business breakfast meeting with an abundance of croissants and pastries, don't continue to overeat the rest of the day. Simply acknowledge that you ate part (or all) of your lunch calories early. Come noontime, listen to your body, which is likely still feeling well fed, and notice you really don't need a full lunch because you aren't very hungry. Discard the bad mental voices that encourage "last-chance" eating: "You blew your diet at breakfast, so keep eating all day; this is your last chance to indulge before The Diet starts again tomorrow."

The Number One Breakfast for Champions

My clients commonly ask what I recommend for breakfast. In general, my answer is any combination of wholesome choices from three food groups. More specifically, my answer is cereal because it's a simple way to get those three types of foods—whole grains, low-fat milk, and fruit—plus a host of other benefits. By eating a bowl of whole-grain cereal topped with fruit, you can get half of the recommended daily fruit and whole-grain servings before you even get out of your pajamas.

What's So Great About Cereal?

I'm big on cereals because they are all these positive things:

- **Quick and easy.** People of all ages and cooking abilities can easily pour a bowl with no cooking or messy cleanup.
- **Convenient.** By simply stocking the cupboard, gym bag, or desk drawer, breakfast will be ready for the morning rush. A plastic bag of dry cereal is better than nothing.
- **Rich in carbohydrate.** Your muscles need carbohydrate for energy. Cereal, a banana, and juice constitute a superior carbohydrate-based meal; milk offers a protein accompaniment.
- **Rich in fiber.** When you select bran and whole-grain cereals, you reduce your risk of becoming constipated, an inconvenience that can certainly interfere with enjoyment of exercise. You also consume a health-protective food.
- **Rich in iron.** By selecting fortified or enriched brands, you can easily boost your iron intake and reduce your risk of becoming anemic. Drink orange juice or another source of vitamin C with the cereal to enhance iron absorption from the cereal.
- **Rich in calcium.** Cereal is rich in calcium when it's eaten with low-fat milk or yogurt or calcium-fortified soy milk. Women and children, in particular, but also men benefit from this calcium

booster that helps maintain strong bones and protects against osteoporosis.

- **Low in saturated fat and cholesterol.** Cereals are a heart-healthier choice than the standard breakfast alternatives of buttered toast, a bagel slathered with cream cheese, or bacon and fried eggs.

- **Versatile.** Rather than becoming bored by always eating the same brand, try mixing cereals to concoct endless varieties of flavors. I typically have 10 to 18 varieties in my cupboard. My friends laugh when they discover this impressive stockpile. I further vary the flavors by adding different mix-ins, such as banana, raisins, dried blueberries, slivered almonds, cinnamon, nutmeg, maple syrup, or vanilla extract.

- **Helpful for weight control.** A survey of 17,881 male physicians who were followed for eight years found that the doctors who ate cereal most often for breakfast weighed less than those who ate less cereal (Bazzano et al. 2005). In another survey of 4,218 women, those who ate cereal for breakfast were 30 percent less likely to be overweight than those who skipped breakfast or ate something else for breakfast (Song et al. 2005). Does this mean cereal aids in weight control? Hard to say. But a cereal breakfast does provide milk and calcium, and some researchers believe that helps control weight (Zemel et al. 2004).

The Scoop on Cereal

Cereal, in general, is a breakfast for champions, particularly if it is a whole-grain, high-fiber cereal that contributes to lower blood pressure and reduced risk of heart attacks. However, some brands offer far more nutritional value than others. Here are five tips to help you make wise choices as you romp through the cereal aisle.

1. Choose iron-enriched cereals. An iron-rich diet is particularly important for active people because iron is the part of the red blood cell that carries oxygen from your lungs to your muscles. If you are anemic (have iron-poor blood), you will feel tired and fatigue easily during exercise. Iron-rich breakfast cereal is a handy way to boost your iron intake, particularly if you eat little or no red meat (the best source of dietary iron).

You can tell which cereals have iron added to them by looking for the words *fortified* or *enriched* on the label or by checking the nutrition facts panel. You should choose a brand that supplies at least 25 percent of the daily value. Table 3.1 provides information that can help you select the brands enriched with iron to supplement the small amount naturally occurring in grains.

Table 3.1　Nutritional Value of Commonly Eaten Cereals

Cereal	Amount	Cal	Sugar (g)	Fat (g)	Fiber (g)	Sodium (mg)	Iron (%DV)
All-Bran Extra Fiber	1/2 cup	50	0	1	13	120	25
Cap'n Crunch	3/4 cup	110	12	1.5	1	210	25
Cheerios	1 cup	110	1	2	3	210	45
Complete Bran Flakes	3/4 cup	90	5	0.5	5	210	100
Corn Flakes, Kellogg's	1 cup	100	2	Trace	1	200	45
Cracklin' Oat Bran	3/4 cup	200	15	7	6	150	10
Crispix	1 cup	110	3	—	1	210	45
Fiber One	1/2 cup	60	0	1	14	105	25
Froot Loops	1 cup	120	15	1	1	150	25
Frosted Flakes	3/4 cup	120	12	—	1	150	25
Frosted Mini-Wheats	24 biscuits	200	12	1	6	5	90
Golden Grahams	3/4 cup	120	11	1	1	270	25
Grape-Nuts	1/2 cup	200	5	1	6	310	90
Great Grains	1/2 cup	210	13	5	4	150	50
Honey Nut Cheerios	1 cup	110	9	1.5	2	190	25
Kashi Go Lean	1 cup	140	6	1	10	85	10
Kashi Heart to Heart	3/4 cup	110	5	1.5	5	90	10
Life	3/4 cup	120	6	1.5	2	160	45
Puffed Rice, Quaker	1 cup	50	0	Trace	Trace	Trace	20
Puffins	3/4 cup	130	5	1	5	190	2
Quaker Oatmeal Squares	1 cup	210	10	2.5	5	250	90
Quaker 100% Natural	1/2 cup	210	15	6	6	30	6
Raisin Bran, Kellogg's	1 cup	190	19	1.5	7	350	25
Rice Krispies	1 1/4 cup	120	3	Trace	0	320	10
Smart Start	1 cup	190	14	0.5	3	280	100
Special K	1 cup	110	4	—	1	220	45
Total	3/4 cup	100	5	0.5	3	190	100
Uncle Sam	3/4 cup	190	<1	5	10	135	10
Wheaties	3/4 cup	100	4	0.5	3	190	45

Nutrition information from food labels, July 2007.

If you prefer all-natural or organic cereals with no additives, remember that "no additives" means there is no iron added, as is often the case with Kashi, Puffins, granola, Shredded Wheat, Quaker 100% Natural, and other all-natural brands. If you like, you can mix all-natural cereals with iron-enriched varieties (e.g., granola with Cheerios, Shredded Wheat with Wheat Chex), or you can choose iron-rich foods at other meals or take an iron supplement.

Because the iron in cereal is often poorly absorbed, you can enhance iron bioavailability—your body's ability to absorb iron—by drinking some orange juice or eating fruit rich in vitamin C along with the cereal (try oranges, grapefruit, cantaloupe, and strawberries).

2. Choose cereal fortified with folic acid. The B vitamin folic acid is found in small amounts in grains but in higher amounts (100 to 400 micrograms, 25 to 100 percent of the daily value) in fortified foods such as breakfast cereals. Folic acid is associated with a lower risk of certain types of birth defects. Folic acid had been thought to reduce the risk of heart disease, but results of the latest vitamin therapy trials have been disappointing (Lichtenstein et al. 2006).

3. Choose high-fiber bran cereals. Cereal with at least 4 grams of fiber per ounce (30 g) is the best breakfast choice. Fiber is beneficial for people with constipation. Research suggests that fiber also has protective qualities that may reduce your risk of heart disease as well as curb your appetite and assist with weight loss.

Bran cereals can provide far more fiber than most fruits and vegetables. High-fiber cereals include Kashi Good Friends, All-Bran, Fiber One, Raisin Bran, Oat Bran, Bran Flakes, and any of the multitudes of cereals with *bran* or *fiber* in the name (see table 3.1). You can also boost the fiber content of any cereal by simply sprinkling Kashi, All-Bran, or Fiber One on it.

4. Choose wholesome cereals. By "wholesome cereals," I mean those with sugar not listed among the first ingredients. (Ingredients are listed by order of weight, from most to least.) By reading the nutrition facts on box labels, you can learn the amount of sugar in a cereal. Simply multiply grams of sugar (listed under Total Carbohydrate) by 4 calories per gram to determine the calories of sugar per serving. Quaker Toasted Oatmeal Squares, for example, has brown sugar and sugar listed as the third and fourth ingredients. A 1-cup serving contains 10 grams of sugar (10 g sugar × 4 cal/g = 40 cal) in 210 calories. That means almost 20 percent of the calories are from added sugar.

Some kids' cereals are 45 percent sugar, or more dessert than breakfast. Although sugar does fuel the muscles and is not the poison it is reputed to be, sugary cereals tend to pamper your sweet tooth rather than promote your health.

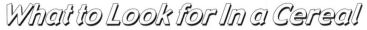

What to Look for In a Cereal

If your favorite cereal doesn't meet these criteria, combine it with others to achieve a healthy mix.

3 GRAMS OR LESS OF FAT PER SERVING

LESS THAN 250 MILLIGRAMS OF SODIUM PER SERVING

5 GRAMS OR MORE OF FIBER PER SERVING

8 GRAMS OR LESS OF SUGAR PER SERVING

AT LEAST 25% DAILY VALUE OF IRON

SUGAR NOT LISTED AMONG THE FIRST FEW INGREDIENTS

IRON ENRICHED

Nutrition Facts

Serving Size 1 Cup (1 oz)
Servings Per Container About 12

Amount Per Serving

Calories 110   Calories from fat 5

	%DV*
Total Fat 0.5g	1%
Saturated Fat 0g	0%
Trans Fat 0g	
Cholesterol 0 mg	0%
Sodium 210 mg	9%
Total Carbohydrate	23g
Dietary Fiber 5g	0%
Sugars 2g	
Protein 3g	

Vitamin A	25%	Vitamin C	15%
Calcium	0%	Iron	50%
Vitamin D	10%	Thiamin	25%
Riboflavin	25%	Niacin	25%
Vitamin B_6	25%	Folate	25%
Vitamin B_{12}	25%	Phosphorus	15%
Magnesium	10%	Zinc	25%
Copper	8%		

Percent Daily Values (DV) are based on a 2000 calorie diet.

INGREDIENTS: Corn; Oat and Wheat Flour; Wheat Germ; High Fructose Corn Syrup; Ascorbic Acid; Iron and Zinc (Mineral-Nutrients); Alphato-copherol Acetate (E); Vitamin A Palmitate; Folic Acid; Vitamin B_{12}; and Vitamin D.

Maya, a flight attendant and avid exerciser, avoided all cereals with sugar listed among the ingredients, even the lightly sweetened ones such as Total, Wheaties, or Bran Flakes. She restricted herself to the sugar-free

Puffed Wheat and Corn Flakes, cheating herself of variety and enjoyment. She failed to recognize that sugar is a carbohydrate that fuels, not poisons, the muscles.

The small amount of sugar in cereal is relatively insignificant in comparison to the sugar Maya ate in frozen yogurt, Twizzlers, and gummy bears. I encouraged her to focus more on a cereal's fiber and whole-grain content than on its sugar content. The overall healthfulness of a breakfast cereal far outweighs those few nutritionally empty sugar calories. I told Maya that 10 percent of daily calories can appropriately come from sugar. Hence, the 4 grams (16 calories) of sugar in Wheaties could certainly fit into her day's 240-calorie sugar budget. Given this perspective, she decided to relax her sugar rules to include more variety, especially brands with health-protective fiber and iron.

   5. Choose low-fat cereals. Rather than fret about a cereal's sugar content, you should focus more on its fat calories. Fat is the bigger health threat because it's linked with weight gain, heart disease, and cancer. If you like the higher-fat cereals, such as granola or Cracklin' Oat Bran, use them for a topping sprinkled on a foundation of a lower-fat cereal.

Cereal Alternatives

Cereal may be one breakfast of champions, but it's not the only one. For you non-cereal-eaters, rest assured that other breakfasts can fuel you for a high-energy day. See the recipes in part IV for some wholesome high-carbohydrate breakfast breads and muffins you might want to enjoy with a glass of low-fat milk and some fruit or juice.

   Dimitri, a businessman and breakfast skipper who needed to lose the 20 pounds (9 kg) of fat that had crept on since his years as a collegiate soccer player, decided to eat dinner for breakfast. He loved his chicken and potatoes, so instead of trying to have small portions at dinnertime, he ate his full dinner in the morning and then had cereal for supper. He lost weight easily and happily. Although few people are willing or able to make the effort to prepare dinner for breakfast, the point is that any breakfast is better than no breakfast, a bigger breakfast is preferable to a skimpy breakfast, and a hearty breakfast that includes wholesome foods is best for your health and performance.

Fast-Food Breakfasts

If you are destined to eat breakfast at a fast-food restaurant, be sure to make wise food choices.

- Rather than high-fat bacon, sausage, croissant, or biscuit combinations, choose the egg and English muffin or wrap. Pancakes, hot or cold cereal, juice, bagels (with light cream cheese), English muffins (with jam), low-fat muffins, and fruit–yogurt–granola parfaits are other options.

- Because fresh fruits can be hard to find on the menu, remember to tuck an apple or orange into your pocket. Or, take a big swig of juice before you leave home.

- Treat yourself to a latte (with low-fat milk), instead of coffee with cream, for more protein and calcium.

- Find a deli with fresh bagels, fruit, juice, and yogurt.

- Skip the breakfast temptations (Cinnabons, doughnuts, croissants) and bring a box of cereal to the office. On your way to work, pick up some milk and a banana, along with your coffee, if desired. If you are traveling and staying at a hotel, you can save yourself time, money, and temptation by bringing your own cereal and dried fruit (and spoon). Bring powdered milk, or buy a container of low-fat or nonfat milk at the corner store. A water glass or milk carton can double as a cereal bowl.

Nontraditional Breakfasts

If you skip breakfast because you don't like breakfast foods, just eat something else. Who said you have to eat cereal or toast? Any food you eat at other times of the day can be eaten at breakfast. I happen to love leftover pizza or Chinese food for a morning change of pace.

You might even want to eat most of your treats at breakfast. One of my clients learned that by enjoying a chocolate croissant in the morning, she killed her desire for sweets the rest of the day. No longer did she want cookies for an afternoon snack. Rather, she enjoyed the bowl of cereal that seemed humdrum at 8:00 a.m.

Your goal is to eat one-quarter to one-third of your daily calories in the morning. Some acceptable choices are planned leftovers from dinner, a baked potato with cottage cheese, a peanut butter and honey sandwich, a yogurt "sundae" with sliced fruit and sunflower seeds, tomato soup with crackers, or even special holiday foods. Why not enjoy for breakfast such high-calorie treats as leftover birthday cake or Thanksgiving pies? You're better off eating them during the day and burning off their calories than holding off until evening, when you may succumb to overconsumption in a moment of weakness.

Coffee: The Morning Eye-Opener

Coffee is a universally loved morning beverage. Every culture the world over enjoys some type of caffeinated beverage, be it tea in England and China, espresso in Italy, or a "coffee regular" in the United States. Questions abound about the role of coffee in a healthy diet. Here are some answers to commonly asked questions.

Q: **Is coffee bad for me? That is, will it hurt my health?**

A: Because coffee is so widely consumed, it has been extensively researched. On the positive side, coffee drinkers might actually have a lower risk of diabetes and Parkinson's disease. To date, there is no obvious negative connection between caffeine and heart disease, cancer, or blood pressure. Hence, the general answer, according to leading medical and scientific experts, is normal coffee consumption produces no adverse health effects.

The average American consumes about 200 milligrams of caffeine per day, the equivalent of about 10 to 12 ounces—a large mug—of coffee. For the 10 percent of Americans who ingest more than 1,000 milligrams of caffeine per day and sustain themselves on the cream and sugar in coffee (plus a few cigarettes alongside), heart disease is indeed more common—and linked to the poor diet and unhealthful lifestyle.

In addition to smokers, those who should abstain from caffeine are ulcer patients and others prone to stomach distress (caffeine stimulates gastric secretions and may cause "coffee stomach"). Athletes with anemia should also avoid caffeine. Substances in coffee and tea can interfere with the absorption of iron (Zijp, Korver, and Tijburg 2000). If you have anemia and routinely drink coffee or tea with meals or up to one hour after a meal, you might be cheating yourself nutritionally. A cup of coffee consumed with a hamburger can reduce by about 40 percent the absorption of the hamburger's iron. However, drinking caffeinated beverages up to an hour before eating seems to have no negative effect on iron absorption.

The biggest health worries about coffee have to do with the following habits surrounding that beverage:

○ Adding cream or coffee whiteners containing coconut or palm oils. These add saturated fat that contributes to heart disease. At least switch to milk or powdered milk for whitening your coffee.

○ Drinking coffee instead of eating a wholesome breakfast. A large coffee with two creamers and two sugars contains 70 nutritionally empty calories. Multiply that by three mugs, and you could have had a nourishing bowl of cereal for the same number of calories. Table 3.2 provides the fat content of some common coffee beverages. Many people who say they "live on coffee" could easily drink much less if they would eat a satisfying breakfast and lunch. Food is better fuel than caffeine.

○ Drinking coffee to stay alert. A good night's sleep might be a better investment. You could also try drinking a tall glass of ice water to perk yourself up. Sometimes dehydration contributes to fatigue.

Table 3.2   Gulp! It's a Calorie Cafe!

Beware of the calories in the popular beverages that are readily available at coffee-houses. A survey of 41 college women who drank one gourmet coffee a day suggests they consumed about 200 calories and 32 grams of sugar more than nonconsumers (Shields, Corrales, and Metallinos-Katsaras 2004). A large Coffee Coolatta can blow half the day's recommended fat allowance (for a person eating 2,000 calories, a low-fat diet offers 55 to 65 grams of fat). Using low-fat or nonfat milk instead of whole milk or cream can save considerable calories.

Beverage	Calories	Fat (g)
Dunkin' Donuts coffee, black	0	0
Iced coffee with cream and sugar, 16 oz (480 ml)	120	6
Coffee Coolatta with skim milk, 16 oz (480 ml)	170	0
Coffee Coolatta with 2% milk, 16 oz (480 ml)	190	2
Coffee Coolatta with cream, 16 oz (480 ml)	350	14
Coffee Coolatta with cream, 32 oz (960 ml)	700	28
Strawberry Fruit Coolatta, 16 oz (480 ml)	290	0
Vanilla chai, 10 oz	230	8
Hot chocolate, 10 oz (300 ml)	230	7
Mocha Swirl Latte, 10 oz (300 ml)	220	8
Strawberry Banana Smoothie, 24 oz	550	4
Starbucks Latte with whole milk, 12 oz (360 ml)	210	11
Latte with skim milk, 12 oz (360 ml)	120	0.5
Coffee Frappuccino, 12 oz (360 ml)	200	2
Coffee Frappuccino, 24 oz (720 ml)	405	5
Java Chip Frappuccino with whipped cream, 16 oz (480 ml)	510	22

Nutrition information from www.dunkindonuts.com and www.starbucks.com, July 2007.

These bad habits are more likely to harm your health than the caffeine itself. If you are concerned about caffeine and health, you might want to switch to tea. Tea drinkers tend to have a lower risk of heart disease. That might be because tea is a rich source of flavonoids that protect against heart disease or because tea drinkers, in general, tend to be more health conscious, smoke less, and eat more fruits and vegetables (Geleijnse et al. 2002).

Q: **What does coffee do to my body?**

A: The caffeine in coffee is a mild stimulant that increases the activity of the central nervous system. Hence, caffeine helps you stay alert and enhances mental focus. Caffeine's stimulant effect peaks in about one hour and then declines as the liver breaks down the caffeine. If you are an occasional coffee drinker, you'll tend to be more sensitive to caffeine's stimulant effects as compared with the daily coffee consumer who has developed a tolerance to caffeine.

Although a little coffee offers enjoyable benefits of alertness, enhanced performance, and happier mood, if you drink too much coffee, you start to get adverse effects: caffeine jitters, acid stomach, and anxiety. Drinking more than 32 ounces (1 L) of coffee or 64 ounces (2 L) of tea per day is pushing the limits of "reasonable intake" (CSPI 2006).

Q: **Do people get addicted to coffee?**

A: Although coffee has been a popular beverage for centuries, its sustained popularity fails to classify it as "addictive." Coffee is not associated with the behaviors found with hard drugs (such as a need for more and more coffee, antisocial behavior, severe difficulty stopping consumption). If you are a regular coffee drinker who decides to cut coffee out of your diet, you may develop headaches, fatigue, or drowsiness. The solution is to gradually decrease your caffeine intake rather than eliminate coffee cold turkey. And be aware, if you should get a headache due to caffeine withdrawal, taking caffeine-containing medicines such as Anacin or Excedrin will foil your efforts to reduce your caffeine intake.

Switching to tea reduces caffeine intake (and also increases your intake of a beverage that has potential benefits in terms of reducing heart disease and cancer). Other ways to reduce your caffeine include drinking more of the following caffeine-free alternatives: decaffeinated coffee, decaffeinated tea, herbal teas, hot water with a lemon wedge, low-sodium broth or bouillon,

Swiss Miss, Ovaltine, other hot milk-based drinks, mulled cider, and hot cranberry or apple juice. Without a doubt, the best caffeine-free alternative to an eye-opening cup of coffee is exercise. A quick walk and some fresh air might be far more effective than a cup of brew.

Q: How much caffeine is in espresso?

A: Ounce for ounce, espresso is about twice as strong as coffee (35 versus 17 mg of caffeine per oz—but a Starbucks gourmet espresso has 65 mg of caffeine per oz). Because a serving of espresso is small, however, you end up with less caffeine: 35 milligrams from one shot (one ounce) of espresso versus 135 milligrams from an 8-ounce (240 ml) cup of standard coffee.

Q: How much caffeine do Coke and Pepsi have compared with coffee?

A: A 12-ounce can of cola averages 35 to 50 milligrams of caffeine. This is far less than the typical 12-ounce mug of coffee, which averages 200 milligrams of caffeine. The real kick from soft drinks comes from sugar, not caffeine.

Q: Are there any concerns about women who consume caffeine?

A: Pregnant women should prudently limit their caffeine to less than 300 milligrams per day (less than 15 oz, or 450 ml, of coffee). Caffeine readily crosses the placenta and, in excess, may be associated with premature birth. Women who are breastfeeding should also limit their intake. Caffeine crosses into breast milk and can make babies agitated and poor sleepers. Women who are trying to get pregnant might want to reduce caffeine intake even more, but more research is needed to clarify the controversy over the effects of caffeine on fertility. Women who are worried about getting osteoporosis may have heard that caffeine is linked to low bone density. To help you achieve the recommended intake of at least 24 ounces (720 ml) of milk or other calcium equivalents per day, adding more milk to your coffee or enjoying some lattes are smart choices.

Q: If I drink too much alcohol, will coffee help me sober up?

A: No. Coffee will just make you a wide-awake drunk. Coffee does not speed the time needed for the liver to detoxify alcohol. But coffee does get some water into your body, and that can have a positive effect.

Q: Does coffee count toward my daily fluid needs?

A: Yes. All fluids count—plain water, juice, soup, watermelon, and even coffee. The rumor that coffee dehydrates people lacks scientific support (Armstrong 2002). Yes, coffee might make you urinate more in 2 hours, but not in 24 hours. Even during exercise in the heat, athletes can consume coffee and not be concerned about dehydration.

CHAPTER 4

Lunch and Dinner: At Home and on the Run

If you are old enough to remember when people used to eat three square meals a day, you also remember that eating well was less of a challenge. Unfortunately for our health, today's lifestyles rarely include breakfast and barely accommodate lunch and dinner, even when eaten on the run. Relaxing lunches and dinners—nicely prepared, attractively served, and shared with family and friends—are rare occurrences for many active people and sports families.

My clients commonly express dissatisfaction with their mealtime eating. Yet, when life is full, stress is high, and schedules are crazy, eating well-balanced meals on a predictable schedule can provide the energy you need to better manage stress and prevent fatigue. The purpose of this chapter is to provide meal management tips so you can care for your health while balancing work, workouts, family, and stress.

The Lunch Bunch

For active people who should be in the continuous cycle of fueling up for workouts and refueling afterward, lunch is the second most important meal of the day. Breakfast remains number one. Lunch refuels morning or noontime exercisers and offers fuel to those preparing for an afternoon session. Given that active people tend to get hungry every four hours (if not sooner), if you eat breakfast at 7:00 or 8:00 a.m., you are certainly ready for lunch at 11:00 or 12:00. But if you eat too little breakfast (as commonly happens), you'll be hungry for lunch by 10:00 a.m.—and that throws off the rest of the day's eating schedule.

The solution to the "I cannot wait until noon to eat lunch" predicament is simple: You could either eat a bigger breakfast that sustains you until noon, eat a midmorning snack (more correctly, the second half of your too-small breakfast), or eat the first of two lunches, one at 10:00 and the other at 2:00.

For a nation of lunch skippers, eating two lunches may seem a wacky idea. But why not? Ideally, you should eat according to hunger, not by the clock. After all, hunger is simply your body's request for more fuel. If you've eaten only a light breakfast or have exercised hard in the morning, you can easily be ready for lunch 1 at 10:00 a.m. and for lunch 2 at 2:00. That's what I do, and this system keeps me evenly fueled and helps me arrive home agreeably ready for dinner, but not starving.

In general, when you plan your intake for the day, you should try to divide your calories evenly. Given their tendency to become hungry every four hours, active people can appropriately eat 25 percent of their calories at each of four meals (breakfast, lunch 1, lunch 2, and dinner); this covers a 16-hour time span. By experimenting with this concept of evenly sized and spaced meals, you'll eradicate your afternoon sweet cravings or after-dinner dietary disasters. A hearty lunch (or two) truly invests in a higher-energy day.

Despite the importance of lunch, logistics tend to be a hassle. If you pack your own lunch, what do you pack? If you buy lunch, what's a healthful bargain? If you're on a diet, what's best to eat? Here are some helpful tips to improve your lunch intake.

Brown-Bagging It

If you pack your lunch, the what-to-pack dilemma quickly becomes tiring. Most people tend to pack more or less the same food every day and end up with yet another turkey sandwich, salad, or bagel. As long as you're content with what you choose, fine. But if you're tired of the same stuff, consider these suggestions:

- Strive for at least 500 calories (even if you are on a reducing diet) from three types of food at lunch. This means a bagel, yogurt, and banana or salad, turkey, and pita. Just a bagel or just a salad is likely too little fuel.

- Remember peanut butter. Peanut butter is an outstanding sports food—even for dieters—because it's satisfying and helps you stay fueled for the whole afternoon. Yes, it has 200 more calories than a standard turkey sandwich, but a satisfying peanut butter sandwich allows you to nix the afternoon cookies and snacks that would otherwise sneak into your intake for the day. Refresh your memory of this childhood staple!

- Pack planned leftovers from dinner and heat them in the microwave oven. They're preferable to the cup of noodles or frozen lunches that cost more than they're worth.

If you're lucky enough to have a cafeteria at work or to participate in a business lunch, take advantage of the opportunity to enjoy a hot meal. Eating a dinner at lunch

- fuels you for a high-energy after-work exercise session,
- simplifies the "what's to eat for dinner" routine because you'll feel less hungry and may be content to enjoy a bowl of cereal or a sandwich, and
- reduces the hungry horrors that you might otherwise fight if you were to eat a light lunch. Why not enjoy a substantial meal? You are going to eat the calories eventually, so you might as well honor your hunger and eat now.

Lunch for Dieters

Because most Americans regard meals as fattening, dieters tend to skip or skimp on lunch. As one overweight walker confided, "I have only a very light lunch. I'm fat, so I don't give myself permission to eat lunch because I should be dieting." That sad statement is common in our society. I urged her to take care of herself better and at least eat enough "diet foods" to keep her metabolism going and fuel her muscles for her walking program. Once she started to have a turkey sandwich, yogurt, and orange for lunch, she discovered the benefits of eating this meal. She was more effective at work, less hungry in the afternoon, less likely to raid the refrigerator the minute she arrived home, and better able to lose weight. Eating lunch works!

Super Salads

Salads are a popular lunch and a super way to boost your intake of vegetables. In just one big bowlful you can get your five daily vegetable servings—if not more. Yet lunchtime salads can be either good news or bad news, depending on the salad.

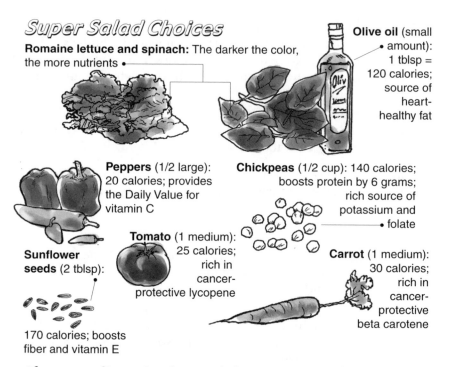

Super Salad Choices

Romaine lettuce and spinach: The darker the color, the more nutrients •

Olive oil (small amount): 1 tblsp = 120 calories; source of heart-healthy fat

Peppers (1/2 large): 20 calories; provides the Daily Value for vitamin C

Chickpeas (1/2 cup): 140 calories; boosts protein by 6 grams; rich source of potassium and folate

Sunflower seeds (2 tblsp): 170 calories; boosts fiber and vitamin E

Tomato (1 medium): 25 calories; rich in cancer-protective lycopene

Carrot (1 medium): 30 calories; rich in cancer-protective beta carotene

If you are a dieter who deems salads an appropriate lunch, take heed. A meager salad offers too few calories. You'll likely end up visiting the vending machine that afternoon. I suggest that dieters have a salad for dinner but eat a substantial meal at lunch. If you take full advantage of a brimming salad bar, take heed. A typical salad-bar meal can easily contain 1,000 calories, with 45 percent of those from fat. This is not a diet meal.

To create a high-energy sports salad that is the mainstay of your lunch or dinner, include enough carbohydrate-rich foods to make it substantial, but limit the fat to control the calories. Here are five tips to help you get the most in your salad bowl.

Tip 1. Boost the salad's carbohydrate content by adding

- carbohydrate-dense vegetables such as corn, corn relish, peas, beets, and carrots;
- beans and legumes such as chickpeas, kidney beans, and lentils;
- cooked rice, pasta, or potato chunks;
- orange sections, diced apple, raisins, banana slices, or berries;
- toasted croutons (limit your intake of buttered croutons that leave you with greasy fingers); and
- thick slices of whole-grain bread and a glass of low-fat milk for accompaniments.

Tip 2. Choose a variety of dark, colorful veggies such as red tomatoes, green peppers, orange carrots, and dark lettuces. Colorful vegetables nutritionally surpass paler lettuces, cucumbers, onions, celery, and radishes. For example, a salad made with spinach has seven times the vitamin C of one made with iceberg lettuce; one made with dark romaine has twice the vitamin C. Plus, colorful vegetables are brimming with the antioxidant nutrients and phytochemicals that protect your health. Cauliflower, although colorless, is a good source of vitamin C (70 mg per cup, raw) and the cancer-fighting nutrients found in the cruciferous vegetable family to which it belongs. See table 4.1 for a ranking of salad fixings.

Table 4.1 Ranking Vegetables

The Center for Science in the Public Interest (CSPI) has developed a system for ranking vegetables in order of their nutritional value and fiber content. The higher the score, the better and more nutrient dense the vegetable.

Vegetable	Nutrition score*
Spinach, 1 cup raw	287
Red pepper, 1/2 medium raw	261
Carrot, 1 medium raw	204
Romaine lettuce, 1 cup shredded	174
Broccoli, 1/2 cup raw florettes	160
Cabbage 1/2 cup raw	135
Boston or Bibb lettuce, 1 cup	134
Green pepper, 1/2 raw	109
Green peas, 1/2 cup frozen	104
Avocado, 1/2 Hass raw	82
Tomato, 1/2 raw	78
Corn, 1/2 cup	67
Green beans, 1/2 cup cooked	65
Cauliflower, 1/2 cup raw	62
Iceberg lettuce, 1 cup	45
Beets, 1/2 cup canned	33
Mushrooms, 1/2 cup cooked	33
Cucumber, 1/2 cup raw	14
Alfalfa sprouts, 1/2 cup raw	7

*Based on six nutrients and fiber.

Copyright CSPI 2002. Adapted from Nutrition Action Healthletter. www.cspinet.org

A Word About Salad Dressings

A few innocent ladles of salad dressing can transform a potentially healthful salad into a high-fat nutrition nightmare. On a large salad, dressing can easily add 800 to 1,000 calories. On even a small side salad, a dressing can drown the salad's healthfulness in 400 calories of fat. These fat calories appease the appetite, add to your waistline, and fail to fuel the muscles with carbohydrate. I advise my clients to educate themselves about salad-dressing calories by reading labels and measuring out the amount of dressing they normally use on a salad—they tend to be shocked by what they learn!

Dressing, 2 tbsp	Calories	Fat (g)
Plain olive oil	240	26
Plain vinegar	5	0
Herbs, sprinkling	5	0
Blue cheese, Wish-Bone, chunky	150	15
Blue cheese, Wish-Bone fat free, chunky	35	0
Ranch, Wish-Bone regular	160	13
Ranch, Just 2 Good	40	2
Ranch, Wish-Bone fat free	30	0
Italian, Newman's Own regular	150	16
Italian, Kraft Zesty Italian	70	6
Italian, Just 2 Good	35	2

Nutrition information from food labels, July 2007.

To reduce the fat and calories from salad dressing, choose low-fat dressings or simply dilute a regular dressing with extra vinegar, lemon juice, water, or milk in creamy dressings. By using only small amounts of this diluted version, you'll get lots of flavor and moisture with fewer calories. You might also want to venture into the world of exotic vinegars. Balsamic is one of my favorites.

At restaurants, always request that the dressing be served on the side so you can control the amount you consume. Add the dressing sparingly, or dip a forkful of salad into the dressing before each bite. And be forewarned: Even fat-free dressings have calories and should be used sparingly. Replacing the fat calories from dressings with more carbohydrate (e.g., an extra dinner roll or a baked potato) can improve your body's capacity for exercise.

Tip 3. Pile on the potassium-rich vegetables. This mineral, which gets lost in sweat, protects against high blood pressure. You should try to get at least 4,700 milligrams of potassium per day, an easy task for salad lovers.

Some of the vegetables richest in potassium are romaine lettuce, broccoli, tomatoes, and carrots (see table 1.1 on page 11).

Tip 4. Include adequate protein by adding low-fat cottage cheese; flaked tuna; canned salmon; or sliced turkey, chicken, or other lean meats. For plant-based protein, toss in diced tofu, chickpeas, kidney beans, walnuts, sunflower seeds, almonds, and peanuts. Too often vegetarians eat just the greens and neglect the protein. They often end up anemic, injured, and chronically sick with colds or the flu.

Tip 5. Remember the calcium. For calcium (and protein), add grated part-skim mozzarella cheese; cubes of tofu; dressing made from plain yogurt seasoned with oregano, basil, and other Italian herbs; or a scoop of low-fat cottage cheese (a better source of protein than of calcium). Drink low-fat milk or nonfat milk along with the salad, or have yogurt for dessert. Don't try to live on lettuce alone!

Dinners at Home and Away

In the United States, dinners are commonly the biggest meal of the day— the reward for having survived yet another busy, stress-filled day. I invite you to start putting dinner at the bottom of the meal priority list and placing more focus on breakfast and lunch. That way, you'll have more energy to cope with daytime stresses, enjoy a good workout, and feel less in need of high-calorie rewards at night. Yes, you can and should still enjoy a pleasant evening meal—but you won't need a humongous feast, followed by endless snacks.

Active people commonly eat a huge dinner because they ate too little during the day. If this sounds familiar, experiment with reorganizing your good-nutrition game plan so that you put more emphasis on breakfast and lunch as a means of fueling up and remaining fueled throughout the busy day. Use the evening meal as a time to refuel, but whenever possible keep it relatively equal in size to breakfast and lunch or lunches.

As Gretchen, a kindergarten teacher, said, "I used to stuff myself at night as a reward for having survived a hectic day. I'd arrive home stressed and tired, then overeat and feel lousy. Now I eat breakfast like a king, lunch like a prince, and dinner like a pauper. I've found that by eating this way, I have lots more energy for my students during the day and for my family in the evening. By eating a lighter dinner, I sleep much better and feel better overall."

Dinner at Home

When dinner is home based, you need a game plan to pull together a team of nutritious foods. The following tips can help you plan for and prepare wholesome dinners without much time or effort—with little or no cooking. The recipes in part IV offer additional tried-and-true menu suggestions.

Tip 1. Don't arrive home too hungry. One prerequisite for successful nighttime dining is to eat a hearty lunch plus a second lunch or afternoon snack. Irina, a busy stockbroker, experimented with my suggestion to eat a heartier lunch plus a preexercise snack before her 5:30 p.m. kickboxing class. In one day, she discovered this food enhanced her energy for exercise and transformed her 7:00 bowl of ice cream for dinner into a bowl of salad. A substantial lunch supports less fatigue in the afternoon, higher-quality afternoon workouts, more physical and mental energy to prepare a nourishing supper, and a greater ability to cope with the day's stresses.

Tip 2. Plan time to shop for food. Good nutrition starts in the grocery store. By stocking your kitchen shelves and freezer with a variety of wholesome foods that are ready and waiting, you will be more likely to eat a better dinner. Kirsten, a 24-year-old dental assistant, used to spend most of her food budget in restaurants on the way home from work because at home she faced bare cupboards and an empty refrigerator. Although she liked to cook, she rarely did so because she simply didn't plan the time to grocery shop. Plus, she got discouraged by meats and vegetables that often spoiled before she got around to cooking them.

I advised Kirsten to enter into her day planner a time to food shop. She kept that appointment and was then able to stock her freezer with individually wrapped chicken breasts, lean hamburger patties, turkey burgers, and frozen vegetables—particularly vitamin-rich broccoli, spinach, and winter squash. Freezing does not destroy a food's nutritional value, so frozen foods provide quick nutrition with less fuss and waste than fresh items do. The frozen broccoli provides far more nutrients than the wilted, five-day-old stalks that Kirsten occasionally dragged from her refrigerator. Once she had stocked her kitchen with frozen foods and other staples, Kirsten discovered that she liked to come home for dinner.

I always stock basic foods that won't spoil quickly. On days when I arrive home to an empty refrigerator, I can either pull together a no-cook meal or quickly prepare a hot dinner. Some of my standard menus include these items:

- English-muffin pizzas
- Stoned-wheat crackers, peanut butter, and milk
- Lentil soup with extra broccoli, leftover pasta, and a tub of yogurt
- Refried beans, salsa, and cheese rolled in a tortilla and heated in the microwave

- Tuna sandwich with tomato soup
- Oatmeal cooked with low-fat milk, banana, and almonds

My standard ingredients include the following:

Cupboard		Refrigerator	Freezer
Spaghetti	Salsa	Low-fat cheese	English muffins
Rice	Minced clams	Shredded mozzarella	Bagels
Potatoes, white	Tuna	Low-fat cottage cheese	Multigrain breads
Potatoes, sweet	Spaghetti sauce	Low-fat yogurt	Strawberries
Wheat crackers	Canned salmon	Low-fat milk	Blueberries
RyKrisp crackers	Kidney beans	Eggs (omega-3)	Winter squash
Pretzels	Refried beans	Oranges	Spinach
Wheaties	Soups (lentil, tomato)	Baby carrots	Broccoli
Oatmeal	Peanut butter	V8 juice	Chicken breasts
Almonds	Raisins	Orange juice	Ground turkey
Bananas	Canned peaches	Tortillas	Extra-lean hamburger

When creating a meal from these staples, I choose items from three of the five food groups, using carbohydrate as the foundation for each meal. The following are sample 650-calorie, 60 percent carbohydrate, well-balanced meals with no cooking. The portions are appropriate for an active woman who needs about 1,800 to 2,000 calories per day; a hungry man may want more.

Food group	Menu 1: crackers with tuna	Menu 2: peanut butter and raisin sandwich
1. Grain	8 stoned-wheat crackers	2 slices multigrain bread
2. Protein	1/2 can tuna with 1 tbsp light mayo	2 tbsp peanut butter
3. Fruit		1/4 cup raisins
4. Vegetable	12 oz (350 ml) can V8 juice	10 baby carrots
5. Dairy	1 cup fruit yogurt	1 cup low-fat milk
Food group	Menu 3: pizza	Menu 4: burrito
1. Grain	2 English muffins	2 tortillas
2. Protein	(cheese)	1 cup vegetarian refried beans
3. Fruit	1 cup orange juice	Canned peaches
4. Vegetable	3/4 cup spaghetti sauce	Salsa
5. Dairy	1/2 cup grated mozzarella cheese	1 cup low-fat cottage cheese

Tip 3. Eat more than just plain pasta at a meal. For active people, pasta in any shape (spaghetti, ziti, twists, whatever) is without question a very popular and easy-to-cook meal. Although carbohydrate-rich pasta does provide muscle fuel for your body's engine, pasta is a marginal source of vitamins and minerals (the "spark plugs" needed for top performance). Whole-wheat pastas offer a little more nutritional value, but wheat and other grains are better respected for their carbohydrate value than their vitamin density. Even spinach and tomato pastas are overrated; they contain very little of the vegetables. Pasta becomes a nutrition powerhouse when it is topped with any combination of the following:

- Tomato sauce (fresh or from a jar)
- Spinach and garlic sauce
- Vegetables (broccoli, spinach, or green peppers from the freezer)
- Canned beans, cottage cheese, or tuna for cook-free protein

Tip 4. Plan cook-a-thons. Lauren, a 53-year-old high school teacher, enjoyed cooking on the weekends when she had the time. She always created a big batch of something on Sunday so it would be waiting for her when she arrived home tired and hungry after work and workouts. She preferred convenience to variety and thrived on beans and rice for a week, then lasagna the next week, split pea soup the third, and so on. When Lauren couldn't face another repetitious dinner, she cooked something else and put the leftovers in the freezer.

Dinner Out

Some people eat in restaurants because the cupboards are empty or they prefer not to cook. Others enjoy dining in restaurants with their friends. And some end up in restaurants because of business meetings. Whatever the situation, every active person who relies on restaurants for a balanced sports diet faces the challenge of finding healthful meals among all the rich temptations. Unfortunately, many people select whatever's fast and happens to tempt their taste buds at the moment, particularly when they are tired, hungry, stressed, anxious, or lonely. Here are some suggestions for what to eat when you are eating out.

Low-Fat and Healthful Choices

The most important first step to selecting healthful restaurant meals is to patronize the restaurants that offer carbohydrate-rich sports foods; don't go to a steak house if you're looking for muscle fuel. Study the menu before you sit down to see if the restaurant offers pasta, baked potatoes, bread, juices, and other carbohydrate-based foods. Try to avoid the places that have only fried items. Also, check to see if they allow special requests. If the menu clearly states "no substitutions," you might be in the wrong place.

When you're in an appropriate restaurant, choose your foods wisely. In general, you should request foods that are baked, broiled, roasted, or steamed—anything but fried. Low-fat poultry and fish items tend to be better choices than items naturally high in fat, such as prime rib, cheese, sausage, and duck. Keep the following foods in mind as you peruse a menu:

- **Appetizers.** Tomato juice, fruit juice, shrimp cocktail, fruit cocktail, melon, and crackers make great starters for your meal.

- **Breads.** Unbuttered rolls and breads are great—particularly if they are whole grain; ask for extras! If the standard fare is buttered (as in garlic bread), request some plain bread also, and enjoy the buttery bread in moderation.

- **Soups.** Broth-based soups (such as vegetable, chicken and rice, and Chinese soups) and hearty minestrone, split pea, navy bean, and lentil soups can be good sources of carbohydrate and are more healthful than creamy chowders and bisques. They are also a source of fluids.

- **Salads.** Enjoy the veggies, but limit the chunks of cheese, bacon bits, parmesan, olives, and other high-fat toppings. Always request that the dressing be served on the side so you can control how much you use. Be extra generous with chickpeas and toasted croutons.

- **Seafood and poultry.** Request chicken or fish that's baked, roasted, steamed, stir-fried, or broiled. Because many chefs add a lot of butter when broiling foods such as fish, you might want to request that your entree be broiled dry (cooked without this extra fat). If the entree is sauteed, request that the chef saute it with very little butter or oil and add no extra fat before serving.

- **Beef.** Many restaurants pride themselves on serving huge slabs of beef or 12-ounce (340 g) steaks. If you order beef, plan to cut this double portion in half and take the rest home for tomorrow's dinner, share it with a companion (who has ordered accordingly), or simply leave it. Trim all the visible fat, and request that any gravy or sauce be served on the side so that you can use it sparingly, if at all. Your goal is to eat meat as the accompaniment to the meal, not as the focus. Your muscles will perform better if two-thirds of your plate is covered with carbohydrate-based potatoes, vegetables, and bread.

- **Potatoes.** Order extra to make this the mainstay of your dinner. Baked potatoes are a great source of carbohydrate, unless the chef loads them up with butter or sour cream. Request that these top-pings be served on the side so you can control how much you eat. Better yet, trade those fat calories for more carbohydrate. Add moisture by mashing the potato with some milk (special request). This may sound a bit messy, but it's a delicious, low-fat way to enjoy what might otherwise be a dry potato.

- **Pasta.** Enjoy a pile! Pick pasta served with tomato sauces (carbo-hydrate) rather than the high-fat cheese, oil, or cream sauces. Also be cautious of cheese-filled lasagna, tortellini, and manicotti. They can be high-fat choices.

- **Rice.** In a Chinese restaurant, you'll be better off filling up on an extra bowl of plain steamed rice, another good source of carbohy-drate, than on egg rolls or other fried appetizers.

- **Vegetables.** Request plain, unbuttered vegetables with any special sauces (hollandaise, lemon butter) served on the side.

- **Chinese food.** Steamed rice with stir-fry combinations such as chicken with veggies or beef with broccoli are the best choices. Ask for extra vegetables. You can also request that the food be cooked with less oil. Be cautious at buffets; the chefs tend to add extra oil so the food is less sticky.

- **Dessert.** Sherbet, low-fat frozen yogurt, angel food cake, a fruit cup, or berries are among the best choices for your sports diet. Fresh fruit is often available, even if it isn't listed on the menu. If you can't resist a decadent dessert, just be sure to enjoy it after you have eaten plenty of carbohydrate. That is, don't eat a carbohy-drate-poor dinner to save room for a high-fat dessert.

When you are faced with a meal that's all wrong for you, try to make the best of a tough situation. For example, you can scoop the sour cream off the potato, drain the dressing from the salad, scrape off the gravy, or remove the fried batter from the chicken. You can also top off a carbohy-drate-poor meal with your own high-carbohydrate after-dinner snacks, such as fig bars, a bagel, pretzels, animal crackers, a banana, graham crack-ers, dried pineapple, raisins, and juice boxes. Take these emergency foods along with you. However, also try to make special requests. Remember, you are the boss when it comes to restaurant eating. The restaurant's job is to serve you the low-fat foods that enhance your health and your performance. Bon appetit!

Fast-Food Choices

Eating at a quick-service restaurant is like visiting Fat City. You have an easy opportunity to select a dietary disaster and choose items that are high in saturated fat and calories but low in carbohydrate, fiber, fruits, and vegetables. Although the occasional burger and fries meal is of little health concern, fast foods that are a common part of your diet need to be balanced with wholesome, lower-fat choices. Fortunately for our health, most of today's quick-service food centers offer healthful, low-fat carbohydrate options. Table 4.2 provides the calories and fat grams found in commonly consumed fast-food items.

Travelers, in particular, need to learn how to fuel themselves wisely, even if on a budget. If you are a 150-pound (68 kg) athlete who needs 2,700 to 3,000 calories a day, the cheapest way to stave off hunger is to fill up on fatty foods—such as tempting value meals. Bad idea. These high-fat meals not only clog the arteries and bulk up the waistline but also fail to adequately fuel the muscles. A better bet is to carry carbohydrate-rich foods with you. Some easy-to-tote choices include bagels, crackers, fig bars, breakfast cereals, and dried fruits.

The following menu ideas can help you healthfully navigate the world of fast foods.

- Any way you look at them, burgers and French fries have high fat content. You'll be better off going to an eatery that offers more than just burgers. Find a menu that offers grilled chicken or roast-beef sandwiches accompanied by soups (brothy or beany ones). Other options include roast or grilled chicken meals with mashed potatoes, rice, vegetables, and salad bars complete with kidney beans, chickpeas, and bread.

- If you order a burger, request a second roll or extra bread. Squish the grease into the first roll, then replace it with the fat-free roll. Boost carbohydrate intake with beverages such as juice, smoothies, or low-fat shakes. Pack supplemental carbohydrate, such as dried fruit or fig bars.

- Shy away from value meals. You'll be better off having a burger and milk than having your money go "to waist" by choosing the meal deal.

- Beware of chicken sandwiches topped with a special mayonnaise-based sauce, which can make the sandwich as fatty as a fried-chicken sandwich. Request that the server hold the sauce, or wipe off the mayo yourself.

- Meals with chicken that is roasted or grilled are generally preferable to fried-chicken meals. If you order fried chicken, get the larger pieces, remove all the skin, and eat just the meat. Order extra rolls, cornbread with honey or jam, corn on the cob, and other vegetables for more carbohydrate.

Table 4.2 Fast-Food Calories and Fat

Menu item	Cal	Fat	Menu item	Cal	Fat
McDonald's (www.mcdonalds.com)					
Hamburger	250	9	McDonaldland cookies	250	8
Quarter Pounder	410	19	Fruit'n'Yogurt Parfait w/granola	160	2
Quarter Pounder with Cheese	510	26	Egg McMuffin	300	12
Big Mac	540	29	Sausage McMuffin with Egg	450	27
Grilled Chicken	420	10	Egg, bacon, cheese McGriddle	460	21
Grilled Chicken Wrap	270	10	Biscuit	230	10
Chicken McNuggets (6)	250	15	Biscuit w/bacon, egg, cheese	440	25
Sauce, sweet'n'sour	50	0	Hash browns	140	8
Filet-o-Fish	380	18	Hotcakes w/2 margarine, syrup	600	17
Grilled chicken Caesar salad, plain	220	6	Hotcakes, plain	340	8
Low-fat dressing	50	2	Breakfast burrito, sausage	300	16
Caesar dressing (1 package)	190	18	Orange juice, 12 oz (360 ml)	140	0
Side salad, no dressing	20	0	Milk, 1%, 8 oz	100	2
French fries, small	250	13	Cola, 21 oz (630 ml)	210	0
French fries, medium	380	20	Shake, chocolate, 16 oz (480 ml)	580	14
French fries, large	570	30	McFlurry, M&M, 12 oz (360 ml)	620	20
Burger King (www.burgerking.com)					
Whopper	670	39	Grilled chicken garden salad	240	9
Whopper, no mayo	510	22	Light Italian dressing, 2 oz (60 ml)	120	11
Whopper, double w/cheese, mayo	990	64	Chicken sandwich, grilled, no mayo	450	10
Whopper, triple with mayo	1130	82	Chicken Tenders (5 pieces)	210	12
BK Broiler Chicken	510	19	Fries, medium	360	20
BK Broiler Chicken, no mayo	390	8	Onion rings, small	150	7
Veggie Burger	420	16	Croissanwich w/sausage, egg, cheese	470	32
Domino's Pizza (www.dominos.com)					
Classic cheese, 1/8 of 14 in. large	290	9	Deep dish, 1/8 of 14 in. large	320	12
Thin crust cheese, 1/8 of 14 in. large	180	9	Buffalo wings, hot (2)	210	14
Brooklyn style, 1/6 of 14 in. large	330	17	Cheesy Bread, 1 of 8 sticks	140	7
Pizza Hut (www.pizzahut.com)					
Personal pan pizza, pepperoni	640	29	Fit'n'Delicious, 1 slice of 14 in.	230	6
Personal pan pizza, supreme	710	34	Hot wings	120	7
Kentucky Fried Chicken (www.kfc.com)					
Original recipe breast, 5.5 oz (175 g)	360	21	Tender Roast sandwich, no sauce	300	5
Extra crispy breast, 6 oz (175 g)	440	27	Corn on the cob, 5.5 oz (14 cm)	150	3
Crispy strips (3)	350	19	Macaroni and cheese	180	8
Wendy's (www.wendys.com)					
Chili, small	220	6	Baked potato, plain	270	0
Mandarin chicken salad (dry)	170	2	Baked potato w/sour cream	370	6
Taco Supreme salad	370	17	Fresh fruit bowl	130	0
Turkey Frescata sandwich	430	15	Frosty Jr., 6 oz (180 ml)	170	4
Taco Bell (www.tacobell.com)					
Taco	170	10	Mexican pizza	550	31
Taco Supreme	260	16	Bean burrito	350	8

Menu item	Cal	Fat	Menu item	Cal	Fat
Taco Bell (continued)					
Soft taco, grilled chicken	190	7	Taco salad	810	46
Gordita, chicken baja	340	18	Nachos Supreme	440	24
Gordita, beef	360	21	Refried beans	140	3
Au Bon Pain (www.aubonpain.com)					
Soup			**Croissant**		
Garden vegetable, 12 oz (360 ml)	80	2	Plain	260	15
Tomato Florentine, 12 oz (360 ml)	120	3	Chocolate	330	17
Vegetarian chili, 16 oz (480 ml)	350	4	Sweet cheese	340	19
Salad without dressing			Spinach and cheese	250	14
Garden, large	110	2	Ham and cheese	350	18
Chicken Caesar, 1 container	300	14	**Cookies**		
Thai chicken salad	190	5	Chocolate chip	260	11
Fresh fruit and yogurt	170	2	Oatmeal raisin	230	8
Breakfast sandwiches			**Muffins, bagels, Danishes**		
Egg on a bagel	400	4	Bagel, plain	290	1
Lox and wasabi on a bagel	490	11	Bagel, raisin	320	1
Sandwiches			Bran muffin	410	9
Classic tuna	550	27	Low-fat triple berry muffin	290	2
Turkey and Swiss, baguette	760	28	Blueberry muffin	510	19
Arizona chicken croissant	680	30	Pecan roll	520	28
Dunkin' Donuts (www.dunkindonuts.com)					
Glazed donut, raised type	180	8	Chocolate chip muffin	630	26
Jelly filled donut	210	8	Bagel, plain	320	2
Powdered sugar donut, cake type	330	19	Bagel, multigrain	380	6
Glazed chocolate donut, cake type	350	19	Bagel sandwich (egg, cheese, bacon)	540	18
Munchkin, cake, cinnamon, 1	65	4	Coffee w/cream, sugar, 10 oz (300 ml)	120	6
Blueberry muffin, large	470	17	Coffee Coolatta w/cream, 16 oz (480 ml)	350	22
Blueberry muffin, reduced fat	400	5	Coffee Coolatta w/skim, 16 oz (480 ml)	170	0
Bran muffin	480	15	Chocolate chunk cookie	540	23
Cinnabon (www.cinnabon.com)					
Cinnabon roll	730	24	Caramel Cinnabon	1,100	56
Subway (www.subway.com					
Roasted turkey, 6 in. (15 cm)	280	5	Roast beef wrap	280	7
Tuna, 6 in. (15 cm)	530	31	Chicken Teriyaki wrap	360	7
Mrs. Fields (www.mrsfields.com)					
Triple chocolate cookie	210	11	Double fudge brownie	360	20
White chunk madadamia cookie	230	12	Peanut butter nibbler (1)	60	3
Panera Bread (www.panerabread.com)					
Bagel, whole grain	340	3	Crispani pizza, tomato and basil	320	13
Panini, portobello and mozzarella, 1/2	370	19	Salad, Asian sesame chicken	450	22
Panini, turkey and artichoke, 1/2	420	19	Honeydew green tea, 16 oz (480 ml)	350	15
Tuscan chicken sandwich, 1/2	370	15	Chai tea latte, 10 oz (300 ml)	190	4

Information from Web sites, August 2007.

- Even though roasted chicken is preferable to fried, be aware that the roasted skin is still fatty. By removing the skin and wing from a KFC Rotisserie Gold quarter breast, you remove 13 grams of fat and 115 calories. Additionally, many of the accompaniments to chicken meals are laden with butter; however, any vegetable tends to be better than no vegetable. Ask if unbuttered, steamed vegetables are an option.

- At a salad bar, be generous with the colorful vegetables and hearty breads, but be careful to choose light dressings. Also, note that a Caesar salad is not a dieter's delight. For example, Boston Market's chicken Caesar salad with dressing totals more than 800 calories. You'd have been better off eating a chicken breast (remove the skin and wing), corn bread, steamed vegetables, and whole-kernel corn for 225 fewer calories and 46 fewer grams of fat.

- Resist the temptation to choose baked potatoes smothered with high-fat toppings. Your best bet is to order an additional plain potato and split the broccoli and cheese topping (14 g of fat) between the two. That way, you end up with a hearty 800-calorie, high-carbohydrate meal, with only 15 percent of the calories from fat. For additional protein, drink a glass of low-fat milk.

- Order thick-crust pizza that has extra crust rather than extra cheese. More dough means more carbohydrate. A slice of Pizza Hut's pan pizza has 10 more grams of carbohydrate than a slice of their thin-crust pizza. Pile on vegetables (green peppers, mushrooms, onions), but shy away from the pepperoni, sausage, and ground beef. Don't be shy about using a napkin to blot the fat that cooks out of the cheese.

- Seek out a deli that offers wholesome breads. Request a sandwich that emphasizes the bread rather than the filling. A large submarine roll (preferably whole wheat) provides far more carbohydrate than half a small pita. Hold the mayo, and add moistness with light salad dressings (if available), mustard, or ketchup. The lowest-fat fillings are turkey, ham, and lean roast beef.

- Hearty bean soups accompanied by crackers, bread, or corn bread provide a satisfying carbohydrate-rich, low-fat meal. Chili, if not glistening with a layer of grease, can be a good choice. For example, a Wendy's large chili with eight crackers provides a satisfying 400 calories, and only 20 percent (9 g) are from fat.

You can eat a high-carbohydrate sports diet even if you are eating fast foods. You simply need to balance the fat with the carbohydrate. Here are some additional suggestions from Joanne "Dr. Jo" Lichten's *Dining Lean: How to Eat Healthy When You're Not at Home* (pages 41-47).

Breakfast Suggestions

- Egg, egg white, or Egg Beaters omelet (nonstick spray) served with mixed fruit and rye toast with jam
- Raisin Bran or Shredded Wheat plus low-fat milk, juice or fresh or canned fruit, and toast with butter on the side
- Au Bon Pain Egg on a Bagel, Jack in the Box Breakfast Jack, or McDonald's Egg McMuffin
- Whole-grain bagel with light cream cheese and a latte (low-fat milk)

Lunch Suggestions

- Chick-fil-A Chargrilled Chicken Sandwich (hold the cheese), Carrot and Raisin Salad, and fruit cup
- McDonald's Premium Grilled Chicken Classic (hold the cheese) and Apple Dippers with Low Fat Caramel Dip
- Bowl of miso or egg drop soup and 10 pieces of sushi with soy sauce, horseradish, and ginger
- Two slices of cheese or onion, pepper, mushroom, ham, and pineapple pizza
- A 12-inch Subway Veggie Delite, Turkey Breast, Ham, Roast Beef, or Club
- Grilled chicken salad (dressing on the side) and roll
- Gardenburger on bun (mustard, ketchup, lettuce, tomato, onion)
- Boston Market quarter roasted white-meat chicken (without skin or wings), green beans, steamed vegetables, and new potatoes
- KFC Tender Roast Chicken Sandwich (no sauce), corn on the cob (small), and BBQ baked beans
- Wendy's plain baked potato topped with small chili

Dinner Suggestions

- Grilled chicken, sirloin steak, pork tenderloin, or fish with baked potato (or rice), steamed vegetables (no butter), and a dinner roll
- Applebee's Tortilla Chicken Melt
- Boston Market quarter white-meat Original Rotisserie Chicken (no skin), mashed potatoes with gravy, and green beans
- Olive Garden Capellini Primavera or Pomodoro and a lightly buttered breadstick

- Red Lobster Roasted Tilapia in a Bag, rice, vegetable, and rolls
- Salad bar: vegetables, chickpeas, kidney beans, and light dressing, plus broth-based soup and cornbread
- Chicken and vegetable stir-fry (prepared with very little oil) and steamed brown rice
- Pasta with tomato sauce, red or white clam sauce, or Bolognese sauce, plus a salad (dressing on the side)
- Mexican chicken fajita meat, tortillas, lettuce, and salsa, plus Mexican rice and bean soup

Reprinted, with permission, from *Dining Lean: How to Eat Healthy When You're Not at Home* (2007) by Joanne "Dr. Jo" Lichten, PhD, RD. www.drjo.com.

CHAPTER 5

Snacks and Snack Attacks

Once upon a time, people ate three square meals a day. They rarely snacked. Today, people are forever seeking a quick energy fix, and snacks commonly make up 20 to 50 percent of total calories. If you are a big-time snacker, I encourage you to redefine snacks as meals so that you are less likely to choose cookies, potato chips, soft drinks, and other traditional energy boosters. In fact, I generally eliminate the word snack when counseling clients. I teach them to think *two lunches* instead of *lunch* and *afternoon snack*. That way, they end up choosing wholesome foods (such as vegetable soup) and not typical snacks (such as sweets) in the afternoon.

Wise Snacking

Many of my clients believe that snacking is bad because they snack on glazed doughnuts, snack cakes, candy bars, cookies, colas, and other lackluster choices that fail to offer the nutrients needed for optimal performance. If this sounds like you, remember that your body needs calories and the vitamins, minerals, and protein found in wholesome foods to function well. If you want to have quality workouts, high energy, and good health, you need to fuel your body with quality calories. You can do this by thinking *second lunch* instead of *sweet snack*.

Some people try not to snack because they believe that eating between meals is sinful and fattening. The truth is that snacking is important. Remember that active people tend to get hungry at least every four hours, so if you have lunch at noon, your body will still want a snack (or a second lunch) by 4:00 p.m., if not sooner. If you will be exercising in the afternoon, you need added fuel to energize your workout. Snacking is good for you and your workouts, and you should plan it as part of your sports diet.

Fast Snacks

When you are eating on the run and grabbing snacks instead of real meals, be sure to choose wholesome foods. You can make wise choices from among many nutritious and conveniently available items. Some popular suggestions include

- a whole-grain bagel with peanut butter and a (decaf) latte;
- a slice of thick-crust pizza with green peppers;
- peanut butter, crackers, and raisins;
- trail mix with granola, nuts, and dried fruit;
- Grape-Nuts with yogurt and berries;
- Chinese takeout—stir-fried chicken with vegetables and steamed rice; and
- instant oatmeal made with low-fat milk and slivered almonds.

Note that each of these mini-meals includes foods from three food groups. Ideally, you'll choose foods from different groups to help balance your diet. That way, even people who graze throughout the day can get a variety of nutrients needed for good health and top performance. The following list provides additional ideas for snacks and grazing at home and on the road:

- **Dry cereal.** Mix your favorite cereal with raisins, dried fruits, cinnamon, or nuts.
- **Instant oatmeal.** Microwave the oatmeal with milk instead of water to boost its nutrition power. Sprinkle with raisins and chopped nuts.
- **Popcorn.** Eat plain or sprinkled with spices such as chili powder, garlic powder, onion powder, or soy sauce. If you like, spray with low-calorie butter-flavor sprays so that the spices stick.
- **Pretzels.** If you wish to reduce your salt intake, knock the salt off or buy salt-free pretzels.

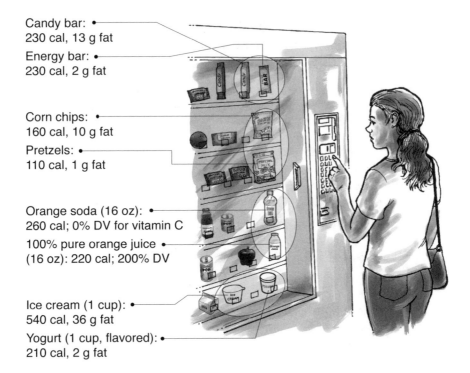

Candy bar:
230 cal, 13 g fat

Energy bar:
230 cal, 2 g fat

Corn chips:
160 cal, 10 g fat

Pretzels:
110 cal, 1 g fat

Orange soda (16 oz):
260 cal; 0% DV for vitamin C

100% pure orange juice
(16 oz): 220 cal; 200% DV

Ice cream (1 cup):
540 cal, 36 g fat

Yogurt (1 cup, flavored):
210 cal, 2 g fat

- **Crackers.** Stoned wheat, sesame, bran, whole grain, and low-fat brands are good choices.

- **Muffins.** Homemade with canola oil are best; wholesome bran or corn muffins are preferable to those made with white flour (see the recipes in part IV). If store bought, choose low-fat muffins.

- **Bagels.** Whole-grain varieties provide more vitamins and minerals than do bagels made with white flour.

- **Fruits.** Choose oranges, bananas, apples, or any fresh fruit. When traveling, pack dried fruit for concentrated carbohydrate. See table 5.1 for some of the best fruit choices.

- **Smoothies.** Whip together milk, yogurt, or juice; fresh or frozen fruit; and wheat germ or flax meal (see information and recipes beginning on page 395).

- **Frozen fruit bars.** You can slowly savor these pleasant treats in good health.

- **Yogurt.** Buy plain low-fat yogurt and flavor it with vanilla, honey, cinnamon, instant decaffeinated coffee, applesauce, fruit cocktail, or berries.

Table 5.1   Ranking Fruits

Vitamin packed and health protective, fruit is a top-notch sports snack. To help you make the best choices, use this list, which orders fruits according to their content of nine vitamins and fiber. The higher the score, the more nutrient dense the fruit.

Fruit	Nutrition score
Watermelon, 2 cups	310
Grapefruit, 1/2 pink or red	263
Papaya, 1/2	223
Cantaloupe, 1/4	200
Orange, 1 average	186
Strawberries, 1 cup	173
Kiwi, 1	115
Raspberries, 1 cup	106
Tangerine, 1 average	105
Mango, 1/2	94
Honeydew, 1/8 melon	85
Apricots, 2 fresh	78
Banana, 1	54
Peach, 1 large	47
Pear, 1 average	44
Apple, with skin, 1	43
Raisins, 1/4 cup packed	24
Pears, canned, 2 halves	20
Apple juice, unsweetened, 1/2 cup	14

Copyright CSPI 2003. Adapted from Nutrition Action Health letter. www.cspinet.org

- **Energy bars, breakfast bars, low-fat granola bars.** Prewrapped and portable, these travel well in pockets and gym bags and can be very handy.

- **Nuts and seeds.** Peanuts, walnuts, almonds, sunflower seeds, pumpkin seeds, and other nuts and seeds are excellent for protein, B vitamins, vitamin E, and healthful fat.

- **Sandwiches.** Sandwiches don't have to be just for lunch; they are great for snacks. Choose peanut butter, turkey, hummus, lean roast beef, or tuna with light mayo.

- **Baked sweet potatoes.** Microwave ovens make these a handy snack. They're tasty warm or cold, a carbohydrate-rich choice for refueling your muscles after a hard workout. Try them with a dash of nutmeg—mmm!

Energy Bars: Costly but Convenient

PowerBars, Luna bars, Zone bars, Balance Bars—energy bars await you at every convenience store, each boasting its ability to enhance your performance. You can spend a fortune on these prewrapped bundles of energy, thinking they offer magic ingredients (not true). Energy bars are far more about convenience than necessity, and they do suit the needs of many hungry people who seek a hassle-free, somewhat nutritious snack. Here is some information to help you decide how much of your food budget to dedicate to these popular snacks.

- **Energy bars are portable.** You can easily tuck these compact and lightweight vitamin-enriched bars into a pocket for "emergency food." Energy bars are handy for runners and bikers who want to carry a durable snack on a long run or ride, for dancers who want fuel without bulk, or for hikers who want a light backpack.

- **Energy bars promote preexercise eating.** Fueling before exercising is a great way to boost stamina and endurance. The energy bar industry has done an excellent job of educating us that preexercise eating is important for optimizing performance. The associated energy boost likely does not result from magic ingredients (chromium, amino acids) but from eating 200 to 300 calories. These calories clearly fuel you better than the zero calories in no snack. Note that calories from tried-and-true fig bars, graham crackers, bananas, and low-fat granola bars are also effective preexercise energizers.

- **Energy bars promote eating during endurance exercise.** Energy bars are also a great way to boost stamina and endurance during extended exercise, such as hikes or bike rides, instead of just relying on what you eat before you exercise.

- **Most energy bars claim to be highly digestible.** One could debate whether energy bars are easier to digest than standard food because digestibility varies greatly from athlete to athlete. As with all sports snacks, you have to learn through trial and error during training what foods work for your system and what foods don't.

Do not try this pricey treat for the first time before a special event, such as a marathon, bike race, or rugby game, only to discover it causes discomfort. One key to tolerating energy bars is to drink plenty of water along with the bar. Otherwise, the product will settle poorly. Energy bars have a very low water content to make them more compact than fresh fruit, for example, which has high water content.

- **Some energy bars boast about a low carbohydrate content.** This is a holdover from the "carbohydrate is fattening" era. As I have said before and will say again, carbohydrate is not fattening; rather, excess calories are fattening. You want to snack on carbohydrate-based foods because they are the best sources of fuel for your muscles.

- **Energy bars are expensive.** You'll have to fork over at least one dollar, if not two, to buy most sports bars. The better value is to buy low-fat granola bars or breakfast bars from the supermarket at a much lower price (see table 5.2). A handful of raisins can also do a great job.

Table 5.2   **Energy Bars Versus Standard Foods**

Sports snack	Cal/oz (cal/30 g)	Carb/oz (carb/30 g)	Cost/100 cal ($)
Raisins	80	20	0.18
Banana	25	7	0.25
NutriGrain cereal bar	105	20	0.30
Nature Valley granola bar	120	19	0.33
Clif Bar	104	18	0.52
PowerBar	105	18	0.53
Balance Bar	114	12	0.60
Luna bar	106	15	0.72

Nutrition information from food labels. Prices based in North Carolina.

Snack Attacks

Snacks prevent not only hunger sensations but also cravings for sweets. Many of my clients complain about their constant cravings. They believe they are hopelessly, and helplessly, addicted to sugary snacks. I believe they are not addicted and that they can change their behavior. They are just hungry. When people get too hungry, they crave calorie-dense foods such as cookies, ice cream, chocolate—carbohydrate with fat (Gilhooly et al. 2007).

I've helped many clients resolve their problematic sweet cravings easily and painlessly. The solution is simple: Eat before you get too hungry. When you are ravenous, you tend to crave sweets (and fat) and overeat. An apple won't do the job; you'll want calorie-dense apple pie . . . plus ice cream.

If you frequently experience uncontrollable snack attacks, examine the following case studies and solutions to learn how to tame the cookie monster within you. Remember, snack attacks, not snacks per se, are the problem.

Case 1: Predinner Snack Attack

"I have the worst sweet tooth. I manage to fight sweet cravings until I get home, and then I inevitably attack the chocolate chip cookies. I feel as though I'm powerless and have no control over sweets. I hope you can put me on the straight and narrow."

—David, 47-year-old marathon runner, accountant, and father

Stories like David's are typical among my clients. He came to me feeling guilty about his lack of control over sweets. He required about 3,000 calories per day but ate zero calories at breakfast and barely ate lunch, only a 200-calorie yogurt, because he claimed he had no time. No wonder he was uncontrollably ravenous by the time he got home; he had accumulated a 2,800-calorie deficit! Nature took control by encouraging him to eat more than enough so that he would get adequate energy into his system.

I suggested that David eat his 1,600 cookie calories in the form of wholesome meals during the day. He started eating 800 calories for breakfast (cereal, milk, banana, juice, and bagel) and 1,000 calories of easy-to-eat snack-type foods for lunch and throughout the afternoon (two yogurts, two large bananas, two juices). Within one day he discovered that he wasn't a cookie monster after all. He could come home in a better mood, feel untempted by cookies, and have the energy to enjoy his family rather than be focused on eating cookies. This switch reduced his intake of fat, improved the quality of his overall diet, helped him flatten the spare tire that had been inflating around his middle, and lowered his cholesterol.

Case 2: Premenstrual Snack Attack

"Once a month I feel driven to devour a bag of chocolate kisses. I can easily tell the time of the month by my eating habits. Premenstrual chocolate cravings do me in."

—Charlene, 20-year-old active college student

Charlene, like many women, recognized that her eating patterns change with the stages of the menstrual cycle. In the week before her period, she has overwhelming sweet cravings; the week afterward, she tends to crave more protein foods or have very little appetite. Researchers have verified these eating patterns and report that a complex interplay of hormonal changes seems to influence women's food choices. High levels of estrogen may be linked with the premenstrual carbohydrate cravings.

Women may also crave carbohydrate because they are hungrier. Before menstruation, a woman's metabolic rate may increase by 100 to 500 calories (Barr, Janelle, and Prior 1995). That addition can be the equivalent of another meal. But when Charlene felt bloated and fat because of premenstrual water weight gain, she, like most women, would put herself on a reducing diet. The result was double deprivation. She had a physiological need for extra calories just when she put herself on the calorie-deficient reducing diet. No wonder she experienced overwhelming hunger and craved sweets.

I told Charlene not to diet but instead, when she felt hungry in the week before her period, to give herself permission to eat up to 500 additional wholesome calories. She started adding a slice of toast and jam to her standard breakfast, a hot cocoa at lunch, and an afternoon snack of some raisins. She successfully curbed the nagging hunger that had previously plagued her, and she was less irritable. Even her friends and family noticed a difference in her moods. She also lost interest in chocolate and was thrilled to survive a menstrual cycle without gaining weight from chocolate gluttony. Other clients have chosen to enjoy these extra premenstrual calories in the form of brownies or chocolate chip cookies—but within 500 calories.

Case 3: Chocolate Snack Attack

"Chocolate is my favorite food. I fight the urge to feed myself chocolate bars for lunch, M&Ms for snacks, and chocolate ice cream for dinner."

—Jocelyn, 17-year-old high school basketball player

Some folks simply love sweets. They need no excuse to indulge in sugary goo. They eat sweets daily, three times if not more, starting with chocolate doughnuts for breakfast, cookies for lunch, sweet-and-sour pork for dinner, and then ice cream for dessert. Naturally, this high consumption of sweets results in a poor diet because sugar lacks vitamins and minerals.

As a healthy, active teen, Jocelyn had space in her diet to fit in some sweets without jeopardizing her health. For people eating an overall wholesome diet, about 6 to 10 percent of the calories can appropriately come from refined sugar, if desired (Institute of Medicine 2002). Because Jocelyn required 2,800-plus calories per day, she could certainly fit in 280 calories of sugar, a reasonable amount.

Sweets abusers are more at risk for nutrition problems than those who enjoy an occasional treat. Eating a little chocolate as a fun food for dessert after a nourishing meal is far different from eating a box of chocolates to replace that meal. Chocoholics commonly skip breakfast because they're not hungry in the morning after eating a whole bag of chocolate chip cookies the night before. They would nourish themselves better by eating one or two cookies for dessert and then waking up hungry for a wholesome breakfast the next morning.

In Jocelyn's case the chocolate problem stemmed from having no time for breakfast, disliking school lunch, and having easy access to the vending machine. I encouraged her to eat breakfast on her way to school, which helped her consume less chocolate during the day.

Is Chocolate a Health Food?

Dark chocolate might help reduce blood cholesterol and offer heart-health benefits, specifically improved blood vessel health and lower blood pressure (Taubert et al. 2007). Although you need not eat a perfect diet to have a good diet, you also need not add chocolate to your diet for health benefits (despite what you might see advertised by the candy industry).

Chocolate is made from cocoa, a plant food. It contains health-protective compounds called flavonoids that help relax and dilate blood vessels, reduce blood pressure, and increase blood flow to the brain. These flavonoids are also found in other plant foods, such as green tea, red wine, apples, and onions, so think twice before you plan to replace an apple with a chocolate bar.

Because pure cocoa is bitter and unpalatable, it needs a lot of added sugar to transform it into a delicious candy bar. Labeling this sugar-coated cocoa a "health food" is a stretch of the imagination. Yet, if you are destined to eat chocolate, dark chocolate does contain more flavonoids than does milk chocolate.

Mars, the maker of the fortified chocolate bar CocoaVia, suggests that eating two bars a day offers "full benefits"; this potentially displaces 200 calories of healthier snacks (fruit, nuts, yogurt) that might have offered better health protection. The better bet is to eat chocolate for pleasure, not health. There's little wrong with savoring a small piece of dark chocolate after a meal, when a little bit will satisfy you, and even this small amount has been shown to slightly reduce blood pressure (Taubert et al. 2007).

CHAPTER 6 ———————————

Carbohydrate to Fuel Muscles

Without question, wholesome forms of carbohydrate are the best choices for fueling your muscles and promoting good health. People of all ages and athletic abilities will benefit from nourishing themselves with abundant carbohydrate-rich fruits, vegetables, and whole-grain foods, along with adequate protein and healthful fat balanced into their meals and snacks.

Unfortunately, confusion about carbohydrate—what it is and how much to eat (if any)—keeps people from properly balancing their diets. As one runner questioned, "Is carbohydrate good or bad? Fattening or fuel? How much is too much? If I have a bagel for breakfast, can I also have bread at lunch—or is that too fattening?" Like many active people, he was confused by the plethora of myths and misconceptions about the role of carbohydrate in a sports diet. The purpose of this chapter is to eliminate this confusion so you can make choices that best promote your health, desired weight, and performance.

Simple and Complex Carbohydrates

All forms and sources of carbohydrate are not alike. The carbohydrate family includes both simple and complex carbohydrates. The simple carbohydrates are monosaccharides and disaccharides (single- and double-sugar molecules). Glucose, fructose, and galactose are monosaccharides, the simplest sugars. Monosaccharides can be symbolized like this:

The disaccharides can be symbolized like this:

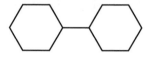

Four common sources of disaccharides are table sugar (sucrose), milk sugar (lactose, a combination of glucose and galactose), corn syrup, and honey.

Table sugar, corn syrup, and honey all contain glucose and fructose but in differing amounts. With digestion, table sugar breaks apart into 50 percent glucose and 50 percent fructose. The high-fructose corn syrup commonly used in soft drinks breaks down to about 55 percent fructose and 45 percent glucose. Honey contains about 31 percent glucose, 38 percent fructose, 10 percent other sugars, 17 percent water, and 4 percent miscellaneous particles. Your body eventually converts all monosaccharides and disaccharides to glucose, which travels in the blood (blood glucose) to fuel your muscles and brain.

Fruits and vegetables offer a variety of sugars in differing proportions. Because you absorb different sugars at different rates and by differing pathways, research indicates that consuming a variety of sugars allows for better absorption during exercise. This means you should read the ingredient label on your sports drink to be sure it offers more than one type of sugar.

Fructose, in the form of high-fructose corn syrup (HFCS), has come under scrutiny as a possible culprit contributing to the obesity epidemic (Wylie-Rosett, Segal-Isaacson, and Segal-Isaacson 2004). HFCS is made using chemical processes that first convert cornstarch to corn syrup and then convert 42 to 55 percent of the glucose in the corn syrup to fructose as a way to make it taste sweeter. Animal research suggests that fructose can lead to weight gain because of changes in insulin and leptin, two hormones that influence appetite. Whether or not HFCS promotes obesity in humans requires more study. Some research hints that fructose is digested, absorbed, and metabolized differently than glucose in ways that favor fat production (Bray, Nielsen, and Popkin 2004; Vertanian, Schwartz, and Brownell 2007).

Until we have a definitive answer, the safest bet is to simply drink less soda. The most likely answer is that the excess calories associated with drinking too many soft drinks made with high-fructose corn syrup are the fattening culprit, more so than the HFCS itself. I'm sure you can find a far better way to spend the 150 calories—the equivalent of 10 teaspoons of sugar—in each can of soft drink!

Honey has been mistakenly described as being superior to HFCS or refined white sugar. If you prefer honey because of the pleasant taste, fine. But it's not superior in terms of vitamins or performance. Sugar in any form—honey, corn syrup, brown sugar, raw sugar, maple syrup, or jelly—has insignificant nutritional value, and your body digests any type of sugar or carbohydrate into glucose before using it for fuel.

Another type of sugar that is found in many engineered sports foods is glucose polymers, also called maltodextrins. Polymers are chains of about five glucose molecules. Sports drinks sweetened with polymers can provide more energy with rapid absorption and less sweetness than regular sugar provides. Some sports drinks that use polymers include Powerade and HydraFuel.

Complex carbohydrates, such as starch in plant foods and glycogen in muscles, are formed when sugars link together to form long complex chains, similar to a string of hundreds of pearls. They can be symbolized like this:

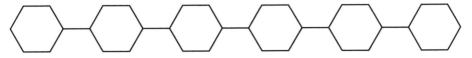

Plants store extra sugar in the form of starch. For example, corn is sweet when it's young, but it becomes starchy as it gets older. Its extra sugar converts into starch. In contrast to corn and other vegetables, fruits tend to convert starch into sugar as they ripen. A good example is the banana:

- A green banana with some yellow is 80 percent starch and 7 percent sugar.
- A mostly yellow banana is 25 percent starch and 65 percent sugar.
- A spotted and speckled banana is 5 percent starch and 90 percent sugar.

The potatoes, rice, bread, and other starches you eat are digested into glucose and then are burned for energy or stored for future use. Humans store extra glucose mostly in the form of muscle glycogen and liver glycogen (but generally not as body fat). This glycogen is readily available for energy during exercise.

Sugars and starches have similar abilities to fuel muscles but different abilities to nourish them with vitamins and minerals:

- The carbohydrate in sugary soft drinks provides energy but no vitamins or minerals.
- The carbohydrate in polymer sports drinks provides energy but no vitamins or minerals, unless the drink is fortified.
- The carbohydrate in fruits, vegetables, and grains provides energy, vitamins, minerals, fiber, and phytochemicals—the fuel and spark plugs that your body's engine needs to function best.

Is Carbohydrate Fattening?

Stacey, a personal trainer, wanted to eat carbohydrate for fuel but also wanted to maintain a lean weight. Like many weight-conscious people who exercise, Stacey considered carbohydrate-based foods to be fattening, and she was frustrated. "I don't keep crackers, bread, cereal, or bagels in the house, because when they are there, I eat them—too many of them! I want to lose weight, not gain it from all that fattening carbohydrate."

Fad diets preach the message that carbohydrate is fattening. Wrong! Carbohydrate is not fattening. Excess calories are fattening; in particular, excess fat calories—butter on bread, oil on pasta, mayonnaise on sandwiches, cheese on crackers—are fattening. Fat provides 36 calories per teaspoon compared with 16 for carbohydrate. Additionally, the conversion of excess carbohydrate into body fat is limited because you burn carbohydrate when you exercise. Your body preferentially burns the carbohydrate and stores the fat because the metabolic cost of converting excess carbohydrate into body fat is 23 percent of the ingested calories. Excess dietary fat, on the other hand, is easily stored as body fat; the metabolic cost of converting excess dietary fat into body fat is only 3 percent of ingested calories (Sims and Danforth 1987).

If you are destined to be gluttonous, your better bet is to overeat pretzels (carbohydrate) rather than peanuts (fat). You'll fuel your muscles better, and the next day you'll have a high-energy workout with muscles well loaded with carbohydrate. But be aware that a continuous intake of excess calories from carbohydrate will eventually contribute to weight gain. When your glycogen stores are filled, the excess calories will be stored as body fat (Hill et al. 1992).

Rather than try to stay away from breads, bagels, and other grains, remember these points:

- Carbohydrate-based foods are less fattening than fatty foods.
- You need carbohydrate to fuel your muscles.

- You burn carbohydrate during hard exercise.
- Carbohydrate is a friendly fuel; the enemy is excess calories from fat.
- When dieting to lose weight, you should energize with fiber-rich cereal, whole-grain breads, potatoes, and other carbohydrate-dense vegetables but reduce your intake of the butter, margarine, and mayonnaise that often accompany them.

Quick and Slow Forms of Carbohydrate

Just as carbohydrate is referred to as simple or complex and sugars or starches, it can also be categorized as quick or slow. The quick or slow refers to a complex system called the glycemic index (GI). The glycemic index is theoretically based on how 50 grams (200 calories) of carbohydrate (not counting fiber) in a food will affect blood sugar levels. For example, white bread is a carbohydrate high on the glycemic index and supposedly causes a rapid spike in blood sugar, while beans are considered low on the glycemic index and cause a more gradual increase in blood sugar levels. Table 6.1 provides the glycemic index and glycemic load (glycemic response to a standard serving of food) of popular sports foods. That is, a person might eat 200 calories of carbohydrate from pasta in a sitting,

Table 6.1 Glycemic Index and Glycemic Load of Popular Sports Foods

Food	Glycemic index	Glycemic load	Serving size
Coca-Cola	63	16	8 oz (240 ml)
Apple juice	40	12	8 oz (240 ml)
Gatorade	78	12	8 oz (240 ml)
Chocolate milk (1.5% fat with Nesquik)	41	5	8 oz (240 ml)
Rice cakes	78	17	1 oz (30 g)
Bagel, white Lenders	72	25	2.5 oz (75 g)
Wonder Bread	73	10	1 oz (30 g)
Spaghetti	58	28	6 oz (175 g)
Cheerios	74	15	1 oz (30 g)
Oatmeal, cooked	69	16	1 cup
Banana, underripe	42	10	4 oz (125 g)
Orange	42	5	4 oz (125 g)
Snickers bar	68	23	2 oz (60 g)
PowerBar, chocolate	56	24	2.3 oz (67 g)

Created from data in K. Foster-Powell, S.H. Holt and J.C. Brand-Miller, 2002, "International table of glycemic index and glycemic load values: 2002," *American Journal of Clinical Nutrition* 76(1):5–56.

but most people do not eat 200 calories of carbohydrate from rice cakes at one time. Hence, the actual glycemic load of a food differs from its glycemic index.

The glycemic index was initially developed to help people with diabetes better regulate their blood glucose. But people with diabetes generally eat foods in combinations (e.g., a sandwich with bread, turkey, and tomato), which alters the glycemic index of the meal (Franz 2003). Athletes, however, commonly eat foods solo (a banana, a bagel). Hence, exercise scientists became curious about the possibility that quick or slow forms of carbohydrate might affect exercise performance because they affect blood glucose in different ways. Could athletes use this ranking system to determine what to eat before, during, and after exercise?

In theory, low-glycemic index foods (apples, yogurt, lentils, beans) provide a slow release of glucose into the bloodstream, and high-glycemic index foods (sports drinks, jelly beans, bagels) quickly elevate blood sugar. Could low-GI foods help endurance athletes perform better by providing sustained energy during long bouts of exercise? Are high-GI foods best to consume immediately after exercise to rapidly refuel the muscles and, thereby, enhance subsequent performance?

Although this seems logical, I tell my athletes to disregard all the hype about the glycemic index and simply enjoy fruits, vegetables, and whole grains without fretting about their glycemic effect. Too many factors influence a food's glycemic index, including where the food was grown, the amount eaten, added fat, the way the food is prepared, and whether the food is eaten hot or cold. To make the glycemic index even less meaningful, each of us has a differing daily glycemic response that can vary approximately 43 percent on any given day (Vega-Lopez et al. 2007). Also, keep in mind that well-trained muscles can readily take up carbohydrate from the bloodstream. Hence, athletes secrete less insulin than do unfit people. This means most athletes don't get the blood sugar spikes seen in unfit people. Athletes also don't commonly get type 2 diabetes; exercise is an excellent way to manage blood sugar.

All things considered, you, as an athlete, have little need to obsess about a food's glycemic effect because you don't even know your personal response to the food. Plus, the sports nutrition research fails to clearly show performance benefits from these theories (Burke, Collier, and Hargreaves 1998). The research does indicate that the best way to enhance endurance is to consume carbohydrate before and during exercise—tried-and-true choices that taste good, settle well, and digest easily. You need not choke down low-glycemic index kidney beans thinking they will offer sustained energy, when they actually might only create digestive distress. To enjoy sustained energy, simply eat a tried-and-true preexercise meal or snack and then, after the first hour, consume about 200 to 250 calories of carbohydrate per hour of endurance exercise. (See chapters 9 and 10 for more information about fueling before and during exercise.)

For athletes who train hard or compete within 4 to 6 hours of the first session, choosing high-glycemic index recovery foods is a smart choice. High-GI foods provide glucose quickly and refuel depleted glycogen stores quicker than a lower glycemic index choice. Yet, 24-hour research suggests a low-GI diet might actually contribute to better performance the second day (109 versus 99 minutes of running to exhaustion) (Stevenson, Williams, and Biscoe 2005; Stevenson et al. 2005). The low-GI diet might facilitate better replacement of intramuscular fat stores (important for endurance) as well as enhance the use of fat for fuel, instead of the limited (and limiting) glycogen stores.

The bottom line: If you have to rapidly refuel from one bout of exhausting exercise to prepare for a second bout of exercise, eat *enough* easy-to-digest carbohydrate—at least 0.5 gram of carbohydrate per pound (1 g per kg) of body weight, or about 300 calories for a 150-pound (68 kg) person every two hours for four to six hours—and enjoy a balance of healthy fat and protein to take care of all the recovery needs, not just carbohydrate for glycogen. (See chapter 10 for more information about recovery.)

Insulin and Fat Storage

What about the popular notion that high-glycemic index foods are fattening because they create a rapid rise in blood sugar, stimulate the body to secrete more insulin, and thereby (supposedly) promote fat storage? Not so simple. Excess calories are fattening, not excess insulin. Insulin can stimulate the appetite, as well as fat deposition, and that's where high-GI carbohydrate gets a bad reputation.

We need more research to determine whether physically fit people will lose weight more easily with a diet based on low-GI foods. Indeed, even the research on low-GI foods and weight loss in overweight people is unclear. In one study of obese people (ages 18 to 35) with high insulin secretion, a low-GI diet (that lowered the insulin response) contributed to about 13 pounds (6 kg) of weight loss in 18 months—more than the 2.5 pounds (1 kg) lost by a comparison group who ate a higher-carbohydrate, lower-fat diet (Ebbeling et al. 2007). Yet, in another yearlong study of overweight adults (average age 35 years), a low-GI diet resulted in no differences in weight loss, hunger, or satiety compared with those who ate high-GI meals (Das et al. 2007). Stay tuned!

Is White Bread Poison?

White bread fails to offer the whole-grain goodness found in whole-wheat, rye, or other whole-grain breads. But white bread is neither poison nor a bad food. It can be part of an overall wholesome diet. As I mentioned in chapter 1, at least half of your grains should be from whole grains. So if you have oatmeal for breakfast and brown rice for dinner, your diet can accommodate a sandwich made on white bread (or pita or wrap) for lunch, if desired.

The reputation of white bread as being unhealthful is partially because of its high glycemic effect. That is, 200 calories of carbohydrate from white bread—if you eat just plain bread without the butter or sandwich filling that dampens the glycemic response—digest quickly and cause the blood glucose and insulin to rise higher than would the same amount of a whole-grain, fiber-rich bread.

Remember, if you are physically fit, your muscles readily store the sugar from the digested bread as glycogen, with much less insulin than required by a sedentary person. Hence, active people can better handle high-GI foods such as white bread and have less need to worry about the glycemic effect of the food.

Sugar Highs and Lows

Some athletes claim to be sugar sensitive; that is, after they eat sugar they report an energy spike followed by a crash. If that sounds familiar, the trick is to combine carbohydrate with protein or fat, such as bread plus peanut butter or an apple plus low-fat cheese. This changes the glycemic index of the carbohydrate. By experimenting with various types of snacks, you might notice you perform better after eating 200 calories of yogurt (a low-GI food) as compared with 200 calories of jelly beans (a high-GI food). Honor your personal response when choosing foods to support a winning edge for your body.

I suggest you experiment with a variety of fuels before, during, and after exercise to determine which ones taste best, settle well, and enhance your performance. Consider yourself an experiment of one. If you are unable to consume calories during endurance exercise, such as a swimmer who finds it difficult to eat while exercising or a person with a finicky stomach who prefers to abstain from taking anything but water during exercise, choosing a low-GI preexercise snack (such as yogurt or a bagel with peanut butter) might provide sustained energy that enhances your endurance and stamina.

If you can fuel your muscles during exercise with sports drinks, gels, fruit, or some form of carbohydrate, the energizing power of those snacks taken during exercise will be stronger than any potential benefits from eating a low-GI food preexercise (Burke, Collier, and Hargreaves 1998). And keep in mind that a bowl of low-GI lentils might look like a good idea on paper, but it would likely "gas propel" you to the portable toilets.

Carbohydrate for Glycogen

If you are trying to stay away from forms of carbohydrate such as bagels, pasta, and breads because you mistakenly believe carbohydrate to be fattening, think again. If you are dieting and exercising, you'll want to include carbohydrate foods in your diet. They are not fattening, and you need them to fuel your muscles so that you can enjoy your exercise program.

The average 150-pound (68 kg) male has about 1,800 calories of carbohydrate stored in the liver, muscles, and blood in approximately the following distribution:

Muscle glycogen	1,400 calories
Liver glycogen	320 calories
Blood glucose	80 calories
Total	**1,800 calories**

The carbohydrate in the muscles is used during exercise. The carbohydrate in the liver gets released into the bloodstream to maintain a normal blood glucose level and feed the brain (as well as the muscles). These limited carbohydrate stores influence how long you can enjoy exercising. When your glycogen stores get too low, you hit the wall—that is, you feel overwhelmingly fatigued and yearn to quit. In a research study, cyclists with depleted muscle glycogen stores were able to exercise only 55 minutes to fatigue (as measured by inability to maintain a specified pedaling speed on a stationary bicycle), as compared with more than twice as long—about 120 minutes—when they were carbohydrate loaded (Green et al. 2007). Food works!

In comparison to the approximately 1,800 calories of stored carbohydrate, the average lean 150-pound man also has 60,000 to 100,000 calories of stored fat—enough to run hundreds of miles. Unfortunately, for endurance athletes, fat cannot be used exclusively as fuel because the muscles need a certain amount of carbohydrate to function well. Carbohydrate is a limiting factor for endurance athletes.

During low-level exercise such as walking, the muscles burn primarily fat for energy. During light to moderate aerobic exercise, such as jogging, stored fat provides 50 to 60 percent of the fuel. When you exercise hard, as in sprinting, racing, or other intense exercise, you rely primarily on glycogen stores.

Biochemical changes that occur during training influence the amount of glycogen you can store in your muscles. The figures that follow indicate that well-trained muscles develop the ability to store about 20 to 50 percent more glycogen than can untrained muscles (Costill et al. 1981; Sherman et al. 1981). This change enhances endurance capacity and is one reason why a novice runner can't just load up on carbohydrate and run a top-quality marathon.

Muscle Glycogen per 100 Grams (3.5 oz) of Muscle

Untrained muscle	13 g
Trained muscle	32 g
Carbohydrate-loaded muscle	35-40 g

Because of the unfounded fear that carbohydrate is fattening or that high protein intake is better for muscles, many athletes today are skimping on carbohydrate foods. The resulting low-carbohydrate diet can potentially hurt performance; it contrasts sharply with the diet of 3 to 5 grams of carbohydrate per pound of body weight (6 to 10 g per kg)—or 55 to 65 percent carbohydrate—recommended by most exercise and health professionals.

A case in point is ice hockey, an incredibly intense sport that relies on both muscular strength and power. During a game, carbohydrate is the primary fuel; muscle carbohydrate (glycogen) stores decline between 38 and 88 percent. Muscle glycogen depletion relates closely to muscular fatigue. A motion analysis of elite ice-hockey teams showed that the players with a high-carbohydrate (60 percent) diet skated not only 30 percent more distance but also faster than the players who ate their standard low-carbohydrate (40 percent) diet. In the final period of the game, when a team often either wins or loses, the high-carbohydrate group skated 11 percent more distance than they did in the first period; the low-carbohydrate group skated 14 percent less. The researchers reached the following conclusions:

- Low muscle glycogen at the start of the game can jeopardize performance at the end of the game.
- Three days between games (with training on two of those days) plus a low (40 percent) carbohydrate diet does not replace normal muscle glycogen stores (the players with the high-carbohydrate diet had 45 percent more glycogen).
- The differences in performance between the well-fueled players and those who ate inadequate carbohydrate was most evident in the last period of the game (Ackermark et al. 1996).

Train Low, Compete High?

Train low, compete high (i.e., train with low glycogen stores, and compete with high glycogen stores) is a fueling practice that some serious athletes use— sometimes unknowingly when they do double workouts and fail to refuel well after the first workout. After being trained half the time in a glycogen-depleted state, the (fueled) muscles of 10 (initially untrained) men responded with greater endurance (Hansen et al. 2005). But questions arise: Does this same response happen with trained athletes? Can you train as well when your muscles are glycogen depleted? Do your form and technique suffer? Are you more prone to injuries? Are you able to enjoy the workout? The research is still too sparse to justify recommending this technique without caution.

Whether your sport is ice hockey, soccer, rugby, football, basketball, or any intense sport, remember to eat responsibly, with carbohydrate as the foundation of each meal and protein as the accompaniment.

Consuming carbohydrate also allows for the replenishment of muscle glycogen after exercise. In a landmark study by exercise physiologist Dr. J. Bergstrom and his colleagues (Bergstrom et al. 1967), researchers compared the rate at which muscle glycogen was replaced in subjects who exercised to exhaustion and then ate either a high-protein, high-fat diet or a high-carbohydrate diet. The subjects on the high-protein, high-fat diet (similar to an Atkins-type diet with abundant steak, eggs, hamburgers, tuna salad, peanut butter, and cheese) remained glycogen depleted for five days (see figure 6.1). The subjects on the high-carbohydrate diet

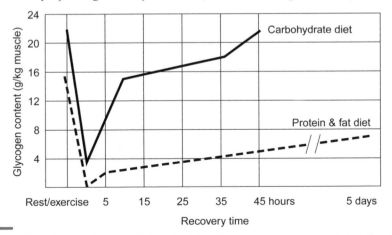

Figure 6.1 A carbohydrate diet replenishes the glycogen content of muscles more quickly than a protein and fat diet.

Reprinted, by permission, from J. Bergstrom et al., 1967, "Diet, muscle glycogen and physical performance," *Acta Physiologica Scandinavica* 71:140.

totally replenished their muscle glycogen in two days. This result shows that protein and fat aren't stored as muscle glycogen and that carbohydrate is important for replacing depleted glycogen stores.

Carbohydrate Loading for Endurance Exercise

If you are preparing for an endurance event that lasts more than 90 minutes—a competitive marathon, triathlon, cross-country ski race, or long-distance bike race—you should saturate your muscles with carbohydrate. Although carbohydrate loading sounds simple (just stuff yourself with pasta, right?), the truth is that many endurance athletes make food mistakes that hurt their performance. Here is my nine-step carbohydrate-loading plan to help all endurance athletes fuel optimally for their events.

   1. **Carbohydrate load daily.** Your daily diet should be carbohydrate based and balanced with adequate protein and healthful fat. A daily carbohydrate intake of about 3 to 5 grams of carbohydrate per pound of body weight (6 to 10 g per kg) prevents chronic glycogen depletion and allows you to not only train at your best but also compete at your best. Divide your target grams of carbohydrate into three parts of the day: breakfast plus snack (7:00 a.m. to 12:00 p.m.), lunch plus snack (12:00 p.m. to 5:00 p.m.), and dinner plus snack (5:00 p.m. to 10:00 p.m.).

Your weight	Total g carb/day	Target g carb/5 hours
100 lb (45 kg)	300 to 500	100 to 175
125 lb (57 kg)	375 to 625	125 to 210
150 lb (68 kg)	450 to 750	150 to 250
175 lb (79 kg)	525 to 875	175 to 290

   The philosophy that "if some carbohydrate is good, then more will be better" does not hold true for carbohydrate loading. If you eat too much, you will likely experience intestinal distress, and your muscles will be no better fueled than if you'd eaten an adequate amount (Rauch et al. 1995). As one marathoner said after stuffing herself the night before her first marathon, "I felt heavy and bloated . . . not the way I wanted to feel at the start of the race."

   2. **Taper your training.** Forget any plans for last-minute training sprees. Do your final hard training three weeks before race day, and start

tapering your training at least two weeks out. Although hard training builds you up, it also tears you down, and you need time to heal any damage that occurred during training and to completely refuel with carbohydrate. Some exercise scientists suggest reducing your exercise time to 30 percent of normal, doing little exercise in the last 7 to 10 days before the event other than some short, intense speed intervals to keep you sharp (Houmard et al. 1990).

Correct tapering requires tremendous mental discipline and control. Most athletes are afraid to taper for such a long time. They are afraid they will get out of shape because they are exercising less. Worry not. The proof will come when you perform better—perhaps 9 percent better. Swimmers, for example, maximized their performance when they tapered for two

Rapid Loading

Some athletes prefer not to taper their exercise for two to three weeks before an endurance event; they are barely willing to take off one day for rest. To satisfy the needs of these intense athletes, researchers developed the following rapid-load program (Fairchild et al. 2002):

1. One day before the event, the subjects cycled very hard (130 percent $\dot{V}O_2max$) on stationary bikes for two and a half minutes, and then in the last half minute they did an all-out effort to total exhaustion and depletion of muscle glycogen.

2. As soon as tolerable, they started to consume a very high carbohydrate diet, targeting about 5 grams of carbohydrate per pound (10 g per kg) of body weight, eaten over the course of the day. This means that an athlete who weighed 150 pounds (68 kg) needed to eat about 750 grams of carbohydrate, which is the equivalent of 3,000 calories of carbohydrate. Because they were filling up on so much carbohydrate, they had little room for fat or protein in that day's diet (only 10 percent of total calories, as opposed to a standard day with 45 percent of calories from protein and fat).

3. Throughout the day they rested and consumed carbohydrate-loading beverages, juices, gels, and other forms of carbohydrate-dense products. By resting, the athletes gave their muscles the opportunity to superload using the abundance of carbohydrate that flooded the system. The athletes were able to achieve levels of glycogen as high as those reached by athletes who carbohydrate loaded for three to six days.

If this rapid-load protocol sounds enticing to you, be sure to practice it before the event. The drastic change in diet may lead to intestinal problems. And the intense exercise before the event may leave you tired.

weeks (Costill et al. 1985). Research suggests that a 10- to 13-day taper can be better than a 7-day taper (Zarkadas, Carter, and Banister 1994).

Because you will be exercising less during the preevent taper, you do not need to eat hundreds of additional calories when carbohydrate loading. Simply maintain your standard intake (this should be about 3 to 5 g of carbohydrate per pound of body weight, or 6 to 10 g per kg). The 600 to 1,000 or so calories that you generally burn during training will be used to give your muscles extra fuel. By saving the calories that you otherwise would have burned during training, you can approximately double your glycogen stores and will be able to exercise harder during the third hour of your event (Rauch et al. 1995).

You'll know you have carbohydrate loaded properly if you gain 2 to 4 pounds (1 to 2 kg) of water weight. With each ounce (30 g) of stored glycogen, you store about 3 ounces (90 ml) of water. This water becomes available during exercise and reduces dehydration.

3. Eat enough protein. Because endurance athletes burn some protein for energy, they should take special care to eat two small servings every day of protein-rich foods in addition to getting protein from two or three dairy servings. Even when carbohydrate loading, your diet should include about 0.6 to 0.7 gram of protein per pound (1.3 to 1.6 g per kilogram) of body weight.

4. Do not fat load. To reduce your fat intake to 20 to 25 percent of your calories, choose toast with jam rather than with butter, pancakes moistened with maple syrup rather than with margarine, and pasta with tomato sauce rather than with oil and cheese. A little fat is OK, but don't fat load.

To achieve a carbohydrate-based diet with about 4 grams of carbohydrate per pound (600 g of carbohydrate for a 150 lb person, or 2,400 calories of carbohydrate), you need to trade some of the fat calories to make room for more carbohydrate. For example, trade the fat calories in two pats of butter and a dollop of sour cream for a second plain baked potato. When you trade fat for more carbohydrate, you need to eat a larger volume of food to obtain adequate calories. A 1-pound (500 g) box of spaghetti cooks into a mountain of pasta but provides only 1,600 calories. That's a reasonable calorie goal for a hefty premarathon meal, but it may be more volume than anticipated. See table 6.2 for a sample carbohydrate-loading menu.

5. Choose fiber-rich foods. Fiber-rich foods promote regular bowel movements and keep your system running smoothly. Bran cereal, whole-wheat bread, oatmeal, fruits, and vegetables are some good choices. If you carbohydrate load on too much white bread, pasta, rice, and other refined products, you're likely to become constipated, particularly if you are doing less training. Yet the day before an event, some athletes (who

Table 6.2   Sample Carbohydrate-Loading Menu

The following high-carbohydrate diet provides about 4.5 grams of carbohydrate per pound (9 grams per kilogram) of body weight for a 150-pound (68 kilogram) marathoner. The menu includes adequate protein (0.8 grams per pound, or 1.8 grams per kilogram) to maintain muscles.

Food	Calories	Carbohydrate (g)
Breakfast	**800**	**152**
Oatmeal, 1 cup dry, cooked in	300	55
Milk, 1%, 16 oz (480 ml)	200	25
Raisins, 1/4 cup	130	30
Brown sugar, 1 1/2 tbsp	50	12
Apple juice, 8 oz (240 ml)	120	30
Lunch	**980**	**155**
Sub sandwich roll, 6 in. (4 oz)	320	60
Lean meat, 4 oz (125 g)	200	–
Fruit yogurt, 8 oz (230 g)	240	40
Grape juice, 12 oz (360 ml)	220	55
Snack	**480**	**103**
Fig Newtons, 6	330	65
Jelly beans, 15 large	150	38
Dinner	**940**	**188**
Spaghetti, 2 cups cooked	400	80
Spaghetti sauce, 1 cup (240 ml)	250	40
Italian bread, 2 slices	150	30
Root beer, 12 oz (360 ml)	140	38
Snack	**200**	**48**
Canned peaches in syrup, 1 cup	200	48
Total	**3,400**	**646 g**

do not worry about constipation) prefer to eat very low fiber diets so that they have less intestinal fullness. They carbohydrate load on pretzels, juices, gelatin, sherbet, white breads, rice, and pasta. Through trial and error, you'll learn what works for your body. If you are worried about diarrhea, avoid fiber-rich foods before an event.

   6. **Plan meal times carefully.** NYC Marathon queen Grete Waitz once said she never ate a very big meal the night before a marathon because it usually would give her trouble the next day. She preferred to eat a bigger lunch. You, too, might find that pattern works well for your intestinal tract. That is, instead of relying on a huge pasta dinner the night before

the event, you might want to enjoy a substantial carbohydrate fest at breakfast or lunch. This earlier meal allows plenty of time for the food to move through your system—and reduces the stress of fretting about portable toilets. Plus, you also might sleep better. And if you are a traveling athlete, you'll be able to more easily get a table at a restaurant that might be overcrowded at dinner time.

You can also carbohydrate load two days before if you will be too nervous to eat much the day before the event. (The glycogen stays in your muscles until you exercise.) Then graze on crackers, chicken noodle soup, and other easily tolerated foods the day before your competition.

You'll be better off eating a little bit too much than too little the day before the event, but don't overfeed yourself. Learning the right balance takes practice. Each long training session leading up to the endurance event offers the opportunity to learn which food—and how much of it—to eat. You need to train your intestinal tract as well as your heart, lungs, and muscles. Remember to practice your preevent carbohydrate-loading meal during training so you'll have no surprises on the day of the event.

7. Drink extra fluids. To reduce your risk of starting the event dehydrated, be sure to drink extra water and juice. Abstain from too much wine, beer, and alcoholic beverages; they are not only poor sources of carbohydrate but also dehydrating. Drink enough alcohol-free beverages to produce a significant volume of urine every two to four hours. The urine should be pale yellow, like lemonade. Don't bother to overhydrate; your body is like a sponge and can absorb only so much fluid.

On the morning of competition, drink another two or three glasses of water up to two hours before the event (to allow plenty of time to excrete the excess) and then another cup or two 5 to 10 minutes before race time. See chapters 8 and 10 for more information about proper hydration tactics.

8. Be sensible about your selections. Do not carbohydrate load on fruit only; you're likely to get diarrhea. Do not carbohydrate load on refined white bread products only; you will likely become constipated. Do not carbohydrate load on beer; you'll become dehydrated. Do not do too much last-minute training; you'll fatigue your muscles. And do not blow it all by eating unfamiliar foods that might upset your system. Change your exercise program more than your diet.

9. Eat breakfast on event day. Carbohydrate loading is just part of the fueling plan. Eating enough breakfast before the endurance event is very important; it will prevent hunger and help maintain normal blood sugar level. Equally important is choosing food you're familiar with. As I mentioned before, you should determine which foods in what amounts work best for you long before the day of your event.

Don't try any new foods. That festive pancake breakfast may settle like Mississippi mud, and so may the unfamiliar energy bar you've been saving for the occasion. See chapters 8, 9, and 10 for more information about preexercise fueling, as well as fueling during the event. With wise eating, you can enjoy miles of smiles.

Against the Grain: Carbohydrate Loading Without Pasta

Not every athlete can carbohydrate load on pasta, breads, and cereals. About 1 in 133 people has celiac disease, a disorder in which the body can't tolerate gluten, a protein found in wheat, rye, barley, and sometimes oats (if the oats get contaminated with wheat during processing). In these people, gluten triggers intestinal inflammation and eventually can interfere with the absorption of nutrients, including iron and calcium. Gluten intolerance easily leads to anemia (if iron is not absorbed) and osteoporosis (if calcium is not absorbed).

Celiac disease can be difficult to diagnose because the symptoms vary from person to person. Some people experience diarrhea; others complain about constipation and bloating. Your best bet is to talk with your doctor if you are having intestinal problems or have other niggling health concerns including unexplained fatigue, infertility, and lactose intolerance.

For athletes, fueling without gluten can be a challenge. You can still carbohydrate load, however, on rice, corn, potatoes, yams, chickpeas, bananas, fruits, vegetables, juices, and numerous other sources of carbohydrate. To help you with your gluten-free diet, I highly recommend that you meet with a local sports dietitian and read *Gluten-Free Diet: A Comprehensive Resource Guide* (2006) by Shelley Case, RD. See appendix A for more information sources.

Bonking

Whereas depleted muscle glycogen causes athletes to hit the wall, depleted liver glycogen causes them to bonk, or crash. Liver glycogen feeds into the bloodstream to maintain a normal blood sugar level essential for "brain food." Despite adequate muscle glycogen, an athlete may feel uncoordinated, light-headed, unable to concentrate, and weakened because the liver is releasing inadequate sugar into the bloodstream.

You already know that your muscles and brain require glucose for energy. What you may not be aware of is that although the muscles can store glucose and burn fat, the brain does neither. This means that for the brain to function optimally, you must consume food close enough to strenuous events to supply sugar into the blood so the brain has fuel. Athletes with low blood sugar tend to perform poorly because the poorly fueled brain limits muscular function and mental drive. They also tend to be grumpy, be easily irritated, and have less fun.

Carbohydrate for Building Muscles?

"I know runners should eat carbohydrate to fuel their muscles. But what about weightlifters? Shouldn't I eat a lot of protein to build up my muscles?" Perhaps, like Steve, a 34-year-old salesman who lifts weights to bulk up, you are confused about what to eat for energy, strength, and top performance—carbohydrate or protein. This is what I recommend:

- Eat carbohydrate-rich breakfasts, such as oatmeal, rather than eggs.
- Focus your lunches and dinners on whole-grain breads, potatoes, brown rice, fruits, and vegetables. Wholesome forms of carbohydrate should cover two-thirds of your plate.
- Eat fish, chicken, lean meats, low-fat cheeses, and other forms of protein as an accompaniment to lunch and dinner, not as the focus. Alternatively, you could eat carbohydrate-rich plant sources of protein such as beans and rice, lentil soup, chili, hummus, and other vegetarian choices.

Carbohydrate is fundamental for both runners and bodybuilders, because unlike protein or fat, carbohydrate is needed to fuel muscle-building exercise. Adequate protein is also important, but you should dedicate only one-third of your dinner plate to protein-rich foods. To optimally perform the strength training for building muscles, bodybuilders need a carbohydrate-rich diet. Research suggests that three sets of biceps curls (8 to 10 repetitions per set) reduce muscle glycogen by 35 percent (Martin, Armstrong, and Rodriquez 2005). With repeated days of low carbohydrate and high repetitions, the muscles of bodybuilders can soon become depleted.

Gianni, a 28-year-old runner and banker, faithfully carbohydrate loaded his muscles for three days before his first Boston Marathon. On the evening before the marathon, he ate dinner at 5:00 and then went to bed at 8:30 to assure himself a good night's rest. But, as often happens with anxious athletes, he tossed and turned all night (which burned a significant amount of calories). Gianni got up early the next morning and chose not to eat breakfast, even though the marathon didn't start until 10:30. By that time, he had depleted his limited liver glycogen stores. He lost his mental drive about 8 miles (13 km) into the race and quit at 12 miles (19 km). His muscles were well fueled, but energy was unavailable to his brain, so he lacked the mental stamina to endure the marathon.

Gianni could have prevented this needless fatigue by eating some oatmeal, cereal, or other form of carbohydrate at breakfast to refuel his liver glycogen stores. Athletic success depends on both well-fueled muscles and a well-fueled mind.

Recovery From Daily Training

Carbohydrate is important on a daily basis for those who train hard day after day and want to maintain high energy. If you habitually eat a low-carbohydrate diet, your muscles will feel chronically fatigued. You'll train, but not at your best.

Figure 6.2 illustrates the glycogen depletion that can occur when athletes eat an inadequate amount of carbohydrate and still try to exercise hard day after day (Costill et al. 1971). In this landmark study, on three consecutive days the subjects ran hard for 10 miles (16 km) at a pace of 6 to 8 minutes per mile. They ate their standard meals: a diet that provided about 45 to 50 percent of calories from carbohydrate, not the 55 to 65 percent required in a top-performance sports diet. The subjects' muscles became increasingly glycogen depleted. Had the runners eaten larger portions of carbohydrate (and smaller portions of protein and fat), they would have better replaced their glycogen stores and better invested in top performance.

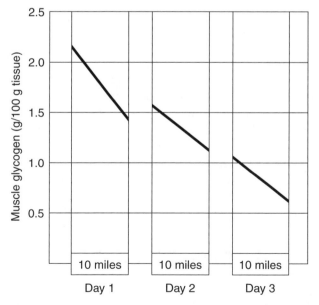

Figure 6.2 A proper diet is needed to prevent the cumulative effects of glycogen depletion.

Adapted from D.L. Costill et al., 1971, "Muscle glycogen utilization during prolonged exercise on successive days," *Journal of Applied Physiology* 31(6): 836. Used with permission.

This study emphasizes the need not only for a daily carbohydrate-rich diet but also for recovery days with light or no training. If you are doing daily hard workouts, take heed: Your depleted muscles need at least one day, if not two, to refuel after exhaustive sessions. (If you are a casual exerciser who uses significantly less glycogen during, let's say, a half-hour walk or a gentle swim, recovery days are less essential.)

Maria, a 28-year-old nurse practitioner and dedicated exerciser, learned the importance of recovery days and adequate carbohydrate through a sports nutrition experiment. When she first came to see me, she insisted on training every day to get in shape for her first marathon. I recommended that she take one or two days off a week.

Maria decided to experiment with her two-hour Sunday run to determine if her running improved with running less and eating better. She discovered she could train at her best when she did little or no training the day before her long run (to rest her muscles), followed by a day off after her long run (to refuel). She stopped forcing herself to do the obligatory daily training run any day when her muscles felt fatigued. Instead, she planned at least one or two rest days per week and started focusing on *quality* training rather than *quantity* training. Her running improved, as did her mental outlook and enthusiasm for her sport. She ran a personal best in the marathon, cutting seven minutes off her time.

Many athletes hesitate to exercise less because they are afraid of getting out of shape. If this sounds like you, remember that rest will enhance, not hurt, your performance. You won't lose fitness but rather will enhance your strength and endurance with better-fueled muscles. Athletes who underestimate the value of rest and instead train relentlessly set the stage for injuries, chronic glycogen depletion, chronic fatigue, and reduced performance. These athletes often hope that vitamin supplements, special sports foods, and other pills and potions will boost their energy. All they really need to perform better is less exercise.

If you are severely overtrained, you may need weeks, if not months, to recover. One study with swimmers showed that a two-and-a-half-week taper was inadequate for recovery from the staleness acquired during a six-month season (Hooper et al. 1995). Don't underestimate the value of rest.

Carbohydrate-Rich Foods

All too often, I talk with athletes who think they eat a carbohydrate-rich diet when they really don't. Eric, a 33-year-old store manager and triathlete, intended to carbohydrate load the night before his first triathlon. Because of inadequate nutrition knowledge, he "carbohydrate loaded" with a pepperoni pizza with double cheese. Little did he know that of the 1,800 calories in the pizza, 1,200 were from the protein and fat in the double cheese and pepperoni. Only 35 percent of the calories, from the thin crust and tomato sauce, were from carbohydrate (160 g). No wonder he felt sluggish during the event. I gave Eric a list of carbohydrate in common foods (see table 6.3) to post on his refrigerator. With this tool he learned to select high-carbohydrate foods.

In addition, I taught Eric how to make better selections based on the nutrition-facts panel on food labels. You, too, can use labels to guide your selections. The nutrition-facts panel lists the number of grams of carbohydrate, protein, and fat (and alcohol if present) per serving. The panel also lists, as I have listed here, the calories per gram:

$$1 \text{ g carbohydrate} = 4 \text{ calories}$$

$$1 \text{ g protein} = 4 \text{ calories}$$

$$1 \text{ g fat} = 9 \text{ calories}$$

$$1 \text{ g alcohol} = 7 \text{ calories}$$

Using this information, you can make some simple calculations. To determine the number of carbohydrate calories in a food item, multiply the number of grams of carbohydrate by four (calories per gram). Next, compare the carbohydrate calories to the total calories per serving to determine the percentage of calories that are from carbohydrate. For example, a half-cup serving of a gourmet vanilla ice cream might have 200 total calories and 20 grams of carbohydrate.

$$20 \text{ g carb} \times 4 \text{ cal/g} = 80 \text{ cal carb}$$

$$80 \text{ cal carb} / 200 \text{ total cal} = 40\% \text{ carb}$$

Using food-label information, you can determine that ice cream contains relatively fewer grams of carbohydrate than frozen yogurt does. For example, for every 100 calories of vanilla ice cream (two spoonfuls), you get only 10 grams of carbohydrate. This is equal to 40 calories of carbohydrate, which is 40 percent of total calories. On the other hand, for every 100 calories of frozen yogurt (four spoonfuls), you get about 22 grams of carbohydrate. This is roughly 88 calories of carbohydrate and 88 percent of total calories.

Your diet should provide carbohydrate as the foundation of each meal—about 3 to 5 grams of carbohydrate per pound (6 to 10 g per kg) for endurance athletes and 2 to 3 grams (1 to 1.5 g per kg) for fitness exercisers (ACSM, ADA, and Dietitians of Canada 2000). For example, a 160-pound (73 kg) endurance athlete should consume 480 to 800 grams, or about 60 percent of a 3,200- to 5,300-calorie diet—a range of fuel appropriate for an active person of that weight. (Note that this

Table 6.3 Carbohydrate in Common Foods

Food	Amount	Carbohydrate (g)	Total calories
Fruits			
Raisins	1/3 cup	40	150
Banana	1 medium	25	105
Apricots, dried	10 halves	20	85
Apple, dried	1 medium	20	80
Orange	1 medium	15	65
Vegetables			
Spaghetti sauce, Prego	1/2 cup	22	120
Corn, canned	1/2 cup	15	70
Winter squash	1/2 cup	15	60
Peas	1/2 cup	10	60
Carrot	1 medium	10	40
Green beans	1/2 cup	5	20
Broccoli	1/2 cup	5	20
Zucchini	1/2 cup	2	10
Bread-type foods			
Hoagie roll	1	75	400
Bagel, Thomas'	1	54	300
Pita	1 average (3 oz)	46	240
Tortilla	1 large (2.5 oz)	36	220
English muffin	1	25	120
Bread, rye	1 slice	15	80
Waffle, Eggo	1	14	90
Saltine crackers	5	10	60
Graham crackers	2 squares	10	70
Breakfast cereals			
Grape-Nuts	1/2 cup	48	210
Raisin Bran, Kellogg's	1 cup	45	190
Granola, low fat	1/2 cup	40	190
Oatmeal, maple instant	1 packet	33	160
Cheerios	1 cup	20	100
Beverages			
Cola	12 oz (360 ml)	39	155
Apricot nectar	8 oz (240 ml)	35	140
Cran-raspberry juice	8 oz (240 ml)	35	140
Apple juice	8 oz (240 ml)	30	120
Orange juice	8 oz (240 ml)	25	105
Milk, chocolate	8 oz (240 ml)	25	180
Gatorade	8 oz (240 ml)	14	50
Beer	12 oz (360 ml)	13	145
Milk, 2%	8 oz (240 ml)	12	120

Food	Amount	Carbohydrate (g)	Total calories
Grains, pasta, starches			
Baked potato	1 large	50	220
Baked beans	1 cup	50	260
Rice, cooked	1 cup	45	200
Lentils, cooked	1 cup	40	230
Stuffing, bread	1 cup	40	340
Spaghetti, cooked	1 cup	40	200
Ramen noodles	1/2 package	25	190
Entrees, convenience foods			
Macaroni and cheese, Kraft	1 cup	47	390
Bean burrito, frozen	5 oz (150 g)	45	350
Spaghettios	1 cup	37	180
Lentil soup, Progresso	12 oz (350 ml)	33	210
Refried beans, canned	1 cup	31	180
Sweets, snacks, desserts			
Frozen yogurt	1 cup	44	240
Pop-Tart, blueberry	1	36	220
Fruit yogurt, Dannon	6 oz (175 g)	26	150
Honey	1 tbsp	15	60
Cranberry sauce	2 tbsp	14	60
Maple syrup	1 tbsp	13	50
Strawberry jam	1 tbsp	13	50
Fig Newton	1	11	55
Oreo	1	8	50

Nutrient data from food labels and J. Pennington, 1998, *Bowes & Church's Food Values of Portions Commonly Used*, 17th ed. (Philadelphia: Lippincott).

method of calculating carbohydrate needs works best for active athletes with high calorie needs, not for sedentary people.) Although you need not get obsessed about counting grams of carbohydrate (unless that is of interest), you do want to choose more starches and grains and fewer fatty or greasy foods. Replace muffins with bagels, granola with muesli, and Alfredo sauce with tomato sauce on pasta.

Learning about the composition of your training diet is important. The Internet offers several options for calculating grams of carbohydrate, and this can be easier than gathering the information from food labels. Many of my clients are shocked at how easily fat creeps into their diets. For example, Pedro, a health-conscious fitness exerciser, simply indulged in too many helpings of peanuts, almonds, and sunflower seeds, his favorite snacks. By trading them in for higher-carbohydrate items—baked pita chips, raisins, dried apricots, and bananas—he easily boosted his carbohydrate intake. "You know, my training has improved since I made that switch. My muscles feel springier, and I have greater endurance. I feel great. I'm glad I learned this simple solution to my needless fatigue." He soon learned he could compete better because he was able to train better.

CHAPTER 7

Protein to Build and Repair Muscles

Traditionally, protein-rich foods have been synonymous with muscular athletes. The (misguided) theory is that if you eat a lot of protein, you will build a lot of muscle. The truth is that heavy weightlifting, push-ups, and other forms of resistance exercise—not excess protein—build and strengthen muscles. If you consume more protein than you need, you will simply burn more protein as a fuel source (Bolster et al. 2005).

Confusion exists about the best diet for building muscles. When you work out in the weight room at the gym, you likely hear you need to consume lots of chicken breasts and egg whites and drink protein shakes between meals to be stronger. But when you hang around in the cardio area, you hear that carbohydrate-rich pasta, cereal, and grains should be the foundation of your meals. And you are left wondering, what's the right balance?

Carbohydrate-rich grains, fruits, and vegetables are indeed the best foundation for every type of training program. Even bodybuilders need a carbohydrate-based diet because carbohydrate is stored in the muscles for energy. You can't lift weights and demand a lot from your workout sessions if your muscles are carbohydrate depleted. Protein-based diets low in carbohydrate provide inadequate muscle fuel for you to exercise hard enough to build to your potential.

The best sports diet contains adequate, but not excessive, protein to build and repair muscle tissue, grow hair and fingernails, produce hormones, boost your immune system, and replace red blood cells. Most people who eat moderate portions of protein-rich foods daily get more protein than they need. Any excess protein is burned for energy or, as a last resort, stored as glycogen or fat. Humans do not store excess protein as muscle, protein, or amino acids, so we need to consume adequate protein each day. Daily protein is particularly important for dieters who are restricting calories, because protein is burned for energy when carbohydrate and calories are scarce.

When it comes to protein intake, athletes seem to fall into two categories. First are those who eat too much—the bodybuilders, weightlifters, and football players who can't seem to get enough of the stuff. Those in the second group eat too little—the runners, dancers, and weight-conscious athletes who never touch meat and trade most protein calories for more salads and vegetables. Individuals in either group can perform poorly because of dietary imbalances.

Josh, for example, was a protein pusher. A college hockey player, he routinely snacked after practice on a big protein bar and a protein shake. That one snack satisfied more than half his protein needs for the whole day. As an athlete, he has a slightly higher protein need than a sedentary person, but he overcompensated for that need with the generous servings of chicken and fish he devoured at meals, never mind his high-protein snack.

Paulo, a vegetarian marathon runner who ate spaghetti with tomato sauce seven nights a week, downplayed his need for protein. "Most Americans get way too much protein; I'm sure I get plenty, too." He consumed few protein-rich foods of any types—plant or animal products. He was humbled when he learned that his food intake was deficient not only in protein but also in iron (for red blood cells), zinc (for healing), calcium (for bones), and several other nutrients. No wonder he became anemic, suffered a lingering cold and flu, and performed poorly despite consistent training.

Defining Protein Needs

Research has yet to define the exact protein requirements of sports-active people because individual needs vary. People in the following groups have the highest protein needs:

- **Endurance athletes and others doing intense exercise.** About 5 percent of energy can come from protein during endurance exercise, particularly if muscle glycogen stores are depleted and blood glucose is low.

- **Dieters consuming too few calories.** The protein is converted into glucose and burned for energy instead of being used to build and repair muscles.
- **Growing teenage athletes.** Protein is essential for both growth and muscular development.
- **Untrained people starting an exercise program.** They need extra protein to build muscles.

In scrutinizing the protein needs of athletes, exercise scientists have found that athletes need slightly more protein than other people do to repair the small amounts of muscle damage that occur with training, to provide energy (in very small amounts) for exercise, and to support the building of new muscle tissue.

In general, pinpointing exact protein requirements is almost a moot point because many athletes eat more protein than they require just through standard meals. That is, a 150-pound (68 kg) recreational athlete who burns 3,000 calories can easily consume 300 to 450 protein calories, or 75 to 112 grams of protein. This equates to 0.5 to 0.7 gram of protein per pound (1 to 1.5 g of protein per kg), which is more than the RDA of 0.4 gram per pound (0.8 g per kg).

Table 7.1 provides safe and adequate recommendations for protein intake for a range of individuals. These recommendations include a margin of safety and are not minimal amounts. If you are overfat, base your protein needs on your ideal body weight.

In contrast to the belief that a little more protein is good so a lot more will be better, no scientific evidence to date suggests that protein intakes exceeding 0.9 gram of protein per pound (2.0 g per kg) will provide an additional advantage (Lemon 1995). Nor is there evidence that taking a protein supplement on top of an adequate diet (with about 0.5 g of protein per pound, or 1 g per kg) will enhance muscle strength or size (Godard, Williamson, and Trappe 2002). And don't fret about how the protein is packaged—as whey powder, chicken, egg whites, or chocolate milk; all protein can build muscles. The advantage of getting protein from natural foods (as opposed to supplements) is that natural foods contain protein the way nature intended as well as yet-unknown bioactive compounds that might influence muscle growth.

The physiques of bodybuilders are not attributable to the excessively high protein diet they commonly consume but rather to their intense training. Bodybuilders work incredibly hard. They prefer a high-protein diet because protein not only builds and protects their muscles but also keeps them from feeling hungry when they are cutting calories—lean protein is harder to overconsume.

Table 7.1 Protein Recommendations

Type of individual	Grams of protein per body weight pound	Grams of protein per body weight kilogram
Sedentary adult	0.4	0.8
Recreational exerciser, adult	0.5-0.7	1.0-1.5
Endurance athlete, adult	0.6-0.7	1.2-1.6
Growing teenage athlete	0.7-0.9	1.5-2.0
Adult building muscle mass	0.7-0.8	1.5-1.7
Athlete restricting calories	0.8-0.9	1.8-2.0
Estimated upper requirement for adults	0.9	2.0
Average protein intake of male endurance athletes	0.5-0.9	1.1-2.0
Average protein intake of female endurance athletes	0.5-0.8	1.1-1.8

Data compiled from American College of Sports Medicine, American Dietetic Association, and Dietitians of Canada Joint Position Statement. Nutrition and Athletic Performance. *Medicine and Science in Sports and Exercise* 32 (12): 2130-2145, 2000; R. Maughan and L. Burke, editors. *Sports Nutrition* (part of the Handbook of Sports Medicine and Science series, an IOC Medical Commission Publication) Malden, MA: Blackwell Publishing, 2002; Institute of Medicine. *Dietary Reference Intakes for Energy, Carbohydrate, Fiber, Fat, Fatty Acids, Cholesterol, Protein and Amino Acids.* Food and Nutrition Board, Washington, DC: National Academy Press, 2002.

Your Protein Needs

To learn if you are meeting your protein needs in your current diet, follow two easy steps. First, using table 7.1, identify which category you belong to. For example, if you are a 140-pound (64 kg) bike racer, you would fit the category of an "endurance athlete, adult" and would need about 85 to 100 grams of protein per day:

$$140 \text{ lb} \times 0.6 \text{ g/lb} = 84 \text{ g protein}$$
$$140 \text{ lb} \times 0.7 \text{ g/lb} = 98 \text{ g protein}$$

Second, keep track of your protein intake by listing everything you eat and drink for one 24-hour period. The information on food labels provides protein information, and table 7.2 lists the amount of protein in some common foods. You can also use a variety of Web sites (see Dietary Analysis in appendix A) to analyze your diet and assess your protein intake. Note that you need to eat a generous portion (more calories) of beans and other forms of plant protein to equal the protein in animal foods. Most fruits and vegetables have only small amounts of protein, which may contribute a total of 5 to 10 grams of protein per day, depending on

Table 7.2 Protein in Common Foods

Animal sources	Grams of protein per standard serving	Grams of protein per 100 cal (amount)
Egg white	3.5 / 1 large egg	20 / 6 egg whites
Egg	6 / 1 large egg	8 / 1.3 eggs
Cheddar cheese	7 / 1 oz (30 g)	6 / 0.9 oz (27 g)
Milk, 1%	8 / 8 oz (240 ml)	8 / 8 oz (240 ml)
Yogurt	11 / 1 cup	8 / 6 oz (175 g)
Cottage cheese	15 / 1/2 cup	15 / 1/2 cup
Haddock	27 / 4 oz (125 g) cooked	21 / 3 oz (90 g)
Hamburger	30 / 4 oz (125 g) broiled	10 / 1.5 oz (45 g)
Pork loin	30 / 4 oz (125 g) roasted	10 / 1.5 oz (45 g)
Chicken breast	35 / 4 oz (125 g) roasted	18 / 2 oz (60 g)
Tuna	40 / 6 oz (175 g)	20 / 3 oz (90 g)
Plant sources	Grams of protein per standard serving	Grams of protein per 100 cal (amount)
Almonds, dried	3 / 12 nuts	3.5 / 14 nuts
Peanut butter	4.5 / 1 tbsp	4.5 / 1 tbsp
Kidney beans	6 / 1/2 cup	6 / 1/2 cup
Hummus	6 / 1/2 cup	3 / 1/4 cup
Gardenburger (original)	6 / 2.5 oz (75 g) patty	6 / 2.5 oz (75 g) patty
Refried beans	7 / 1/2 cup	7 / 1/2 cup
Lentil soup	11 / 10.5 oz (315 ml)	6.5 / 6 oz (175 ml)
Tofu, extra firm	11 /3.5 oz (110 g)	12 / 4 oz (125 g)
Baked beans	14 / 1 cup	7 / 1/2 cup
Boca burger	13 / 2.5 oz (75 g) patty	13 / 2.5 oz (75 g) patty

Data from food labels and J. Pennington, 1998, *Bowes & Church's Food Values of Portions Commonly Used*, 17th ed. (Philadelphia: Lippincott) and food labels.

how much you eat. Butter, margarine, oil, sugar, soda, alcohol, and coffee contain no protein, and most desserts contain very little.

An easier way to assess whether you are getting adequate, but not excessive, protein in your daily diet is to use this rule of thumb: Consume daily 16 ounces (2 cups, or 480 ml) of milk or yogurt plus a moderate serving of protein-rich foods at two meals a day. This, along with the small amounts of protein in grains and vegetables, will likely fulfill your daily protein requirement. Here's a sample of one day's worth of protein-rich foods for an active 150-pound (68 kg) adult. Of course, you'll need to eat other foods to round out your calorie and nutrition requirements, and those foods will offer a little more protein, as well.

Breakfast	1 cup milk on cereal
Lunch	2 oz (60 g) sandwich filling (tuna, roast beef, turkey), 1 cup yogurt
Dinner	4 oz (125 g) meat, fish, poultry, or the equivalent in lentils or other beans and legumes

Growing teenagers and novice bodybuilders with high protein needs can get additional protein and calcium by drinking another 2 cups of milk. If you think you need supplements that advertise better "protein digestibility" and "bioavailability," think again. In an overall well-balanced diet, engineered protein offers no advantages over standard protein-rich foods. As long as you are healthy and have a functioning digestive tract (as opposed to patients in the hospital with intestinal disease), you need not worry about your ability to digest or utilize protein. Digestibility and bioavailability are an issue in developing countries where protein and calorie intakes are inadequate and every amino acid counts—but not in the more developed countries, where protein and calorie excesses are more common than deficiencies. (Adequate calories are needed in order to spare protein from being burned for fuel.)

Note that you have a daily need for protein. Some people eat protein-rich foods only once or twice per week and live on salads and pasta for most of their meals. They cheat themselves of an optimal training diet.

Too Much Protein

Contrary to what most people think, too much protein can create problems with health and performance. Jasper, an aspiring bodybuilder, chowed down on chicken and beef yet avoided pasta and potatoes, much to the detriment of his athletic aspirations. He tired easily and asked me if this high-protein diet might be hurting his performance. Here's what I told him:

- If you fill your stomach with too much protein, you won't be fueling your muscles with carbohydrate.
- Protein breaks down into urea, a waste product eliminated in the urine. Anyone who eats excess protein should drink extra fluids. Frequent trips to the bathroom may be an inconvenience during training and competition.
- A diet based on animal protein takes its toll on both your wallet and the environment. You can save money and the environment by eating smaller portions of beef, lamb, pork, and other forms

of animal protein. Use that money to buy more sources of plant protein (beans, lentils, tofu) and more fruits, vegetables, grains, and potatoes.

- A diet high in protein can easily be high in fat (juicy steaks, bacon and fried eggs, pepperoni pizza, and so on). For the sake of your heart and for improved athletic performance, you should reduce your intake of the saturated fat found in animal protein. This kind of diet may also reduce your risk of certain cancers.

I encouraged Jasper to reduce his meat portions at dinner to one-third of his plate and to fill two-thirds with potatoes, vegetables, and whole-grain bread. Within two days, he noticed an improvement in his energy level. He then changed his breakfast from a four-egg ham and cheese omelet to cereal and a banana, and lunch became chili or pasta rather than burgers. His diet gradually became a winner. "I'm amazed," he now says, "at the power of food. Eating carbohydrate-based foods that fuel my muscles definitely enhances my sports performance!"

Healthful and Convenient Meat Choices

"I rarely eat meat except when I go home to visit my family," commented Christina, a college student who lived off campus and was responsible for her own food. "I like meat, but it's expensive and seems to spoil before I get around to cooking it for dinner." She cooked mostly pasta and consequently wondered if she consumed too little protein.

If you, like Christina, think you eat too little protein and its accompanying nutrients iron and zinc, and you are willing to eat animal protein, eating a small amount of lean red meat two to four times per week can enhance the quality of your sports diet. Here are some tips to keep in mind for health-promoting, low-fat meat eatery:

- Take advantage of the deli. For precooked meats, buy rotisserie chicken or slices of lean roast beef, ham, and turkey in the deli section at the grocery store.
- Buy extra-lean cuts of beef, pork, and lamb to reduce your intake of saturated fat. Forgo cuts with a marbled appearance, and trim the fat off steaks and chops before cooking them.
- Get rid of more fat. After browning ground beef, drain it in a colander and rinse it with hot water to remove the fat before adding it to spaghetti sauce.
- At a cafeteria, request two rolls when you order one hamburger. Use one roll to absorb the grease. Eat the second roll with the degreased burger, and throw the greasy roll away.

- Integrate meat into a meal as an accompaniment. Add a little extra-lean hamburger to spaghetti sauce, stir-fry a small piece of steak with lots of veggies, serve a pile of rice along with one lean pork chop, make a savory potato-rich stew with a little lean lamb, or buy deli roast beef for sandwiches made on hearty bread.

Protein and the Vegetarian

Many active people choose not to eat animal protein. Some just eat no red meat; others eat no chicken, fish, eggs, or dairy foods. They may think that animal protein is hard to digest, bad for the health, unethical to eat, or harmful to the environment. Whatever their reason for abstaining, they often overlook the fact that they still need to eat adequate protein to maintain good health. And a balanced vegetarian diet is indeed a good investment in good health.

The trick to eating a balanced vegetarian diet is to make the effort to replace meat with beans. If you eliminate meat, you need to add a source of plant protein. You can easily get adequate protein to support your sports program by including kidney beans, chickpeas, peanut butter, tofu, nuts, and other forms of plant protein in your daily diet. Some non-meat-eaters, however, simply fuel up only on carbohydrate and neglect their protein needs.

Peter, a 150-pound (68 kg) runner, is a typical example of an athlete with a protein-deficient diet. He consumed only 0.3 gram of protein per pound (0.7 g per kg), or half the recommended intake for athletes. A typical day of eating for Peter looked something like this:

Food	Protein (g)*	Calories
Breakfast		
1 large bagel	4	400
2 cups orange juice	2	220
Lunch		
2 large bananas	3	300
12 oz (360 ml) tropical fruit drink	—	240
1 large bagel	4	400
Dinner		
3 cups cooked pasta	20	660
1 cup tomato sauce	2	100
16 oz (480 ml) sweetened iced tea	—	200
Snack		
1 cup dried fruit	5	480
Total	**40**	**3,000**

*Recommended protein intake: 90 to 135 grams of protein (0.6 to 0.9 gram of protein per pound of body weight, depending on calorie intake)

To improve his protein intake, he simply needed to add peanut butter to the bagel, replace the fruit drink with yogurt, add beans or tofu to the spaghetti at dinnertime, and mix in some nuts with the dried fruit for a snack. All these changes were easy to make; Peter just had to be more responsible with balancing his diet. Yes, he could have added some protein shakes and bars to boost his protein intake, but real food offers a more complete nutrition package that includes all the health-enhancing compounds, some of which we may not even know about.

Female Vegetarians and Amenorrhea

Female athletes commonly choose to eat a meatless diet. They may refer to themselves as vegetarians, but many fit into the non-meat-eater category. That is, they eat too much fruit, too many salads, and sometimes abundant jellybeans—but too little beans, tofu, yogurt, or plant sources of protein. This protein deficiency, in conjunction with an overall calorie-deficient diet, is associated with medical problems, specifically loss of regular menstrual cycles.

Some athletic women, in their obsession to lose weight, consume a very low-calorie and low-protein "vegetarian" diet. This drastic restriction of food intake can lead to amenorrhea; that is, they stop having regular menstrual periods. Research suggests that amenorrheic athletes have a two to four times higher risk for suffering a stress fracture than do regularly menstruating athletes (Clark, Nelson, and Evans 1988; Nattiv 2000; ACSM 2007). Eating a balanced diet with adequate calories can enhance resumption of menses, provide adequate protein for building and protecting muscles, and enhance overall health. (See chapter 16 for more information on amenorrhea.)

Jessica, now a healthy gymnast, used to live on melon for breakfast, a salad for lunch, and steamed vegetables with brown rice for dinner. Once or twice a week, she'd sprinkle a few garbanzo beans on a salad or add some soy cheese to the vegetables. She thought her vegetarian diet was great, when in fact it was deficient in several nutrients. At one point she suffered a stress fracture that healed very slowly. She had spindly arms and legs with tiny muscles (despite her exercise program), and her menstrual period was absent, a sign of a malfunctioning body.

Jessica needed to understand that a well-balanced sports diet includes adequate protein—either small portions of lean beef, pork, and lamb or generous portions of tofu, beans, and nuts. (Because plant protein is less concentrated than animal protein, you must eat larger portions to get the same amount of protein.) Dark meats are also important sources of two minerals—iron and zinc.

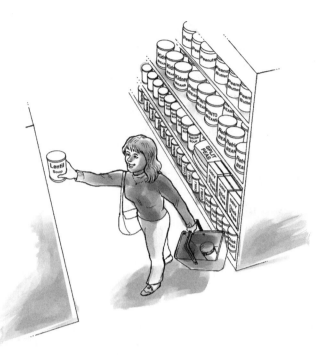

Iron and Zinc Requirements

Iron is a necessary component of hemoglobin, the protein that transports oxygen from the lungs to the working muscles. If you are iron deficient, you are likely to fatigue easily upon exertion. The recommended iron intake for men is 8 milligrams, for women 18 milligrams until menopause, and for women thereafter 8 milligrams. This target iron intake is set high because only a small percentage is absorbed. See table 7.3 for the iron content of some foods. The best iron sources are animal products and fish; the body absorbs far less iron from plant foods.

Athletes with the highest risk of developing iron-deficiency anemia include the following:

- Female athletes who lose iron through menstrual bleeding
- Vegetarians who do not eat red meat (the best dietary source of iron) or iron-enriched breakfast cereals
- Marathon runners who may damage red blood cells by pounding their feet on the ground during training
- Endurance athletes who may lose iron through heavy sweat losses.
- Teenage athletes, particularly girls, who are growing quickly and may consume inadequate iron to meet expanded requirements

Table 7.3 Iron and Zinc in Food

Foods	Iron (mg)	Zinc (mg)
Animal sources*		
Alaskan king crab, 4 oz (125 g)	1	9
Beef, 4 oz (125 g) top round	3	6
Chicken thigh, 4 oz (125 g)	1.5	3
Egg, 1 large	1	0.5
Haddock, 4 oz (125 g)	1	0.5
Oysters, 6 medium raw	5	75(!)
Pork loin, 4 oz (125 g)	1	3
Shrimp, 12 large	2	1
Swordfish, 4 oz (125 g)	1	2
Tuna, 3 oz (90 g) light canned	1	1
Turkey, 4 oz (125 g) breast	2	2
Fruit and juice		
Apricots, 5 halves dried	0.8	0.2
Dates, 10 dried	1	0.2
Prune juice, 8 oz (240 ml)	3	0.5
Raisins, 1/3 cup	1	0.1
Vegetables and legumes**		
Broccoli, 1/2 cup	0.5	0.3
Peas, 1/2 cup	1	1
Refried beans, 1 cup	4	3
Spinach, 1/2 cup cooked	3	1
Soy sources		
Boca Burger, original vegan	1	13
Edamame, 1/2 cup	1	0
Gardenburger, original	1	5
Soy nuts, 1/4 cup	1	2
Tofu, 3 oz (90 g) firm	1	2
Dairy		
Cheddar cheese, 1 oz (30 g)	0.2	1.0
Nonfat milk, 1 cup (240 ml)	0.1	1.0
Grains		
Bread, 1 slice enriched	1	0.2
Brown rice, 1 cup cooked	1	1.2
Raisin Bran, Kellogg's, 1 cup	4.5	1.5
Cereal, Total, 3/4 cup	18	15
Cream of Wheat, 1 cup cooked	9	trace
Pasta, 1 cup cooked, enriched	2	1
Wheat germ, 1/4 cup	2	1.5
Other		
Molasses, 1 tbsp blackstrap	3.5	0.2

*Animal sources of iron and zinc are absorbed best (except for iron from eggs).
**Vegetable sources of iron and zinc are poorly absorbed.
Nutrient data from food labels and J. Pennington, 1998, *Bowes & Church's Food Values of Portions Commonly Used*, 17th ed. (Philadelphia: Lippincott).

Even marginal iron deficiency (found in about 12 percent of women in the United States) can hurt athletic performance. Hence, you want to eat iron-rich foods each day. Apart from taking a multi-vitamin and mineral pill with iron, you can boost your iron intake in several easy ways:

- If you eat meat, consume lean cuts of beef, lamb, pork, and the dark meat of skinless chicken or turkey three or four times per week.

- Select breads and cereals with the words *iron enriched* or *fortified* on the label. This added iron replaces that lost in processing or supplements the small amount that naturally occurs in grains. Eat these foods with a source of vitamin C (e.g., orange juice with cereal, tomato on a sandwich), which may enhance iron absorption. Note: Cereals that are all natural or organic are not fortified with iron or zinc. Mix them with fortified or enriched cereals to boost the iron content of your breakfast.

- Use cast-iron skillets for cooking. These vessels offer more nutritional value than do stainless-steel cookware. The iron content of spaghetti sauce simmered in a cast-iron skillet for three hours may increase from 3 to 88 milligrams per half cup (120 ml).

- Don't drink coffee or tea with every meal, particularly if you are prone to being anemic. Substances in these beverages can interfere with iron absorption. Drinking them an hour before a meal is better than drinking them afterward.

- Combine poorly absorbed vegetable sources of iron (nonheme iron, 10 percent absorption rate) with animal sources (heme iron, 40 percent absorption rate) if you eat meat. For example, eat broccoli with beef, spinach with chicken, chili with lean hamburger, and lentil soup with turkey.

To identify if your fatigue is caused by iron deficiency, you must get your blood tested for not only hemoglobin and hematocrit (the standard tests for anemia) but also serum ferritin. Ferritin measures the iron stores in your body; you want a level of 20 micrograms per deciliter (μg/dl) or higher. If the stores are low, you may be pre-anemic; this can hurt performance (Burke 2007). If you are diagnosed with iron-deficiency anemia, you will need to take iron supplements, typically in the form of ferrous sulfate or ferrous gluconate. You may need about four months of supplementation to resolve the problem.

However, you should not take iron supplements unless recommended by your physician, because too much iron can be linked to heart disease. About 1 in 250 people has a genetic condition that makes him or her susceptible to iron overload. Men and postmenopausal women are most susceptible because they have relatively low iron requirements. The best way to identify iron overload is by having a blood test for serum ferritin, to measure the amount of iron stored in your body. A level of 200 micrograms or higher signals danger.

In addition to iron, your body needs zinc. This mineral is part of more than 100 enzymes that help your body function properly. For example, zinc helps remove carbon dioxide from your muscles when you exercise. Zinc also enhances the healing process. Because the zinc from animal protein is absorbed better than zinc from plants, vegetarian athletes are at risk of eating a zinc-deficient diet.

The recommended intake for zinc is 8 milligrams for women and 11 milligrams for men (see table 7.3 for foods that provide zinc). Like the target for iron, this target is also set high and may be hard to consume. But athletes who sweat heavily and incur zinc losses through sweat should try to hit the target intake.

The Balanced Vegetarian Diet

Without question, a diet based on plant foods can contribute to good health. A plant-based diet tends to have more fiber, less saturated fat and cholesterol, and more phytochemicals—active compounds that are health protective. Foods rich in phytochemicals include not only fruits and vegetables but also the protein-rich foods common to a plant-based diet: nuts, legumes, dried beans, and peas.

But some vegetarians (who for health reasons choose to not eat red meat) often turn to cheese for protein. They thrive on cheese-filled omelets, cheesy lasagna, salads frosted with shredded cheese, and slices of whole-grain bread bubbling with melted cheese. They are unaware, though, that cheese has far more saturated fat than lean meats and that eating a cheese sandwich is, in that respect, worse for your health than a lean roast-beef sandwich without mayonnaise. As I have mentioned before, lean meat, eaten in small portions as the accompaniment to lots of carbohydrate, is not the health culprit it is deemed to be.

Tofu (soybean curd) and other soy products, such as soy burgers and soy milk, are excellent healthful additions to a meat-free diet. They contain a source of high-quality protein that is similar in value to animal protein. Note that a soyburger has less protein than a hamburger, however.

If you want to omit animal protein from your diet, or if you already do, you are making a potentially healthful lifestyle change. The trick is to choose a balanced vegetarian diet and choose enough vegetable protein to satisfy your protein requirements. Doing this can be easier for a man who is eating 3,000 or more calories than for a woman dieter who eats half that amount.

Protein and Amino Acids

The need for protein is actually a need for amino acids. All proteins are made up of amino acids that your body needs to build tissue, hence their nickname "building blocks." There are 21 of these amino acids, and every protein in your body is made up of some combination of them. Your body can make some amino acids itself, but 8 of them (9 for children), called the essential amino acids, must come from the foods you eat.

Taking extra amino acids, such as large doses of ornithine or arginine, will not make your muscles bigger or stronger. To date, no scientific evidence indicates that individual amino acids have a bodybuilding effect. Your body needs all the essential amino acids to make new muscles. Natural food provides the proper balance of all the amino acids, works well, tastes better, and costs less than amino acid supplements. Standard foods, along with regular exercise, can help you achieve your athletic goals.

Lisa, a vegetarian dieter who would spend an hour a day working out at the gym, thought she was eating adequate protein when she included a tablespoon of peanut butter (only 4 g of protein) on a slice of whole-wheat toast for breakfast, a half-cup of hummus (6 g of protein) in a wrap at lunch, and one-quarter cake of tofu (only 9 g of protein) at dinner. These 19 grams of protein fell far short of the daily 50 to 70 grams of protein she needed. No wonder she wasn't building muscle the way she wanted.

When Lisa recognized that her diet was deficient in plant protein, she traded in calories from the protein-poor wrap, pasta, and fruits for more calories from higher-protein nuts and beans. This boosted her intake of the amino acids she needed to build muscles. She had better workouts and felt better overall. I noticed a visible change in her facial complexion—from splotchy and grayish to clearer with rosy cheeks.

Milk, other dairy foods, fish, poultry, meat, and all animal sources of protein contain all the essential amino acids and are often referred to as complete proteins. The protein in soy foods such as tofu, tempeh, and soy milk are also complete proteins. The protein in rice, beans, pasta, lentils, nuts, fruits, vegetables, and other plant foods are incomplete because they have low levels of some of the essential amino acids. Therefore, vegetarians must know how to combine incomplete proteins to make them complete. Vegetarians who drink milk can easily do this by adding dairy to each meal, such as by combining milk with oatmeal or sprinkling grated low-fat cheese on beans.

Vegans (strict vegetarians who eat no dairy, eggs, or animal protein) need to choose complementary vegetable protein that is high in the particular limiting amino acid. One key is to eat a variety of foods to optimize the intake of a variety of amino acids. The following combinations work well together and can be consumed over the course of the day:

- **Grains plus beans or legumes,** such as rice and beans; bread and split-pea soup; tofu and brown rice; cornbread and chili with kidney beans
- **Legumes plus seeds,** such as chickpeas and tahini (as in hummus); tofu and sesame seeds

Non-vegans can choose to add milk products to any meal to boost the protein value, such as cereal and milk, pasta and cheese, or bread and cheese.

By following these guidelines, vegetarian athletes can consume an adequate amount of complete proteins every day. Note that although most vegetarians can get the right amount of protein, they may lack iron and zinc, minerals found primarily in meats and other animal products. Vegans, who eat only plant foods, also need to be sure they get adequate riboflavin, calcium, vitamin B_{12}, and vitamin D, either through a supplement or from carefully selected food sources.

Protein Powders, Shakes, and Bars

Sometimes power athletes forget that food can supply all the protein and amino acids needed to build muscles. These athletes are easily swayed by the powerful advertisements in bodybuilding magazines and start to believe that protein supplements are essential for optimal muscle development. While training in the power gyms, they hear enticing conversations about products with tantalizing names such as Russian Bear and Muscle Milk. The protein-praising bodybuilders who come to me for advice often lug gym bags bulging with assorted powders and potions. They wonder if these supplements are better than the protein in standard food, if they are worth the price, and if they work. Some are avid believers in the stuff, and others are skeptical.

Bulking up is a matter of dedicating yourself to extra exercise and extra calories, not to extra supplements. The protein or amino acids in supplements are no more effective than protein in ordinary foods. If you are struggling to develop bigger muscles, change your body image, and improve your strength, chapter 14 addresses how to gain weight healthfully. This section addresses the role of protein in the gaining process. Heed the following tips:

- **Exercise, not extra protein, is the key to developing bigger muscles.** In theory, if you want to gain 1 pound (0.5 kg) of muscle per week, you need only 14 extra grams of protein per day, the amount in 2 ounces of meat—a mere forkful (Benardot 1992). By eating a small amount of protein in your preexercise snack (milk with cereal, yogurt with granola, half a turkey sandwich), you can optimize the muscle-building process (Rasmussen et al. 2000).

- **Beware of extra fat.** If you are currently eating large amounts of protein-rich foods such as cheese omelets, fried chicken, and cheeseburgers, you may be consuming an excessive amount of calories from saturated fat, which can easily become stored as body fat, not as bulging biceps.

- **Expensive muscle-building supplements are not the answer.** The amount of protein in these formulas is often less than what you might easily get through foods, but costs two to four times as much (see the following chart). In addition, real foods provide a balanced package of vitamins, minerals, and other nutrients that are often missing in engineered food.

Protein source	Cost*	Protein (g)	Cost/g protein
Met-Rx Big 100 Bar	$2.98	26	11.5¢
PowerBar ProteinPlus	$2.19	23	9.5¢
Clif Builder's Bar	$1.89	20	9.5¢
Tuna, 6 oz can white	$1.79	40	4.5¢
Tuna, 6 oz can light	$1.19	32	4.0¢
Nonfat milk, 1 qt	$1.30	32	4.0¢
Nonfat milk, 1/2 gallon	$2.50	64	4.0¢
Nonfat milk, 1 gallon	$4.29	128	3.5¢
Peanut butter, 2 tbsp	$0.15	8	2.0¢

*Prices in Boston July 2007.

Few athletes need to spend money on protein supplements. Even vegetarians can get enough protein through foods. But sometimes, with high school and collegiate athletes, as well as triathletes and others doing double workouts, the need for calories can outweigh the ability to easily consume them because of lack of appetite or time. And at other times, a supplement is just more convenient. But for the most part, I recommend commercial protein supplements in only a few medical situations, such as for malnourished patients with AIDS or cancer.

Protein supplements are also helpful for my clients with anorexia who claim to be vegetarian (a politically correct way of eliminating yet another source of calories from their diets) but commonly are just fat-phobic non-meat-eaters. For example, one "vegetarian" student refuses to eat animal products and also dislikes tofu and beans. Her only acceptable source of protein is a fat-free protein supplement. This case contrasts with the 160-pound (73 kg) protein fanatic who eats a six-egg-white omelet for breakfast, two cans of tuna for lunch, and two chicken breasts for dinner and drinks nonfat milk by the quart, totaling more than 190 grams of high-quality protein. And he wonders how many protein shakes and bars he needs for in-between meals. He needs more carbohydrate for optimal muscle fueling, not more protein.

Questions Bodybuilders Ask

For years, bodybuilders have fed themselves a traditional diet based on egg whites, chicken breasts, canned tuna, and protein shakes. Historically, we've had inadequate science to debate those rigid dietary rules. But today, exercise physiologists are intently researching the best ways to build muscles—without steroids, that is. In particular, they are examining the role of nutrient timing—the impact of when and what you eat in relation to resistance exercise. Rather than focusing on eating large amounts of protein, I recommend paying more attention to when you eat it. Eating small amounts at the right times offers results.

If you are strength trained and in calorie balance, consuming 0.7 to 0.8 gram of protein per pound of body weight per day (1.6 to 1.8 g per kg) is more than sufficient. Given that most athletes eat in excess of the current recommendations, consuming enough protein is generally a moot point, unless you are restricting calories to lose weight. For detailed information on nutrition for bodybuilding, I recommend the book *Nutrient Timing* by exercise physiologists John Ivy and Robert Poortman.

Q: **What should I eat before I lift weights?**

A: By eating carbohydrate before exercise, you'll provide fuel for a stronger workout (even just 5 to 10 minutes beforehand offers benefits). By eating a little protein along with the carbohydrate, you'll start to digest the protein into amino acids, which get used by the muscles during and after exercise. Good choices for a preexercise snack include fruit yogurt, low-fat chocolate milk, cereal with milk, a poached egg with toast, and soy milk and an energy bar.

Q: **I've heard I should eat as soon as I finish lifting weights, but I'm not feeling hungry then. Why is immediate refueling so important?**

A: After a hard gym workout, your muscles are primed for getting broken down: Their glycogen (carbohydrate) stores are reduced, cortisol and other hormones that break down muscle are high, the muscle damage that occurred during exercise causes inflammation, and the amino acid glutamine that provides fuel for the immune system is diminished. If you just guzzle some water after your workout and dash to work, you'll miss the 45-minute postexercise window of opportunity to optimally nourish, repair, and build muscles. You can switch out of the muscle breakdown mode by eating a carbohydrate–protein combination as soon as tolerable after you exercise.

Q: **My friend who is into bodybuilding tells me I need to eat protein every three to four hours. Is that true?**

A: If you want to get the most benefits from your workout, yes. Just as eating protein before and after exercise optimizes muscle development, so does eating protein throughout the day. When the amino acid levels in the blood are above normal, the muscles take up more of these building blocks; this enhances muscle growth. Thus, eating several protein-containing meals and snacks is preferable to eating one big dinner at the end of the day. But don't get overzealous. I've had more than one client wake up every three hours during the night to consume a protein drink. The body does have a pool of amino acids to draw from, so such extreme measures are not necessary.

Q: **Why are protein supplements so popular? Are they better than real foods?**

A: In today's fast-food society, a mindless way to get healthful (no cholesterol, low fat) protein is through supplements. Plus, the label tells you exactly how much protein you are eating and takes away the guesswork. But protein supplements are not a whole food and fail to offer the complete package of health-protective nutrients found in natural foods. Use them to supplement wise eating, if desired, but not to replace it.

Q: **What's all the hype about whey protein?**

A: Whey makes up 20 percent of the protein found in milk; casein makes up the other 80 percent. The two are separated during cheese making. (Remember Little Miss Muffet who sat on her tuffet, eating her curds and whey?) Whey used to be discarded, but today it is made into whey powder and used in a variety of protein supplements.

Whey is digested and absorbed into the bloodstream faster than other forms of protein such as casein. Whey and casein are rich sources of the branched-chain amino acids (BCAAs) leucine, iso-leucine, and valine. BCAAs are taken up directly by the muscles instead of having to be first metabolized by the liver. Hence, whey is "fast acting" and a good source of raw materials for protecting muscles from getting broken down during exercise and for build-ing muscles after exercise.

So does this mean everyone who wants to build muscle needs to rush out to buy whey protein powder? No. Casein supplies a longer-lasting and sustained source of amino acids, and it's also important in the muscle-building process (Tipton et al. 2004). Additionally, whey protein powder can be expensive. The 20 grams of protein in 16 ounces (480 ml) of protein-fortified skim milk offers 1.9 grams of the branched-chain amino acid leucine at $0.40 per gram, and a serving of Met-Rx Ultramyosyn Whey Powder offers 2.1 grams of leucine for a 50 percent higher price of $0.62 per gram.

Milk and powdered milk are good alternatives that offer protein the way nature intended, as well as possible bioactive growth-promoting compounds that are yet to be discovered. Milk offers both rapid and extended protein activity in the body. And remem-ber, whey powders are often void of the carbohydrate needed to refuel muscles. Chocolate milk has been shown to be a popular and effective recovery food (Karp et al. 2006).

If you are a casual exerciser, you need not get obsessed about the type of protein in each meal. People of all ages and athletic abilities have been building muscles for centuries with standard food. If you are an aspiring champion who wants every possible edge, you may want to experiment with protein supplements to see if you achieve any benefits. Does short-term stimulation of muscle growth result in long-term advantages? That has yet to be determined. We do know that muscles have a maximum size that is influenced by genetics.

CHAPTER 8

Replacing Sweat Losses

During hard exercise, your muscles can generate 20 times more heat than when you are at rest. You dissipate that heat by sweating. As the sweat evaporates, it cools the skin. This in turn cools the blood, which cools the inner body. If you did not sweat, you could cook yourself to death. A body temperature higher than 106 degrees Fahrenheit (41 degrees Celsius) damages the cells. At 107.6 degrees Fahrenheit (42 degrees Celsius), cell protein coagulates (as egg whites do when they cook), and the cell dies. This is one serious reason why you shouldn't push yourself beyond your limits in very hot weather.

Some people sweat a lot. For example, James had to put a towel under the exercise bike to mop the sweat that dripped from his body. Although it was a source of embarrassment, I reminded James that sweating is good. It's the body's way of dissipating heat and maintaining a constant internal temperature (98.6 degrees Fahrenheit; 37 degrees Celsius).

James, like many men, produced more sweat than he needed to cool himself. He'd sweat large drops of water, which dripped off his skin rather than evaporate, resulting in a reduced cooling effect. In comparison, women tend to sweat more efficiently than men. But both men and women need to be equally diligent about replacing sweat losses.

James wondered how much he needed to drink to replace his sweat loss. I suggested he learn his sweat rate by weighing himself nude before and after an hour of exercise. For every pound (16 oz, or 0.5 kg) he lost, he needed to drink about 80 to 100 percent of that loss (13 to 16 oz, or 400 to 480 ml) while exercising; this would require training his gut to handle this volume. I also suggested he figure out how many gulps of water equated to 16 ounces (480 ml).

By knowing his sweat rate (4 lb [almost 2 kg], or 64 oz, per hour), he was able to practice "programmed drinking" during exercise in order to minimize sweat losses. James started to drink 16 ounces (16 gulps; half of a 32 oz, or 1 qt, water bottle) every 15 minutes; this matched his thirst and more than doubled what he had previously consumed. His programmed drinking required having the right quantity of enjoyable fluids (chilled, palatable) readily available and even setting an alarm wristwatch to remind him to drink on schedule. He felt so much better after his workout that the extra effort was worthwhile.

Thirst, as defined by a conscious awareness of the desire for water and other fluids, usually controls water intake. The sensation of thirst is triggered when body fluid concentrations are abnormally high. When you sweat, you lose significant amounts of water from your blood. The remaining blood becomes more concentrated and has, for example, an abnormally high sodium level. This triggers the thirst mechanism and increases your desire to drink. To quench your thirst, you need to replace the water losses and bring the blood back to its normal concentration.

Unfortunately for athletes, this thirst mechanism can be an unreliable signal to drink. Thirst can be blunted by exercise or overridden by the mind. Hence, you should plan to drink before you are thirsty. By the time your brain signals thirst, you may have lost 1 percent of your body weight, which is the equivalent of 1.5 pounds (3 cups, or 24 ounces) of sweat for a 150-pound (68 kg) person. This 1 percent loss corresponds with the need for your heart to beat an additional three to five times per minute (Casa et al. 2000). A 2 percent loss fits the definition of *dehydrated*. A 3 percent loss can significantly impair aerobic performance (Coyle and Montain 1992). Remember, you will voluntarily replace only two-thirds of sweat losses. To be safe, drink enough to quench your thirst, perhaps a little more—but stop drinking if your stomach is sloshing. Enough is enough!

Young children, in particular, have a poorly developed thirst mechanism. At the end of a hot day, children often become very irritable, which may be partially due to dehydration. If you are going to spend the day with children at a place where fluids are not readily available, such as at the beach or a baseball game, bring a cooler stocked with lemonade, juice, and ice water, and schedule frequent fluid breaks to increase everyone's enjoyment of the whole day.

Senior citizens also tend to be less sensitive to thirst sensations than are younger adults. Research with active, healthy men aged 67 to 75 years shows that they were less thirsty and voluntarily drank less water when water deprived for 24 hours compared with similarly deprived younger men aged 20 to 31 years (Phillips et al. 1984). In another study, older hikers became progressively dehydrated during 10 days of strenuous hill walking. The younger hikers remained adequately hydrated (Ainslie et al. 2002). Athletic seniors who participate in any sports should monitor their fluid intake.

Fluid Physiology 101

To help you understand the importance of balancing fluids correctly in your sports diet, here are some of the key points from the American College of Sports Medicine's position stand on exercise and fluid replacement (ACSM 2007).

Fluid and Electrolyte Requirements

Fluid needs vary greatly from person to person, so it's hard to make a one-size-fits-all recommendation. Sweat rates commonly range between 1 and 4 pounds (0.5 to 2 quarts, or 480 ml to 2 L) per hour, depending on your sport, body size, intensity of exercise, and clothing; the weather conditions (hot or cold); whether or not you are heat acclimatized; and how well trained you are. Sweat rates for a 110-pound (50 kg) slow runner might be 1 pound (16 oz, or 480 ml) of sweat per hour, while a 200-pound (91 kg) fast runner might lose about 4 pounds (2 qt, or 2 L) per hour. Even fast swimmers sweat—almost a pound per hour of training. Football players wearing full equipment in the summer heat might lose more than 16 pounds (2 gal, or 8 L) of sweat in a day.

On a daily basis, the simplest way to tell if you are adequately replacing sweat loss is to check the color and quantity of your urine. If your urine is very dark and scanty, it is concentrated with metabolic wastes, and you need to drink more fluids or eat more foods with a high water content such as cooked oatmeal, yogurt, and fruit. (Most people get 20 to 30 percent of their fluids from foods; some people actually eat all their daily water requirement.) When your urine is pale yellow, your body has returned to its normal water balance. Your urine may be dark if you are taking vitamin supplements; in that case, volume is a better indicator than color. For specific colors, search the Web for "urine color chart."

In addition to monitoring urine and weight loss, you should also pay attention to how you feel. If you feel chronically fatigued, headachy, or lethargic, you may be chronically dehydrated. This is most likely to happen during long hot spells in the summertime. Dehydration can be cumulative.

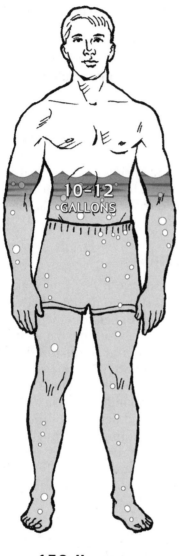

150 lb man

Water and You

Water...

◊ in blood transports glucose, oxygen, and fats to working muscles and carries away metabolic by-products such as carbon dioxide and lactic acid.

◊ in urine eliminates metabolic waste products. The darker the urine, the more concentrated the wastes.

◊ in sweat dissipates heat through the skin. During exercise water absorbs heat from your muscles, dissipates it through sweat, and regulates body temperature.

◊ in saliva and gastric secretions helps digest food.

◊ throughout the body lubricates joints and cushions organs and tissues.

Sweat contains more than just water; it has electrically charged particles that help keep water in the right balance inside and outside of cells. The amount of electrolytes you lose via your sweat depends on how much you sweat, your genetics, your diet, and how well you are acclimatized. The following chart shows the electrolyte loss that can occur with sweating.

Electrolyte	Average amount/2 lb (1 L, ~1 qt) sweat	Food comparison
Sodium	800 mg (range 200-1,600)	1 qt Gatorade = 440 mg sodium
Potassium	200 mg (range 120-600)	1 med banana = 450 mg potassium
Calcium	20 mg (range 6-40)	8 oz (230 g) yogurt = 300 mg calcium
Magnesium	10 mg (range 2-18)	2 tbsp peanut butter = 50 mg magnesium

Muscle cramps are believed to be associated with dehydration, electrolyte deficits, and muscle fatigue. If you sweat profusely, are left caked with salt, and experience cramps, take extra care to drink plenty of sodium-containing fluids while exercising. If your diet has a high salt content, you can likely replace sodium losses after exercise with standard postexercise meals. But consuming extra salt on your food if you had high sweat losses can be a smart way to enhance recovery, retain fluid, and stimulate thirst.

Dehydration and Performance

Dehydration stresses the body: Body temperature rises, your heart beats faster, you burn more glycogen, your brain has trouble concentrating, and exercise feels harder. Some athletes are more tolerant of dehydration than are others, but for the most part, the more dehydrated you are, the greater the strain.

Whereas fitness exercisers (who work out for 30 to 60 minutes at a moderate pace three or four times a week) can easily maintain water balance if they are eating and drinking normally, athletes who exercise hard day after day can become chronically dehydrated if they fail to fully rehydrate daily. Football players in full uniform might lose far more fluids than they would think to consume. Having sweat-loss data eliminates the guesswork.

To determine if you are drinking enough to replace sweat losses and maintain normal water balance during days of repeated hard exercise, you should weigh yourself nude each day in the morning, after emptying your bladder and bowels. Your weight should remain stable, assuming the following:

- You are not restricting calories to lose fat weight.
- You have not eaten abnormally high amounts of sodium the night before, such as a water-retaining Chinese dinner.
- You are not experiencing 2 to 4 pounds (1 to 2 kg) of premenstrual bloat.

Most athletes who lose greater than 2 percent of their body weight in sweat losses lose both their mental edge and their physical ability to perform well, especially if the weather is hot. Yet during cold weather, you are less likely to experience reduced performance even at 3 percent dehydration. That is, runners feel less impact of dehydration on performance during cold winter runs as compared to the same run in the summer heat. Dehydration of 3 to 5 percent does not seem to affect either muscle strength or short intense bursts of anaerobic performance, such as weightlifting. Yet, sweat loss of 9 to 12 percent body weight can lead to death. Some warning signs of heat illness include muscle cramps, nausea, vomiting, headache, dizziness, confusion, disorientation, weakness, reduced performance, inability to concentrate, and irrational behavior.

Fluids Before Exercise

The goal of drinking before you exercise is to start exercising when your body is in water balance, not in deficit from the previous exercise session. You might need 8 to 12 hours to rehydrate. The prehydration goal is to drink about 2 or 3 milliliters per pound (5 to 7 ml per kg) of body weight at least 4 hours before the exercise task. For a 150-pound (68 kg) athlete, this comes to 300 to 450 milliliters, or about 10 to 15 ounces of fluid. (One ounce is about 30 ml.) By hydrating several hours preexercise, you have time to eliminate the excess before starting the exercise event.

If you drink a beverage with sodium (110 to 275 mg of sodium per 8 oz) or eat a few salty snacks or sodium-containing meals, the sodium will stimulate your thirst so that you drink more; the sodium also helps retain the fluid so it doesn't go in one end and out the other. There's no need to try to hyperhydrate. As I mentioned before, the body can absorb just so much fluid—and you will end up needing to urinate during the event. Overhydrating can also dilute your blood sodium; if you then continue to aggressively drink fluids during exercise, you can increase your risk of developing hyponatremia (see page 155).

If you like a preexercise caffeine boost to enhance your performance, rest assured that caffeine (in moderate doses—12 ounces coffee, or about 200 mg of caffeine) is unlikely to increase your daily urine output or cause you to become dehydrated. Enjoy it, if desired.

Fluids During Exercise

The goal of drinking during exercise is to prevent excessive dehydration, as defined by more than 2 percent body weight loss from a water deficit. If you are exercising hard enough to risk becoming dehydrated, you should drink periodically during exercise. If you will be exercising for more than three hours, you really should know your sweat rate to prevent the performance decline associated with small cumulative mismatches between how much fluid you need versus how much fluid you are losing via sweat. Because few athletes actually make the effort to learn their sweat rates, a starting point is to drink as desired, according to thirst.

What should you drink during exercise? The recommended fluid replacer contains a little sodium to stimulate thirst, a little potassium to help replace sweat losses, and a little carbohydrate (sugar) to provide energy. More precisely, the drink should contain 110 to 170 milligrams of sodium per 8 ounces (20 to 30 milliequivalents (mEq) sodium/L); 20 to 50 milligrams of potassium per 8 ounces (2 to 5 mEq potassium/L); and about 12 to 24 grams of carbohydrate per 8 ounces (in a 5 to 10 percent sugar solution, for 50 to 95 calories) (ACSM 2007). You can consume these nutrients via standard foods such as pretzels and bananas as well as engineered foods (see chapter 11), which can be more convenient for runners, triathletes, and other endurance athletes.

When you are exercising hard for more than an hour (or doing less intense, longer exercise), consuming 120 to 240 calories of carbohydrate (30 to 60 g) per hour along with your water can help you perform better. Carbohydrate helps maintain normal blood glucose levels so you are able to enjoy sustained energy. Sports drinks are an easy way to get carbohydrate plus water. For example, 16 ounces (480 ml) of Gatorade offers 25 grams of carbohydrate and 100 calories; 16 ounces of Powerade offers 35 grams of carbohydrate and 140 calories. Practice drinking appropriate amounts of fluid during training to help you adapt to the fluid load and prevent stomach sloshing and discomfort during competition.

Fluids After Exercise

After you exercise, your goal is to fully replace any fluid and electrolyte deficit. How aggressively you rehydrate depends on how quickly you need to recover before your next exercise session and how big a fluid–electrolyte deficit you incurred. Most active people can recover with normal meals (that contain a little sodium) and plain water. If you are significantly dehydrated and need to exercise again within 12 hours, then you need to be more aggressive with your rehydration program and sprinkle extra salt on your food if you had high sodium losses through sweat.

Drinking 50 percent more fluid than you lost in sweat will enhance rapid and complete recovery from dehydration. (The extra fluid accounts for what gets lost via urine.) Sipping fluids over time maximizes fluid retention and is preferable to drinking large amounts in one sitting. If you become dehydrated during an unusually long and strenuous bout of exercise, you should drink frequently for the next day or two. Your body may need 24 to 48 hours to replace the sweat losses.

What to Look for in Your Sports Beverage

Numerous niche sports beverages are fighting for shelf space wherever fluids are sold. With so many options to choose from, you might wonder what to look for in a sports drink. Here's a brief summary:

The Basics

- Good taste. If you like the flavor, you'll drink more and be less likely to become dehydrated.
- Carbohydrate. Look for beverages with about 50 to 70 calories of carbohydrate (13 to 18 g of carbohydrate per 8 oz, or 240 ml). Too much carbohydrate slows absorption; too little leaves you lagging in energy. For long, hard, intense exercise, such as bike racing or marathon running, carbohydrate from a variety of sources (glucose, fructose, and sucrose—or dried fruit, bagels, and gummy bears) might be better absorbed and offer an energy advantage.
- Sodium. Important for maintaining fluid balance, sodium stimulates thirst and enhances fluid retention. If you have significant sweat losses, the sodium found in sports drinks helps replace some of the sodium lost in sweat.

Add-Ins With Questionable Value

- Vitamins. The vitamins in sports drinks are not incorporated quickly enough during exercise to be of any benefit.
- Ginseng, guarana, and other herbs. There are only minimal data to support any claimed benefits and probably too little of the substances in the water to make any difference.
- Caffeine. Because of individual responses, caffeine might enhance endurance or cause side effects of anxiety, jitters, and irritability.
- Protein. The addition of protein may alter the taste (less desirable) and slow gastric emptying. More research is needed to determine if protein in a sports drink (more so than just the additional calories when protein is added to a carbohydrate drink) offers a performance benefit during exercise (Saunders, Kane, and Todd 2004). The benefit noticed after exercise is reduced muscle soreness. You can get this same benefit by eating protein before exercise (let's say, by having a preexercise snack of cereal with skim milk) if you prefer to not consume protein during exercise.
- Potassium, calcium, magnesium, and other minerals. In most cases, too little of these minerals is lost in sweat to create problems. The minerals can be easily replenished with fruits, vegetables, and wholesome foods.

What You May Not Want

- Carbonation. Bubbles can make you bloated and fill you up sooner.
- Plastic bottles. They litter the environment if not recycled. How about having just one bottle that you refill daily?

If you become more than 7 percent dehydrated (either by sweat losses, diarrhea, or vomiting), you will likely end up requiring intravenous fluid replacement under a doctor's care. In most cases, there is no advantage to taking fluids by IV, unless for medical necessity. Your best bet is to stay out of the medical tent in the first place by knowing your sweat rate and drinking accordingly.

Hyponatremia and Sodium Loss

There's no need to try to superhydrate preexercise; your body can absorb just so much fluid. The kidneys regulate water balance by adjusting urine output—from a minimum of about a tablespoon to a maximum of about 1 quart (1 L) per hour. If you overdrink, you then may need to (inconveniently) urinate during exercise. A wise tactic is to drink up two or more hours before exercise; this allows time for your kidneys to process and eliminate the excess. Then drink again 5 to 15 minutes preexercise.

For the most part, frequent trips to the bathroom simply inconvenience people who drink too much water. But in some cases, drinking too much water can actually be lethal if it dilutes body fluids and creates a sodium imbalance. A condition known as hyponatremia occurs when blood sodium levels become abnormally low. In general, hyponatremia that occurs in events that last less than four hours is caused by overdrinking water before, during, and even after the event. Hyponatremia that occurs in endurance events that last more than four hours is often related to extreme sodium loss. Athletes affected by extreme sodium loss tend to be those who exercise more than four hours in the heat. During exercise and heat stress, the kidneys make less urine. Therefore, if athletes overhydrate during exercise, their bodies may not be able to make enough urine to excrete the excess volume.

Athletes likely to experience a sodium imbalance caused by extreme sodium loss commonly include slow marathoners, triathletes, ultrarunners, and unfit weekend warriors who have a higher sweat loss of sodium than their fit counterparts. These athletes may diligently consume high amounts of preexercise water plus consistently drink water during the event. As a result, they accumulate too much water by consuming water faster than their bodies can make urine, and they end up with a relative excess of water compared with sodium. The plain water dilutes their electrolyte balance and makes matters worse.

Hence, with extended exercise, be sure to replace sodium losses with more than just sports drinks. Sports drinks generally contain too little sodium to balance sweat loss. Choose endurance sports drinks and salty snacks (e.g., pretzels, V8 juice, olives, and pickles), salt sprinkled on

foods, soup, and even salt tablets. (Note that some salt tablets, such as
Endurolytes, offer only 100 mg of sodium per tablet.) Your target should
be 250 to 500 milligrams of sodium per hour, the amount in 20 to 40
ounces (0.6 to 1.2 L) of Gatorade, for example. Most athletes get too
much salt in their daily diet, so use sports drinks appropriately, before
and during exercise that lasts for more than an hour, not as a standard
mealtime beverage. Also, remember that the more you train in the heat,
the less sodium you lose because your body learns to conserve sodium
as well as other electrolytes (see table 8.1).

Table 8.1   Electrolyte Content of Sweat in Unfit and Fit Subjects

Electrolyte in sweat	Unfit, unacclimatized	Fit, unacclimatized	Fit, acclimatized
Sodium	3.5 g/L	2.6 g/L	1.8 g/L
Potassium	0.2 g/L	0.15 g/L	0.1 g/L
Magnesium	0.1 g/L	0.1 g/L	0.1 g/L
Chloride	1.4 g/L	1.1 g/L	0.9 g/L

Adapted, by permission, from T. Noakes, 2003, *Lore of running*, 4th ed. (Champaign, IL: Human Kinetics), 214.

As you can see, if you are neither fit nor accustomed to exercising in the
heat, you will lose twice as much sodium as you would if you were fit and
familiar with exercising in the heat. Even if you are fit, you should be mind-
ful of sodium losses if you are not used to exercising in the heat—such as
happens if you live in Alaska and run a marathon in Hawaii.

The symptoms of hyponatremia include feeling tired, bloated, nauseated, and headachy. Any of these symptoms may become increasingly
severe. A person with hyponatremia may also experience swollen hands
and feet, undue fatigue, confusion and disorientation (due to progressive
swelling of water in the brain), a decline in coordination, and wheezy
breathing (due to water in the lungs). Blood sodium levels that drop too
low can lead to seizures, coma, and death. To prevent hyponatremia,
people who will be exercising for more than four hours in the heat should
observe the following guidelines:

- Avoid water loading before the event.
- Eat salted foods and fluids (soup, pretzels, salted oatmeal) 90
  minutes before you exercise. This dose of sodium results in water
  retention in your body. This extra fluid not only can help you
  exercise longer but also may make the exercise seem easier and
  more enjoyable (Sims et al. 2007).

- Consume an endurance sports drink with higher sodium amounts than the standard sports drink during extended exercise in the heat that lasts for more than four hours.

- Consume salty foods during the endurance event, as tolerated (V8 juice, broth, pickles, cheese sticks).

- Stop drinking water during exercise if the stomach is "sloshing," as may happen if you drink more than a quart (32 oz, or 1 L) of water per hour for extended periods.

Fluid Choices

Many sweaty athletes wonder what to drink to quench their thirst; they feel confused by the abundant choices of fluids. There's plain ol' water, sports drinks, soft drinks (sugar sweetened or diet), 100 percent fruit juices, juice drinks, milk (chocolate, skim, low fat, or whole), beer, wine . . . the list goes on. As a sports dietitian, I get lots of questions about what's the best (or the worst) to drink, so here's my advice about a variety of liquids with calories.

Orange juice. Many athletes ask whether they should stop drinking orange juice because they're worried it is loaded with (fattening) carbohydrate and sugar. My answer is no. To start, carbohydrate is not fattening, and it is an important fuel for your muscles (see chapter 6). Please do not knock orange juice out of your breakfast (and then, gulp, replace it with an extra-large coffee with sugar and double cream). Eating a whole orange is preferable to drinking its juice, but for eat-and-runners who won't take the time to peel the orange, OJ is better than no-J. Orange juice offers a strong dose of vitamin C, potassium, folate, and other health-protective nutrients. The trick is to balance the calories from orange juice into your daily calorie budget.

Soft drinks. After a hard workout, some athletes like having a Coke or Pepsi but wonder how bad this is for recovery and for their health. Many of these tired athletes welcome cola's combination of sugar, caffeine, and water to refuel, rehydrate, and revive themselves. Although juice would offer far more vitamins and minerals, dietary guidelines indicate that 10 percent of calories can appropriately come from refined sugar. Hence, you can enjoy, if desired, 200 to 300 calories of daily sugar—a can or two of soft drink.

The choice of whether to drink regular soft drinks (sweetened with high fructose corn syrup) or diet soft drinks is a personal decision. I'd vote for water, myself. Regular soda is filled with nutritionally empty sugar calories; diet soda has artificial sweeteners—unnatural substances that have been rumored to cause cancer. That rumor is likely false, however. Two recent studies show no relationship between artificial sweeteners and cancer (Gallus et al. 2007; Lim et al. 2006).

Sugar aside, soft drinks such as colas contain phosphoric acid, and this may be harmful to bone health if your calcium intake is inadequate. The caffeine in colas can also leach calcium, but this is not an issue if your calcium intake is adequate. The main problem is that colas tend to crowd out milk (and calcium) from your diet. If you insist on drinking cola, enjoy it as an occasional snack, and be sure to maintain milk (regular or soy) as your beverage of choice with meals (Tucker et al. 2006).

Many athletes wonder about a possible link between soft drinks and weight gain. Some studies suggest that people who drink sugary beverages tend to be heavier than those who abstain. This might be because fluid calories fail to "register" (i.e., they may not curb one's appetite), so soda drinkers consume more calories per day. Other studies report that soda might trigger the desire to eat more food. Hence, if soda drinking culminates in consuming more calories than you burn off, the result is indeed weight gain (Drewnowski and Bellisle 2007; Vertanian, Schwartz and Brownell 2007).

As an athlete, you can likely enjoy a daily soda without fat gain if you keep the soda calories within your daily calorie budget. (And please, choose wholesome foods for the rest of your sports diet.) If you are concerned about soft drinks being fattening, please pay attention to how much sports drink you consume. Many thirsty athletes overlook the fact that chugging a quart of sports drink after a workout (or during lunch, for that matter) contributes 200 to 300 sugar calories—and these calories do count.

Water. Remember plain old water? Maybe not! Today we can choose from not only bottled spring waters but also designer waters that are flavored, vitamin fortified, and enhanced with herbs and supposed energizers. Many bottled waters come from municipal water supplies—not from the mountain streams pictured on the label—which validates the high quality of our standard municipal tap water. In the United States, municipal water is strictly regulated by the Environmental Protection Agency (EPA), and most municipal water also contains fluoride, a mineral added to reduce dental cavities. In comparison, bottled water is (loosely) regulated by the Food and Drug Administration (FDA)—but only if it is shipped across state lines or is imported.

If you don't trust the safety of your local tap water, you might want to invest in a water filter and refill an empty name-brand water bottle. Otherwise, you likely will buy water in plastic containers. More than a million tons of plastic are used every year to make water bottles, most of which end up as litter or in landfills and are not environmentally friendly.

Vitamin water, a popular new beverage category, has wide appeal to many health-conscious people who equate vitamins with energy. (Wrong. Energy actually comes from carbohydrate.) Some of these beverages are, indeed, high in energy—there are 125 calories in a 20-ounce (600 ml) bottle of Glacéau VitaminWater. That's enough to contribute to undesired weight gain.

It is not likely that vitamin waters will improve your health. Although they will not hurt you, other than in your pocketbook, they may contain too few vitamins (because of aftertaste) to make much of a health difference. Or if they are highly fortified, they still lack the phytochemicals and other health enhancers found in real food. You'd be better off drinking the original vitamin water: orange juice or any other juices.

Energy drinks. Energy comes from calories, and energy drinks, such as Red Bull and Rockstar, tend to be rich in calories from sugar. For example, an 8.3-ounce (250 ml) can of Red Bull has 110 calories, and a 16-ounce can of Rockstar has 240 calories. The drinks also have caffeine, a known ergogenic aid (see chapter 11). Red Bull has 80 milligrams, similar to the 100 milligrams of caffeine in an 8-ounce cup of coffee but far more than the 20 milligrams in a packet of caffeinated Gu. The jury is still out regarding the other ingredients, such as taurine, ginseng, and yerba mate.

If you are looking for a competitive edge, the better bet is to prevent the need for a quick energy fix by fueling your body with appropriate meals and snacks. No "quick fix" will compensate for a suboptimal sports diet.

A concern about energy drinks is that many athletes and sports fans use them as a mixer with alcohol. The caffeine masks the effects of the alcohol, so the consumers may not realize how intoxicated they are. This enhances the possibility of drunk driving (Ferreira et al. 2006; Marczinski and Fillmore 2006).

Green tea. Many athletes I talk with want to know if green tea is health protective. Green tea is made from fresh tea leaves and, compared with black or oolong teas, does have a higher concentration of compounds that may protect against heart disease and cancer, particularly cancer of the breast, stomach, and skin. Many of the green tea studies have been done on animals or in research labs. To date, the FDA says there is not enough scientific evidence with human studies to prove that green tea reduces the risk of cancer. Stay tuned.

We do know that tea drinkers tend to be healthier overall than coffee drinkers, and there appears to be no downside to drinking tea (unless you

Liquid Calories

Be aware of how quickly liquid calories can add up, especially when they come in large portions. Guzzling a quart (32 oz, or 1 L) of any calorie-containing beverage—even a sports drink after a workout—can hinder weight loss. Here are the calorie counts for a number of popular beverages.

Beverage	Calories
Water, any size	0
Diet soda, any size	0
Coffee and tea, black, any size	0
Propel Fitness Water, 16 oz (480 ml)	20
Tea with 2 tsp sugar	30
V8 juice, 11.5 oz (345 ml)	70
Milk, nonfat, 8 oz (240 ml)	80
Coffee with 2 creamers, 2 sugars	70
Gatorade, 16 oz (480 ml)	100
Beer, light, 12 oz (360 ml)	110
Orange juice, 8 oz (240 ml)	110
Apple juice, 8 oz (240 ml)	120
Milk, 2%, 8 oz (240 ml)	120
Starbucks Skinny Latte, 12 oz (360 ml)	120
Glacéau VitaminWater, 20 oz (600 ml)	125
Wine, red, 5 oz (150 ml)	130
Cranberry juice cocktail, 8 oz (240 ml)	140
Regular soda, 12 oz (360 ml)	145
Milk, whole, 8 oz (240 ml)	150
Beer, regular, 12 oz (360 ml)	160
Slim-Fast, 11 oz can (330 ml)	220
Snapple Lemonade, 16 oz (480 ml)	220
Dunkin' Donuts Coffee Coolatta with cream, 16 oz (480 ml)	350
Nesquik chocolate milk, 16 oz (480 ml)	400
Starbucks Vanilla Frappuccino, 16 oz (480 ml)	470

are caffeine sensitive). But use your common sense. I have a client who started drinking Starbucks Green Tea Latte (230 calories—60 from fat and 140 from sugar). This was a questionable way to invest in good health and likely wiped out the possible health benefits of the green tea.

Recently, green tea beverage products have been introduced with claims that they burn calories. These products are unlikely to solve your weight problem. Although the Coca-Cola Company claims that the caffeine plus green tea extracts in three cans of Enviga a day will result in burning 60 to 100 additional calories, you could just as easily create that calorie deficit by drinking less sports drink or eating one fewer cookie. Yet, desperate dieters will try anything. Green tea–enhanced Celsius, another "calorie-burning soda," saw more than $1.5 million in revenue in 2006 and expects to blow past that figure in the next few years.

Alcohol and Athletics

Alcohol and athletics seem to go hand in hand. Competitors gather at the pub after a team workout, celebrate victories with champagne, and quench thirst with a cold beer. One might think that the detrimental effects of alcohol on performance would make athletes less likely to drink it, but that is not the case. Even serious recreational runners drink more than their sedentary counterparts do.

If you are determined to drink alcohol as a part of your recovery diet, keep in mind the following facts:

- Alcohol is a depressant. It slows your reaction time; impairs eye-hand coordination, accuracy, and balance; and, apart from killing pain, offers no edge for athletes. You can't be sharp, quick, and drunk.

- Late-night drinking that contributes to getting too little sleep can wreck the next day's training session. Drinks that contain congeners—red wine, cognac, whiskey—are more likely to cause hangovers than other alcoholic beverages. The best hangover remedy is to avoid drinking excessively in the first place.

- Alcohol is a poor source of carbohydrate. A 12-ounce can of beer has only 14 grams of carbohydrate, as compared with 40 grams in a can of soft drink. You can get loaded with beer, but it will not load your muscles with carbohydrate—unless you consume pretzels, thick-crust pizza, or other carbohydrate-rich foods along with the beer.

- Alcohol is absorbed directly from the stomach into the bloodstream, appearing within five minutes after you drink it. After a hard workout, alcohol on an empty stomach can quickly contribute to a drunken stupor. You'd be better off enjoying the natural high from exercise than being brought down by a few postexercise beers.

- Beer is often a significant source of postexercise fluids; athletes commonly consume larger volumes of beer than they might of water or soft drinks. But the alcohol in beer has a diuretic effect—the more you drink, the more fluids you lose. This process is unhealthy for recovery and often unhealthy for the next exercise bout. One study showed that athletes who drank beer eliminated about 16 ounces (480 ml) more urine over the course of four hours than those who drank low-alcohol (2 percent) beer or alcohol-free beer (Sherriffs and Maughan 1997).

- Your liver breaks down alcohol at a fixed rate—about four ounces (120 ml) of wine or one can of beer (360 ml) per hour. Exercise does not hasten that process, nor does coffee.

- Hot tubs, alcohol, and athletes are a bad combination. The hotter your body, the drunker you may feel. Alcohol impairs your ability to control your body temperature, and the high temperature of the hot tub heightens the response of the body to alcohol.

- Winter sports and alcohol are a dangerous combination. Don't drink while skiing. If you choose to drink alcohol, alternate with soft drinks or juices for carbohydrate and fluids.

- The calories in alcohol are easily fattening. People who drink moderately often consume alcohol calories on top of their regular caloric intake because alcohol stimulates the appetite. These excess calories promote body-fat accumulation, commonly in the trunk area—the well-known spare tire. If you are trying to maintain a lean machine, abstaining is preferable to imbibing.

- If you are destined to drink, drink moderately. The definition of moderate drinking is two drinks per day for men and one for women. And have at least one glass of water for every alcoholic drink you consume.

- Don't start drinking if you can't easily stop. Be conscious of your ability to keep alcohol consumption within socially and medically acceptable bounds.

- If you believe you need to drink in order to "fit in" and "be popular," think again. A college alcohol survey of 117 student-athletes in Texas found that 22 percent abstained from drinking alcohol, 68 percent described themselves as light to moderate drinkers, and 59 percent did not binge drink (Wagner, Keathley, and Bass 2007).

If you think before you drink, you can talk yourself into moderation. That is preferable to dealing with a hangover. Or if you know you will be drinking, at least eat a hearty meal and drink extra water to buffer the impending flood of alcohol. Drink slowly, don't mix liquors, and please have a designated driver.

If you failed to heed this advice, you are likely dealing with the symptoms of a hangover: headache, light-headedness, irritability, anxiety, sensitivity to light and noise, trouble sleeping, difficulty concentrating, nausea, and vomiting. These symptoms generally dissipate over 12 (or more) hours, but you may be looking for a way to hasten the process.

Anecdotal remedies for a hangover include drinking sodium-containing (nonalcoholic) fluids. The sodium helps retain the fluid in your body. Try chicken soup, Gatorade (with or without added Alka-Seltzer), Pedialyte, or more water or sports drink every time you wake up to urinate during the night. Do not take acetaminophen (Tylenol); this combination can be damaging to the liver.

PART II

The Science of Eating for Sports Success

CHAPTER 9

Fueling Before Exercise

I am forever amazed at how little people eat and drink before and during exercise. For example, while on a four-hour 60-mile (96 km) group bike ride, I have observed people who "ride to eat" rather than "eat to ride." They salivate while describing the "reward" they are going to eat after the ride. One woman complained how tired she'd get two hours into a ride—and then added that she'd never eat or drink much on a ride other than a few bottles of sports drink. She preferred to hold off until the postride feast. She thought she was tired because she hadn't been training hard enough (not because she had run out of fuel). Other riders complained about how parched they were by the end of the ride.

My message to those cyclists and to all athletes and everyday exercisers is this: Just as you put fuel in your car before you take it for a drive, you want to put fuel in your body before you exercise. This preexercise snack or meal will help energize your workout. Preexercise fuel has four main functions:

1. It helps prevent hypoglycemia (low blood sugar) and its symptoms of light-headedness, needless fatigue, blurred vision, and indecisiveness—all of which can interfere with top performance.

2. It helps settle your stomach, absorb some of the gastric juices, and ward off hunger.

3. It fuels your muscles, with both carbohydrate that you eat far enough in advance to get stored as glycogen and carbohydrate that

you eat within an hour of exercise, which enters the bloodstream and feeds your brain.

4. It gives you the peace of mind that comes with knowing your body is well fueled.

Yet many people purposefully exercise on empty because they believe that exercising without having eaten beforehand enhances fat burning. True, but they assume that by burning more body fat, they will lose more body fat. False. To lose body fat, you need to create a calorie deficit by the end of the day. Whether you burn carbohydrate or fat is of less importance. The truth is you'll be able to exercise harder and burn more calories if you eat a preexercise snack. The harder exercise might contribute to the desired calorie deficit. See chapter 15 for more information on appropriate methods to lose weight.

Many people are also afraid that preexercise food will result in an upset stomach, diarrhea, and sluggish performance. Of course, eating too much of the wrong kinds of foods can cause intestinal problems (and I will address that issue in this chapter), but embarking on an exercise session when you are underfueled certainly results in sluggish performance. Morning exercisers who work out before breakfast, in particular, need to be sure they have fueled themselves adequately.

Go by Your Gut

Preexercise foods that settle comfortably can enhance stamina, endurance, strength, and enjoyment. But with the possibility that preexercise food can create intestinal chaos, the threat of diarrhea can turn the thought of pancakes into panic. Adverse reactions occur in 30 to 50 percent of endurance athletes. Complaints include stomach and upper gastrointestinal (GI) problems (heartburn, vomiting, bloating, heaviness of food, and stomach pain) and intestinal and lower GI problems (gas, intestinal cramping, urge to defecate, loose stools, and diarrhea).

Of the 362 Hawaii Ironman Triathlon finishers who ended up in the medical tent in 2004, 63 percent experienced one or more GI problems. This represents about 14 percent of the total field. The most common problem was nausea, followed by vomiting, diarrhea, and abdominal cramps. The GI distress did not correlate with race times or gender (Sallis, Longacre, and Morris 2007).

Each person has unique food preferences and aversions, so no one food or magic meal will ensure top performance for everyone. Frank, a competitive runner, avoids any food within four hours of training or competing. Otherwise, he has horrible stomach cramps. Kristin, a loyal exerciser at a health club, thrives best on a plain bagel an hour before her morning routine. "It absorbs the stomach juices and settles my stomach." Sarah, a gymnast and eighth-grade student, snacks on a banana before practice sessions but on nothing before a competition. She gets so nervous that she can't keep anything down. "I make sure I eat extra the day before a competition."

Choices of what to eat before exercising vary from person to person and from sport to sport—there is no single right or wrong choice. My experience has shown that each athlete needs to learn through trial and error during training and competition what works best for his or her body and what doesn't work. Some people can eat almost anything, others want special foods, and then there are the abstainers who have absolutely no desire to eat anything.

Athletes in running sports, in which the body moves up and down, tend to experience more digestive problems than those in sports in which the stomach is relatively stable. Jostling seems to be a risk factor for abdominal distress; food eaten too close to exercise time can often talk back. For that reason, Walter, a 21-year-old triathlete and college student, eats according to his sport of the day. "When I bike, I enjoy a reasonable meal before the ride and munch on goodies during the workout or even stop for a frozen yogurt. When I run, I have to abstain from food for three hours before a workout, or I get diarrhea. That's one reason why I prefer biking to running."

Your job is to train your intestinal tract to tolerate preexercise fuel. You can do this by starting with a cracker or a sip of a sports drink; gradually add more until you can enjoy about 200 to 300 calories within the hour before you work out. Keep in mind the following predisposing factors for GI problems:

- **Type of sport.** Cyclists, swimmers, cross-country skiers, and others who exercise in a relatively stable position report fewer GI problems than do athletes in sports that jostle the intestines.

- **Training status.** Untrained people who are starting an exercise program report more GI problems than do well-trained athletes who have built up tolerance to exercise. If you are a novice who is experiencing GI distress, gradually increase your training volume and intensity so that your body can adjust to the changes.

- **Age.** GI problems occur more frequently in younger athletes than in veterans. The younger athletes may be less trained and possibly have less nutrition knowledge and experience with precompetition eating. Veterans, on the other hand, have had the opportunity to learn from years of nutrition mistakes.

- **Gender.** Women, as compared with men, report more GI problems, particularly at the time of the menstrual period. The hormonal shifts that occur during menstruation can contribute to looser bowel movements.

- **Emotional and mental stress.** Athletes who are tense are more likely to report that food in the stomach lingers longer and settles like a lead balloon.

- **Exercise intensity.** During easy and even moderately hard exercise, the body can both digest food and comfortably exercise. But during intense exercise, the shift of blood flow from the stomach to the working muscles may be responsible for GI complaints.

- **Precompetition food intake.** Eating too much high-protein and high-fat food (such as bacon and eggs or greasy burgers) shortly before exercise can cause GI problems. Tried-and-true low-fat, carbohydrate-rich favorites (such as oatmeal or bananas) that are part of your day-to-day training diet are a safer bet.

- **Fiber.** High-fiber diets intensify GI complaints. If you are eating large amounts of bran cereal or high-fiber energy bars, try cutting back for a week to see if you feel better.

- **Caffeine.** Some athletes seek enhanced performance from drinking a larger-than-usual mug of coffee but end up with an upset stomach, diarrhea, and substandard performance.

- **Gels and concentrated sugar solutions.** Highly concentrated sugar solutions consumed during exercise may cause stomach distress. Don't confuse the high-carbohydrate recovery drinks (about 200 calories per 8 oz, or per 240 ml) with low-carbohydrate fluid replacers.

- **Level of hydration.** Dehydration enhances the risk of intestinal problems. During training, be sure to practice drinking different fluids on a regular schedule (about 8 oz, or 240 ml, every 15 to 20 minutes of strenuous exercise) to learn how your body reacts to water, sports drinks, diluted juice, and any fluids that you will be drinking during competition.

- **Hormonal changes.** The digestive process is under hormonal control, and exercise stimulates changes in these hormones. For example, the postmarathon levels of GI hormones in marathon runners tend to be two to five times higher than resting levels. These hormonal changes can result in food traveling faster through the digestive system and explain why some people experience GI problems regardless of what they eat.

Fuel Before Morning Workouts

Skipping breakfast is a common practice among people who exercise early in the morning. If you roll out of bed and eat nothing before you jump into the swimming pool, participate in a stationary cycling class, or go for a run, you may be running on fumes. You will probably perform better if you eat something before you exercise. During the night, you can deplete your liver glycogen, the source of carbohydrate that maintains normal blood sugar levels. When you start a workout with low blood sugar, you fatigue earlier than you would have if you had eaten something.

How much you should eat varies from person to person, ranging from a few crackers to a slice of bread, a glass of juice, a bowl of cereal, or a whole breakfast. If you had a large snack the night before, you'll be less needy of early-morning food. But if you've eaten nothing since a 6:00 p.m. dinner the night before, your blood sugar will definitely need a boost. Most people get good results from 0.5 gram of carbohydrate (2 calories) per pound (1 g per kg) of body weight one hour before moderately hard exercise, or 2 grams of carbohydrate (8 calories) per pound (4 g per kg) of body weight four hours beforehand. For a 150-pound (68 kg) person, this is 75 to 300 grams (300 to 1,200 calories) of carbohydrate—the equivalent of a small bowl of cereal with a banana to a big stack of pancakes (ACSM, ADA, and Dietitians of Canada 2000).

Defining the best amount of preexercise food is difficult because tolerances vary greatly from person to person. Some athletes get up two hours early just to eat and then go back to bed and allow time for the food to settle. Others have a few bites of a bagel, a banana, or some other easy-to-digest food as they dash out the door. Then there are those who habitually run on empty. If that's you, an abstainer, here is a noteworthy study that might convince you to experiment with eating at least 100 calories of a morning snack before you work out.

Researchers asked a group of athletes to bike moderately hard for as long as they could. When they ate breakfast (400 calories of carbohydrate), they biked for 136 minutes, as compared with 109 minutes after only drinking water (Schabort et al. 1999). Clearly, these athletes were able to train better with some fuel in their tanks. Preexercise morning fuel will likely work for you, too.

Four hundred calories is the equivalent of an average bowl of cereal with some milk and banana; it's not a pile of pancakes. You need not eat tons of food to notice a benefit. Eat what's comfortable for you, and learn what is the right amount of food to fuel your workouts but still settle well.

Steps of Digestion: Food Into Fuel

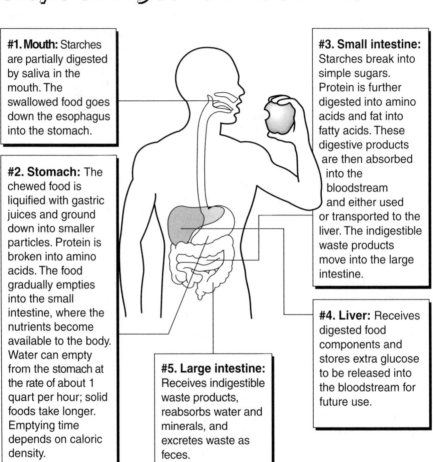

#1. Mouth: Starches are partially digested by saliva in the mouth. The swallowed food goes down the esophagus into the stomach.

#2. Stomach: The chewed food is liquified with gastric juices and ground down into smaller particles. Protein is broken into amino acids. The food gradually empties into the small intestine, where the nutrients become available to the body. Water can empty from the stomach at the rate of about 1 quart per hour; solid foods take longer. Emptying time depends on caloric density.

#3. Small intestine: Starches break into simple sugars. Protein is further digested into amino acids and fat into fatty acids. These digestive products are then absorbed into the bloodstream and either used or transported to the liver. The indigestible waste products move into the large intestine.

#4. Liver: Receives digested food components and stores extra glucose to be released into the bloodstream for future use.

#5. Large intestine: Receives indigestible waste products, reabsorbs water and minerals, and excretes waste as feces.

Fuel Before Afternoon Workouts

Juan, an afternoon runner, wondered if eating a bagel at 3:00 would provide energy for his 4:00 workout or simply sit in his stomach. I explained that, despite popular belief, the food eaten before a workout is digested and used for fuel during exercise. The body can indeed digest food during exercise, as long as you are exercising at a pace you can maintain for more than 30 minutes. Cyclists who ate 300 calories before exercise absorbed all 300 calories during an hour of moderate to somewhat hard exercise (Sherman, Pedan, and Wright 1991).

If Juan were to do extremely intense sprint activity such as a track workout or time trial, the food would be more apt to sit in his stomach and talk back to him. During intense exercise, the stomach shuts down so that more blood can flow to the muscles. Therefore, you need to plan your schedule and eat a hearty lunch at noon if you will be doing a hard workout at 4:00 (with no preexercise snack because of the intensity of the workout).

Here is a second study that demonstrates the importance of eating before you exercise. In this study, cyclists ate either nothing or 1,200 calories of carbohydrate (2 g of carbohydrate per lb of body weight) four hours before an exercise test to exhaustion. When they ate the 1,200-calorie meal, they were able to bike 15 percent harder during the last 45 minutes, as compared with when they ate nothing. Given that road races and many competitive events are won or lost by fractions of a second, to be 15 percent stronger offers a huge advantage (Sherman et al. 1989). The carbohydrate the cyclists ate before they exercised supplied extra fuel for the end of the workout, when their glycogen stores were low.

Although these studies looked at cyclists, who tend to report fewer gastrointestinal complaints than do athletes in running sports that jostle the stomach, the benefits are worth noting. If you've always exercised on an empty stomach, you may discover that you can exercise harder and longer with an energy booster. Experiment during training by eating some carbohydrate-based snacks within a few minutes to four hours before you exercise. If you plan to work out at lunch, eat cereal for breakfast and a yogurt for a 10:00 a.m. snack. If you exercise after work, have a substantial lunch and then a decaf latte and an energy bar for a second lunch later that afternoon.

Eat the Right Food at the Right Time

The trick to completing your workout with energy to spare is to fuel up with the right foods at the right time before the event. The preexercise snack should be predominantly carbohydrate because it empties quickly from the stomach and becomes readily available to be used by the muscles. Eat limited amounts of protein and fat; they take longer to digest. Here are some suggestions for different types of events at different times of the day.

Time: **8:00 a.m. event, such as a road race, swim meet, or stationary cycling class**

Meals: Eat a carbohydrate-rich dinner, and drink extra water the day before. On the morning of the event, about 6:00 or 6:30, have a light 200- to 400-calorie meal (depending on your tolerance), such as yogurt and a banana or one or two energy bars, tea or coffee if you like, and extra water. Eat familiar foods. If you want a larger meal, consider getting up to eat between 5:00 and 6:00.

If your body cannot handle any breakfast before early-morning exercise, eat your breakfast before going to bed the night before. The bowl of cereal, bagel with peanut butter, or packets of oatmeal will help boost liver glycogen stores and prevent low blood sugar the next morning.

Time: **10:00 a.m. event, such as a bike race or soccer game**

Meals: Eat a high-carbohydrate dinner, and drink extra water the day before. On the morning of the event, eat a familiar breakfast by 7:00 to allow three hours for the food to digest. This meal will prevent the fatigue that results from low blood sugar. Popular choices include oatmeal, a bagel, and yogurt.

Time: **11:00 a.m. lightweight crew race, wrestling match, or other weight-class sport that requires a weigh-in one to two hours beforehand**

Meals: Athletes who have crash dieted and dehydrated themselves to reach a specific weight for their sport have only a few hours after weigh-in to prepare for the competition. They need to replace water, carbohydrate, and sodium. An ideal target for a 150-pound (68 kg) depleted athlete would be 700 calories (primarily from carbohydrate), 2,200 milligrams of sodium, and 2 quarts (2 L) of water (Slater et al. 2007). The intake will vary greatly depending on the individual athlete's tolerance for food. Too many wrestlers end up vomiting on the mat after having pigged out after the weigh-in. Food choices might include the following:

- Chicken noodle soup, bread, and lots of water
- V8 juice, pretzels, and water
- Ginger ale or cola, a ham with mustard sandwich, and water
- Gatorade Endurance plus baked potato chips

Time: **2:00 p.m. event, such as a football or lacrosse game**

Meals: An afternoon game allows time for you to have either a big high-carbohydrate breakfast and a light lunch or a substantial brunch by 10:00, allowing four hours for digestion time. As always, eat a high-carbohydrate dinner the night before, and drink extra fluids the day before and up to noon. Popular brunch choices include French toast, pancakes, or cereal and poached eggs on toast.

Time: **8:00 p.m. event, such as a basketball game**

Meals: You can thoroughly digest a hefty high-carbohydrate breakfast and lunch by evening. Plan for dinner, as tolerated, by 5:00, or have a lighter meal between 6:00 and 7:00. Drink extra fluids all day. Two popular dinner choices include pasta with tomato sauce and chicken with a large serving of rice or potato.

Time: **All-day event, such as a hard hike, 100-mile (160 km) bike ride, or a day of cross-country skiing**

Meals: Two days before the event, cut back on your exercise. Take a rest day the day before to allow your muscles the chance to replace depleted glycogen stores. Eat carbohydrate-rich meals at breakfast, lunch, and dinner (see chapter 6 for information about carbohydrate loading). Drink extra fluids. On the day of the event, eat a tried-and-true breakfast depending on your tolerance. Bagels with a little peanut butter are a favorite.

While exercising, plan to eat carbohydrate-based foods (energy bars, dried fruit, sports drinks, gels) every 60 to 90 minutes to maintain normal blood sugar. If you stop at lunchtime, eat a comfortable-sized meal, but in general try to distribute your calories evenly throughout the day. Foods with fat, such as peanut butter, nuts, and cheese, can offer sustained energy; dietary fat takes a few hours to be converted into fat used for fuel. Drink fluids before you get thirsty; you should need to urinate at least three times throughout the day.

Preexercise Fueling Guidelines

To determine the right pretraining or precompetition snack or meal for your body, experiment with the following guidelines:

- On a daily basis eat adequate high-carbohydrate meals to fuel and refuel your muscles so they'll be ready for action. Snacks eaten within an hour before exercise primarily keep you from feeling hungry and maintain your blood sugar; they don't significantly replenish muscle glycogen stores.

- If you will be exercising for less than an hour, simply snack on any tried-and-true foods that digest easily and settle comfortably. Toast, English muffins, a banana, crackers, and granola bars are a few of the most popular high-carbohydrate, low-fat preexercise choices.

- If you will be exercising for more than 60 minutes and will be unable to consume calories during that time, be sure to eat well the day before. Choose a preexercise snack with a little protein and fat for sustained energy, such as a poached egg on toast, a bagel with peanut butter, or oatmeal made with low-fat milk.

- Limit high-fat sources of protein such as cheese omelets, hamburgers, and fried chicken because they take longer to empty from the stomach. Cheeseburgers with French fries, large ice cream cones, and pancakes glistening with butter have been known to contribute to sluggishness, if not to nausea. Note that small servings of lean protein-rich foods (turkey, eggs, low-fat milk), however, can settle well and keep you from feeling hungry.

- Be cautious with sugary foods such as soft drinks, jelly beans, gels, and even lots of maple syrup or sports drinks. Although most athletes perform well after a preexercise sugar fix, a few may experience symptoms of rebound hypoglycemia such as light-headedness and fatigue.

- Allow adequate time for digestion. Remember that high-calorie meals take longer to leave the stomach than do hearty, lighter snacks. The general rule is to allow three to four hours for a large meal to digest, two to three hours for a smaller meal, one to two hours for a blended or liquid meal, and less than an hour for a small snack, according to your own tolerance.

- Allow more digestion time before intense exercise than before low-level activity. Remember, your muscles require more blood during intense exercise than they do at rest, so your stomach may not get the normal blood flow needed for the digestion process. Any food in the stomach jostles along for the ride and may feel uncomfortable or be regurgitated.

- If you have a finicky stomach, experiment with liquid meal replacements to see whether they offer you any advantage. Liquid foods tend to leave the stomach faster than solid foods do. In one research study, a 450-calorie meal of steak, peas, and buttered bread remained in the stomach for six hours. A liquefied version of the same meal emptied from the stomach two hours earlier (Brouns, Saris, and Rehrer 1987). Before converting to a liquid preevent

Sugar Fixes

Is preexercise sugar detrimental to performance? Despite popular belief, most athletes can tolerate a preexercise sugar fix without physical problems (Horowitz and Coyle 1993). Even a candy bar eaten five minutes beforehand is unlikely to hurt performance. But a better solution than consuming preexercise sweets for an energy boost is to maintain a high energy level throughout the day by eating adequate calories of health-promoting foods at breakfast and lunch.

Eating a high-sugar food 15 to 45 minutes before exercise can have a negative effect if you are sensitive to swings in blood sugar. A concentrated dose of sugar (either natural sugar in fruit juice or refined sugar in soft drinks and jelly beans) rapidly boosts your blood sugar but simultaneously triggers the pancreas to secrete a large amount of insulin. Insulin transports excess sugar out of the blood and into the muscles. Exercise, like insulin, similarly enhances this transport. Thus, your blood sugar can drop to an abnormally low level once you start to exercise. In general, though, people who are in good physical condition can regulate their blood sugar with far less insulin than sedentary people and do not experience the "sugar crash."

That was not the case with Jackson, a teacher who liked to take a stationary cycling class after work. Because he was trying hard to lose weight, he ate only small portions at breakfast and lunch. By the time he left work for the 4:00 class, he was drained and searching for a quick energy boost, which he got from drinking a can of soda pop. Within 15 minutes after beginning the exercise class, he felt light-headed, shaky, uncoordinated, and unmotivated to continue. On some days he even had to stop for a rest. The rapid drop in blood sugar interfered with his ability to exercise. I suggested that he trade the 150 calories in his quick-fix soda for more calories at lunch. That change did the trick. He ate an extra half sandwich at lunch (150 calories) instead of an afternoon soda, and he enjoyed a higher energy level.

Without doubt, breakfast and lunch are the best energy boosters. But if for whatever reason you have skipped breakfast or lunch and are hungry and craving sweets before your afternoon workout, eat the sweets within 10 minutes of exercise if you are concerned about experiencing a sugar low. This plan will minimize the risk of a possible hypoglycemic reaction because the insulin will not have greatly increased in that short period.

meal, be it a homemade blenderized meal or a can of a commercial meal replacement such as Boost or Ensure, experiment during training to determine if this new food works well for you.

- If you know that you'll be jittery and unable to tolerate any food before an event, make a special effort to eat well the day before.

Have an extra-large bedtime snack in lieu of breakfast. Some athletes can comfortably eat before they exercise, but others prefer to abstain.

- If you have a "magic food," be sure to take it with you when traveling to an event. Even if it's a standard item such as bananas, pack it so that you will be certain to have it on hand. Even if you have no favorite foods, you still might want to pack a tried-and-true supply in case of an emergency. If you should encounter delays, such as being stuck in traffic or an airplane, you'll still be able to eat adequately. Here are some suggestions for a traveling athlete's emergency food kit:
  - Sealable bags of dry cereal (oat squares, Cheerios, granola)
  - Crackers, tortillas, wraps
  - Meal-replacement bars, granola bars, fig bars
  - Dried fruit, nuts, trail mix
  - Pouches or easy-open cans of tuna or chicken
  - Peanut butter, jam, honey (preferably in single-serve portions)
  - Water, juice, sports drinks
- Always eat familiar foods before a competition. Don't try anything new! New foods always carry the risk of settling poorly; causing intestinal discomfort, acid stomach, heartburn, or cramps; or necessitating pit stops. Schedule a few workouts of similar intensity to and at the same time of day as an upcoming competition, and experiment with different foods to determine which (and how much) will be best on race day. Never try anything new before a competition, unless you want to risk impairing your performance.
- Drink plenty of fluids. You are unlikely to starve to death during an event, but you might become dehydrated. I suggest you drink extra fluid the day before so that your urine is a very pale color. Drink two or three glasses of fluid up to two hours before the event, and drink another one or two glasses 5 to 10 minutes before the start.

Preexercise Caffeine: A Stimulating Topic

Caffeine is a popular preexercise energizer and is known to help athletes train harder and longer. Caffeine stimulates the brain and contributes to clearer thinking and greater concentration. There are many good studies on the use of caffeine for both endurance exercise, such as long runs and bike rides, and short-term, higher-intensity exercise, such as soccer. The vast majority of the studies conclude that caffeine does indeed enhance performance (by about 11 percent) and makes the effort seem easier (by about 6 percent). Endurance athletes notice more benefits than those who do shorter bouts of exercise (Doherty and Smith 2005).

If you rarely drink coffee, you may notice a dramatic caffeine boost because you are not tolerant to caffeine's stimulant effect. A study comparing regular caffeine users to nonusers reports that the nonusers lasted eight and a half minutes longer when biking very hard to exhaustion, as compared with when they had no preexercise caffeine. The regular caffeine users exercised for only four minutes longer when they had the caffeine fix (Bell and McLellan 2002).

Because each person responds differently to caffeine, do not assume you will perform better with a caffeine boost. You might just end up nauseated, coping with a "coffee stomach," or suffering from caffeine jitters at a time when you are already nervous and anxious. And be forewarned: Although a morning cup of coffee can assist with a desirable bowel movement, a precompetition mugful might lead to transit troubles. Experiment during training to determine if a caffeinated beverage or plain water is your best bet.

But doesn't caffeine have a dehydrating effect? According to Dr. Larry Armstrong, an exercise physiologist at the University of Connecticut, caffeine does not contribute to excessive water loss and is OK for athletes, even in hot weather (Armstrong 2002). The military became intensely interested in the physiological effects of caffeine on hydration among soldiers enduring extreme heat. They researched the effects of moderate (approximately 200 mg) and high (approximately 400 mg) doses of caffeine on hydration in soldiers who habitually consumed only one 6-ounce (175 ml) cup of brewed coffee (100 mg caffeine per day). They found no detrimental effects of caffeine. By day's end, the 24-hour urine losses were similar (Armstrong et al. 2005). In another study testing endurance in hot weather (100 degrees Fahrenheit; 37.7 degrees Celsius), the subjects who consumed about 225 milligrams of caffeine—the equivalent of a 12-ounce (355 ml) mug of coffee—exercised for 11 minutes longer (86 versus 75 minutes) compared with the group who had no caffeine (Roti et al. 2006).

Although a cup or two of coffee before exercise may be a helpful energizer, more may be of little value. A 1995 study (Pasman et al. 1995) showed that well-trained cyclists performed equally well with about 350 milligrams of caffeine as they did with 850 milligrams. So if you're tempted to jazz yourself up with a second mugful, think again. You may find that the second mug will do you in with the caffeine jitters. Small doses of caffeine (such as taken socially) may enhance performance, whereas high doses can be counterproductive to performance. A target dose is about 1.5 milligrams per pound (3 milligrams per kilogram)

(Doherty and Smith 2005). For a 150-pound (68 kg) athlete, this comes
to about 225 milligrams of caffeine. Table 9.1 lists the caffeine amounts
in some common perk-me-ups.

Table 9.1   Caffeine Sources

Source of caffeine	Average caffeine content (mg)
Coffee, 16 oz (480 ml) mug	
Brewed, drip method, generic	265 (200-400)
Starbucks brewed, grande	320
Dunkin' Donuts	200
Decaffeinated	10 (6-24)
Other beverages	
Starbucks espresso, doppio (6.5 oz)	150
Espresso, generic, 1 oz (30 ml) shot	40 (30-90)
Hot cocoa, 12 oz (360 ml)	12
Tea	
Tea, brewed, 16 oz (480 ml)	105 (80-240)
Starbucks Tazo Chai Tea Latte, 16 oz (480 ml)	100
Snapple Lemon Tea, 16 oz (480 ml)	42
Snapple Peach Tea, 16 oz (480 ml)	42
Snapple Plain Tea, 16 oz (480 ml)	18
Soft drink, 12 oz (360 ml) can*	
Mountain Dew, regular or diet	71
Pepsi One	54
Mello Yello, regular or diet	53
Pepsi	38
Diet Pepsi	36
Coca-Cola, classic or diet	35
Barq's Root Beer	23
Energy drinks	
Red Bull, 8.3 oz (250 ml)	80
Rockstar Energy Drink, 8 oz (240 ml)	80
Caffeinated sports supplements	
Jolt gum, 1 piece	35
Gu, vanilla, 1 oz (30 g)	20
Drugs	
NoDoz, maximum strength, 1 tablet	200
Dexatrim, 1 tablet	80
Excedrin, 1 tablet	65
Anacin, 1 tablet	32

*Small children who drink a can of cola can receive the equivalent in caffeine to an adult who drinks a cup of coffee.
Copyright CSPI 2007. Adapted from Nutrition Action Healthletter. www.cspinet.org

Many people drink a warm mug of coffee not for an energy boost but because a warm liquid promotes regular bowel movements and helps empty them out before they exercise. This may be the most justifiable reason for some people to include this brew in their preexercise diet. After all, if you are so tired that you seek coffee for its stimulant effect, you should probably be resting and not dragging yourself through a workout. Be sure no trouble is brewing in your desire for caffeine!

CHAPTER 10

Fueling During and After Exercise

Just as what you eat before you exercise greatly affects your energy levels, so does what you eat during and after extensive exercise. Students who practice after-school sports from 3:30 to 5:30, businesspeople who work out at the health club from 5:30 to 7:00 p.m., marathoners who train for one to two hours, and others who exercise for more than 60 minutes need to think about fueling during exercise. Unfortunately, many of these folks are in such a rush to start their workouts that they fail to bring with them the foods and fluids that will enhance their exercise efforts.

This chapter will help you enjoy high energy and enhanced stamina during exercise sessions that last longer than an hour. Standard healthy eating practices should take care of shorter sessions. But when you're pushing the limits, you'll want to pay proper attention to what you eat and drink during and after your hard workouts.

Eating During Extensive Exercise

Ideally, during extensive exercise that lasts for more than 60 minutes, you should try to balance your water and energy output with enough fluid to match your sweat losses and enough carbohydrate to provide energy and maintain normal blood sugar level. You can significantly increase your stamina by consuming about 100 to 250 calories (25 to 60 g) of carbohydrate per hour while performing endurance exercise, after the first hour (ACSM, ADA, and Dietitians of Canada 2000). Research involving cyclists suggests that sports beans, sports drinks, and gels all offer similar performance benefits. (Campbell et al. 2007).

Better yet, mix up your foods and fluids so that you get a variety of types of carbohydrate. Instead of just sports drinks, choose a sports drink and a banana or (part of) an energy bar plus extra water. Because different sugars use different transporters, you can absorb more carbohydrate and have more fuel to support your endurance exercise (Jentjens et al. 2006). Engineered sports foods commonly contain only one or two types of sugar, so don't hesitate to experiment with natural foods that offer more of a variety of carbohydrate.

During a moderate to hard endurance workout, carbohydrate supplies about 50 percent of the energy. As you deplete carbohydrate from muscle glycogen stores, you increasingly rely on blood sugar for energy. By consuming carbohydrate during exercise, such as the sugar in sports drinks, your muscles have an added source of fuel. Sports drinks also help maintain normal blood sugar levels. Because much of performance depends on mental stamina, you should maintain a normal blood sugar level to keep your brain fed and help you think clearly, concentrate well, and remain focused.

Your body doesn't care if you ingest solid or liquid carbohydrate; both are equally effective (Mason, McConell, and Hargreaves 1993). Despite popular belief, even sugar can be a positive snack during exercise (see chapter 6).

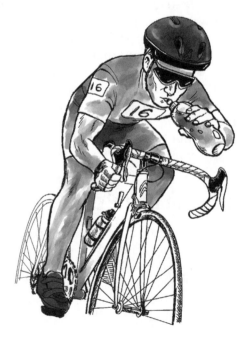

For snacks during exercise, some people prefer the natural sugars from fruits and juices, some choose gels or energy bars, and others prefer sports drinks or hard candy. You need to experiment to determine which foods or fluids work best for you and how much is appropriate.

Is more carbohydrate better? Not if the source of carbohydrate just sits in your stomach. In a study of trained women cyclists who did two hours of moderately hard endurance cycling, consuming a beverage that supplied 60 grams (240 calories) of glucose per hour resulted in the highest amount of carbohydrate being used. When the women drank a beverage with 90 grams of glucose (360 calories) per hour, they did not perform any better—likely because the fuel sat in the stomach unabsorbed and contributed to intestinal distress. With the lower carbohydrate intake, only a few subjects complained about feeling bloated. With plain water, there was only one complaint (Wallis et al. 2007). If the women had consumed a variety of forms of carbohydrate, perhaps they would have had fewer complaints.

Keep in mind that too much sugar or food taken at once can slow down the rate at which fluids leave the stomach and become available to replace sweat losses. Be more conservative with your sugar fixes during intense exercise in hot weather, when rapid fluid replacement is perhaps more important than carbohydrate replacement. In cold weather, however, when the risk of becoming dehydrated is lower, sugar fixes can provide much-needed energy.

Because consuming 100 to 250 calories or more per hour (after the first hour) may be far more than you are used to consuming during exercise, you need to practice eating during training to figure out what foods and fluids do or do not work. That is, you need to train your intestinal tract as well as your heart, lungs, and muscles. Alex, a novice marathoner, tucked hard candies, gummy bears, and chocolate mints in a waist pack that he wore on his long runs. He also hid along his running loop a cooler containing gels, pretzel nuggets, a banana, and bottles filled with water and the sports drink that would be available on the marathon course. Between the snacks and the fluids, he was able to maintain adequate energy during his three-hour training runs and simultaneously learn what he liked to eat during exercise. On marathon day, he assigned friends to specific checkpoints along the route. Their jobs were to keep him well supplied with a variety of these carbohydrate sources. He never hit the wall, and he was pleased with his time.

Whatever the situation, endurance athletes such as marathon runners, ultradistance cyclists, and Ironman triathletes need to make a nutrition plan far in advance of the event and experiment during training to learn if they prefer grape or lemon sports drinks, solid foods or liquids, energy bars or Twizzlers, raisins or bananas.

By developing a list of several tried-and-true foods that taste good even when you are hot and tired, you need not worry about what to eat (and what not to eat) on race day. Ideally, you should have a defined feeding plan for the event and know the following:

- Your fluid targets. You can determine this by weighing yourself naked before and after a workout in different temperatures to determine sweat loss per hour.

- Your calorie targets. By working with a sports nutritionist or exercise physiologist and using the information on calculating calories on pages 270 to 273 you can estimate your calorie needs per hour.

Like Alex, you should also figure out how to have these foods and fluids available for you during your training and competitions. If you have a support crew, instruct them to feed you on a defined schedule so that you can prevent hypoglycemia and dehydration.

Cramping Your Style?

Muscle cramps are often associated with dehydration. If you have ever experienced the excruciating pain of a severe muscle cramp, you may fearfully wonder if it will strike again. Because no one totally understands what causes muscle cramps, these unpredictable spasms are somewhat mysterious. Since cramps occur when muscles are fatigued, the problem may be related to a nerve malfunction that creates an imbalance between muscle excitation and inhibition, which prevents the muscle from relaxing (Schwellnus et al. 2004).

Although cramps are likely related to overexertion, other predisposing factors may include fluid loss, inadequate conditioning, and electrolyte imbalance (Jung et al. 2005). The solution often can be found with massage and stretching. Other times, nutrition may be involved. Although the following nutrition tips are not guaranteed to resolve this malady, I recommend that people who are predisposed to getting cramps rule out these possible contributing causes:

- **Lack of water.** Cramps commonly coincide with dehydration. To prevent dehydration-induced cramps, drink enough fluids before, during, and after you exercise. Always drink enough fluids daily so that your urine is clear, pale yellow, and copious. During a long exercise session, a target for a 150-pound (68 kg) athlete might be about 8 ounces (240 ml) of fluid every 15 to 20 minutes. See chapter 8 for more information on fluid recommendations.

- **Lack of calcium.** Calcium plays an essential role in muscle contractions. Some active people report that their problem with cramping disappears when they boost their calcium intake. For example, one ballet dancer found that once she reintroduced yogurt and skim milk into her diet, her cramping disappeared. A mountaineer resolved his muscle cramps by taking antacid tablets containing calcium when hiking. But some exercise scientists argue that a calcium imbalance seems an unlikely cause of muscle cramps because if a dietary deficiency should occur, calcium would be released from the bones to provide what is needed for proper muscle contraction. Nevertheless, to rule out any possible link between a calcium-poor diet and muscle cramps, athletes plagued by cramps should consume dairy products or other calcium sources (calcium-fortified orange juice or soy milk) at least twice each day.

- **Lack of potassium.** Electrolyte imbalance, such as lack of potassium, may play a role in muscle cramps. But a potassium deficiency is unlikely to occur as a result of sweat losses because the body contains much more potassium than even a marathoner might lose during a hot, sweaty race. Nevertheless, you can rule out this issue by eating potassium-rich foods on a daily basis.

- **Lack of sodium.** Active people who restrict their sodium intake during exercise may be putting themselves at risk of developing a sodium imbalance that could contribute to cramps. This circumstance is most likely to occur in athletes who exercise hard for more than four hours in the heat, such as tennis players, triathletes, or ultrarunners. The risk increases if they consume only water during the event and have eaten no foods or beverages that contain sodium. Endurance sports drinks and salted pretzels would be wise snack choices during exercise.

- **Lack of magnesium.** Just as muscles need calcium to contract, they also need magnesium to relax. Magnesium helps reduce leg cramps that occur in the middle of the night (Roffe et al. 2002). Whether or not magnesium can also help with exercise-related cramps is unclear. Many people do not meet the RDA for magnesium: 320 milligrams per day for women and 420 milligrams per day for men. The richest sources of magnesium include green leafy vegetables, whole grains, nuts, beans, and legumes. One cup of spinach has 155 milligrams of magnesium; a half-cup of All-Bran, 110 milligrams; a cup of brown rice, 85; one whole-wheat pita, 45. I hear marathoners talk about Rolaids as being helpful. One tablet contains 45 milligrams of magnesium and 220 milligrams of calcium.

Although these tips for resolving muscle cramps are only suggestions and not proven solutions, you might want to experiment with these dietary improvements if you repeatedly suffer from muscle cramps. Adding extra fluids, low-fat dairy products, potassium-rich fruits and vegetables, and a sprinkling of salt certainly won't harm you, and it may resolve the worrisome problem. I also recommend that you consult with a physical therapist, athletic trainer, or coach regarding proper stretching and training techniques.

Fueling During Tournaments and Back-to-Back Events

If you are a competitive swimmer, wrestler, tennis buff, or soccer or basketball player, you may frequently face the nutrition challenge presented by back-to-back events and tournaments that require top performance for hours on end, sometimes for days in a row. If you pay careful attention to what you eat, you'll be able to win with good nutrition. Athletes who give no thought to their nutrition game plan for a full day of activity can cheat themselves of the ability to perform well throughout the day.

When engaging in extended periods of exercise, your goals are to maintain proper hydration and normal blood sugar level. You need to plan your strategies for fueling for the upcoming event and for refueling as soon as possible after the first event to prepare for the next session. Knowing your calorie and fluid goals can guide your calorie intake and menu planning. Having tried-and-true sports foods readily available in your gym bag or a cooler can make this an easier task.

Making use of good nutrition can certainly give a team the winning edge. But persuading athletes to dedicate themselves to eating a proper sports diet can be a challenge. One college coach felt frustrated by his team's ritual of preevent high-fat pepperoni pizza and beer parties that filled the stomach but left the muscles unfueled and the players dehydrated. No wonder the team was having a bad season. The coach took a strong stance.

- He hired a sports nutritionist to educate the players about the benefits of proper preevent carbohydrate and fluid intake. The nutritionist gave the players pregame meal suggestions and lists of foods highest in carbohydrate (see chapter 6 and table 6.3 on page 124).
- He instructed all coaches and athletic trainers to enforce appropriate between-game eating. With the financial support of the booster

club, they started to provide bagels, bananas, juices, pretzels, yogurt, chocolate milk, and other high-carbohydrate sports snacks and drinks for tournament days.

- When traveling to a game, the coach preselected an appropriate restaurant that could handle the whole team, and he prearranged an economical buffet with minestrone soup, crackers, spaghetti with tomato sauce, meatballs on the side, green beans, fresh whole-grain rolls, low-fat (chocolate) milk, juice, and frozen yogurt.

- He instructed each player to pack his gym bag with his own favorite sports foods (such as sports drinks, oatmeal raisin cookies, trail mix, oranges, bagels, energy bars) to eat before, during, and between practice sessions and games.

Each player noticed that proper fueling helped him perform better, and the team as a whole respected the value of this "winning nutrition" program. Sure enough, they did start to have greater stamina and strength. Although they didn't always win, they no longer got clobbered in the final minutes, and they felt better about their overall effort.

If you are among the many athletes who give no thought to a sports nutrition game plan during day-long tournaments and repeated events, think again. The right sports diet can indeed enhance your performance. Athletes and teams who are doing well despite poor food choices can do better when they pay attention to their diets. Be responsible. Plan your day-long sports foods, then enjoy your higher energy level.

Pit Stops

Gastrointestinal (GI) problems such as constipation or diarrhea are common among athletes. If you've ever been plagued by one or the other during training or competition, you know how worrisome this is and how much it can interfere with top performance. That's why most athletes go to great extremes to promote regular bowel movements.

If you experience intestinal problems during exercise, try experimenting with what you eat before you work out. Here are some possible solutions:

- Consume liquids, such as a sports drink, instead of solid foods, such as a bagel.

- Decrease the amount of fiber in your daily diet (e.g., limit bran cereal and whole grains).

- Reduce or eliminate suspect foods, such as coffee or milk.

- Exercise in the morning, before you eat much, as opposed to in the afternoon.

- Fuel yourself during morning exercise (e.g., with a sports drink) instead of having an energy bar or other breakfast food before you exercise.

- Eat your breakfast the night before so that you wake up adequately fueled and able to exercise well for a short while without eating or drinking. For longer bouts, consume carbohydrate and water during exercise.

- Eliminate Aspirin, Advil, Motrin, and other similar nonsteroidal anti-inflammatory drugs.

- Experiment with antidiarrheal medication such as Imodium.

People who fear becoming constipated should faithfully eat fiber-rich cereals and breads and plenty of fresh fruits and vegetables to help prevent constipation, drink warm liquids in the morning to encourage regular bowel movements, and drink more than enough fluids. If you struggle with "rapid transit," you should try to determine what triggers the diarrhea by carefully charting for weeks every food and fluid you ingest, as well as the times you exercise and the times you have diarrhea. Be sure to include sugar-free gum and candies that contain sorbitol, a type of sugar that can cause gastrointestinal problems if taken in excess.

You should also try to eliminate suspected problem foods such as milk, broccoli, onions, corn, kidney beans, sugar-free foods with sorbitol, and other possibly hard-to-digest foods for a week to see if the problem goes away. Then look for bowel changes when you reintroduce these foods into your diet.

Some people never do find a simple dietary solution to their intestinal problems. Sometimes they are simply training too much or too fast. Easy exercise of any type can at times stimulate bowel movements. Peter, a jogger, was plagued with diarrhea when he started to increase his training mileage. I recommended that he cut back to his baseline mileage for a week and then gradually add one mile per week rather than four to five. I also advised him to talk with a doctor to determine whether he had a medical problem. For Peter, the solution was to train less intensely. He was trying to run too much, too quickly. Like many novice athletes whose bodies have not yet adapted to the stress of intense exercise, he ended up with diarrhea.

If you have persistent problems with diarrhea, intestinal distress, and GI cramping, consult your physician. He or she may prescribe medication to control the problem. You should also consult a sports nutritionist, especially if you are making radical long-term dietary changes. For example, when Larry, a basketball player, recognized that milk contributed to GI problems, he needed help finding nondairy sources of calcium, riboflavin, and protein—some of the key nutrients in milk. A sports dietitian helped him find substitutes without sacrificing nutrition. To find your local sports dietitian, visit www.SCANdpg.org.

Recovering From Extensive Exercise

When you've exercised hard and feel stiff, sore, and tired, you may wonder, *If I were to eat better, would I recover faster?* Without a doubt, consuming the appropriate foods and fluids can affect your recovery (as can doing light exercise for 10 to 20 minutes while you are cooling down to assist with removal of lactic acid from the blood and muscles). Many of my clients have questions about their recovery diets:

- Football players want to know what they should eat after morning practice to prepare for the afternoon session.
- People who lift weights wonder if they should eat extra protein after workouts to repair muscles.
- Squash players seek foods that will prepare them for the next day's match.
- Swimmers search for the proper foods that will get them through a heavy season of training and competing without deterioration and chronic fatigue.

When you deal with the rigors of a tough training schedule, remember that what you eat after a hard workout or competition affects your recovery. For the serious athlete, foods eaten after exercise require the same careful selection as the meal before exercise. You should not separate your recovery diet from your daily diet. By wisely choosing your foods and fluids both right after you finish exercising and throughout the day, you will recover as best as you possibly can for the next workout.

If you are a recreational exerciser who works out three or four times per week, you need not worry about your recovery diet because you have enough time to refuel your muscle glycogen stores before your next workout. But you should be concerned about your recovery diet if you are a competitive athlete who does two or more workouts per day, such as a soccer player at training camp who practices morning and afternoon, a competitive swimmer who competes in multiple events per meet, a triathlete who trains twice per day, an aerobics instructor who teaches several classes daily, or a basketball player who needs to endure an entire season of intense training and competing. To recover and refuel for the next bout, you should pay particular attention to what you eat right after the first session.

Nutrient Timing

Your muscles break down during a hard workout, but you can stop the breakdown mode by eating as soon as tolerable after you exercise. You'll be taking advantage of the 45-minute postexercise window of opportunity to optimally nourish, repair, and build muscles. Refueling is beneficial in two ways:

- Carbohydrate stimulates the release of insulin, a hormone that helps build muscles as well as transports carbohydrate into the muscles to replenish depleted glycogen stores.

- Carbohydrate combined with a little protein (approximately 10-20 g) creates an even better muscle refueling and building response, and it reduces cortisol, a hormone that breaks down muscle.

Including generous amounts of carbohydrate in the recovery diet enhances glycogen replacement. Having amino acids (from protein) readily available enhances the process of building and repairing muscles (Ivy 2001; Ivy et al. 2002) and reduces muscle soreness (Flakoll et al. 2004). In fact, eating just a little protein before exercise (such as a glass of skim milk or a yogurt) can optimize recovery by providing a ready-and-waiting supply of amino acids after exercise (Zachweija 2002).

Even if you aren't hungry or have a hard time tolerating postexercise food, take note: You don't need to consume a lot of food. As few as 100 calories can make a big difference. In a study with six platoons (387 marines) during 54 days of basic training, the groups who got 100 calories of a postexercise beverage—8 grams (32 calories) of carbohydrate, 10 grams (40 calories) of protein, and 3 grams (27 calories) of fat—experienced significant health benefits compared with the groups that got plain water or the same formula without protein. This first group of marines had an average of 33 percent fewer medical visits, 28 percent fewer visits for bacterial or viral infections, 37 percent fewer visits for muscle or joint problems, 83 percent fewer visits for heat exhaustion, and significantly less postexercise muscle soreness (Flakoll et al. 2004). Pretty impressive, for just 40 calories (10 g) of protein! You can get about 10 grams of protein in 10 ounces (300 ml) of milk, two eggs, 2 tablespoons of peanut butter on a banana, or a cup of yogurt with a little granola. The message is clear: Proper fueling at the right time is worth the effort. Rather than simply dash off to your next obligation, take the time to grab a chocolate milk or a yogurt.

Recovery Fluids and Foods

After you finish a hard workout, your top dietary priority should be to replace the fluids you lost by sweating so that your body can get back into water balance. As discussed in chapter 8, if you will be doing exercise that puts you at risk of becoming underhydrated, you should know your sweat rate. The goal is to drink on a schedule and lose no more than 2 percent of your body weight (e.g., 3 pounds for a 150-pound person). Ideally, you will have minimized dehydration during the event—but that can be hard to do during intense exercise.

One large, muscular man who spent two hours at the gym doing an hour of cardio and an hour of strength training was shocked to discover he'd lost about 8 pounds (3.6 kg) during the morning sessions—5 percent of his body weight and the equivalent of a gallon (4 L) of sweat! (One pound of sweat loss represents 16 ounces of fluid.) By weighing himself, he became aware of the importance of drinking more. He started bringing a gallon of water to the gym. He'd drink one quart every half hour and make sure that he finished the whole gallon. These steps to prevent dehydration helped him recover far more quickly—and he felt much better the rest of the day.

Your second priority is to optimize muscle glycogen replenishment, particularly if you have completed one hard workout and will be exercising again within 4 to 6 hours. As soon as tolerable after your first workout, you want to consume carbohydrate-rich foods and beverages; if they contain a little protein, even better. Your target intake is about 0.5 gram of carbohydrate per pound (1 g per kg) of body weight every hour, taken at 30-minute intervals for four to five hours (Ivy 2001) or until you eat a meal. Let's assume that you weigh 150 pounds (68 kg):

$$150 \text{ lb} \times 0.5 \text{ g carb} = 75 \text{ g carb}$$

Since 1 gram of carbohydrate contains 4 calories, you'll need about 300 calories of carbohydrate within the first hour, or as soon as tolerable after exercise, let's say within 15 minutes after the workout ends, and then again in 15 more minutes. After another 30 minutes, you should consume another dose of the 300 calories of high-carbohydrate foods. Then you can keep grazing for four to five hours.

If you've been exercising so hard that you have concerns about replacing depleted glycogen stores, the chances are good that you are hungry for lots more calories. You can eat more than the calculated amount, but extra carbohydrate will not hasten the recovery process. Choose forms of carbohydrate that taste good, settle well, and help you feel better. Your daily carbohydrate intake should be about 3 to 5 grams per pound (6 to 10 g per kg) of body weight (450 to 750 g of carbohydrate for a 150 lb athlete) or more if you are doing extreme exercise.

Adding a little protein to the carbohydrate can enhance recovery (Ivy 2001). Although engineered sports foods may advertise a 3 or 4 to 1 ratio of carbohydrate to protein, you need not get obsessed about the exact ratio. The idea is to eat primarily carbohydrate with a little protein as the accompaniment.

If exercise diminishes your appetite, you might find liquids more appealing than solid foods. Enjoy some chocolate milk or a fruit smoothie. But, if you are ravenous, there's little wrong with lean roast beef on a kaiser roll, plus some noodle soup with crackers, and a glass of juice or chocolate milk. Think of the roast beef as being an accompaniment to the other carbohydrate-rich choices, and you'll end up with a carbohydrate-rich diet after all.

Your body will naturally want carbohydrate-based recovery meals and repeated snacks, if not initially, then in an hour or so. Liquids and solid foods will refuel your muscles equally well. Some popular carbohydrate-based food suggestions that offer a little protein (and a little sodium) include the following:

- V8 juice and a turkey sub
- A fruit smoothie (made with yogurt or milk) and a handful of pretzels
- Cran-apple juice, string cheese, and some crackers
- A bowl of Cheerios with milk and a banana

Some exhausted athletes seek out protein—hamburgers, steaks. After hours of sugary sports drinks and gels, their bodies want some protein. If that's your case, enjoy the steak—along with potato and rolls.

Recovery Electrolytes

When you sweat, you lose not only water but also some minerals (electrolytes) such as potassium and sodium that help your body function normally. A pound (16 oz) of sweat contains about 80 to 100 milligrams of potassium and about 400 to 700 milligrams of sodium. Assuming that the harder you exercise, the hungrier you'll get and the more you'll eat, you'll consume more than enough electrolytes from standard postexercise foods (see tables 10.1 and 10.2). You won't need salt tablets or special potassium supplements. For example, a marathoner who guzzles a liter of orange juice after completing the event replaces three times the potassium she might have lost. Munching on a bag of pretzels will more than replace sodium losses.

Table 10.1 Potassium in Popular Recovery Foods

Food	Potassium (mg)
Potato, 1 large (7 oz)	840
Yogurt, low fat, 8 oz (230 ml)	520
Orange juice, 8 oz (240 ml)	475
Banana, 1 medium	450
Pineapple juice, 8 oz (240 ml)	335
Raisins, 1/4 cup (40 g)	300
Beer, 12 oz (360 ml) can	90
Cran-apple juice, 8 oz (240 ml)	70
Gatorade, 8 oz (240 ml)	30
Cola, 12 oz (360 ml) can	5
Potential loss in a 2 hr workout	**300**

Nutrition information from food labels and J. Pennington, 1998, *Bowes & Church's Food Values of Portions Commonly Used,* 17th ed. (Philadelphia: Lippincott).

Table 10.2 Sodium in Popular Recovery Foods

Food	Sodium (mg)
Pizza, 1/2 of 12-in. (30 cm) DiGiorno cheese	2,490
Chicken noodle soup, 1 can Campbell's	2,350
Macaroni and cheese, 1 box Kraft (7.25 oz)	1,740
Ramen noodles, Maruchan, 1 packet	1,580
Spaghetti sauce, 1 cup Ragu	1,160
Salt, 1 small packet	590
Pretzels, 1 oz (30 g) Rold Gold thins	560
Bagel, 1 Thomas' New York style (3.7 oz)	540
American cheese, 1 slice Kraft	250
Cheerios, 1 cup multigrain	200
Fruit yogurt, 8 oz (240 ml)	80-150
Bread, 1 slice Pepperidge Farm hearty slices	190
Saltine crackers, 5 (0.5 oz)	180
Potato chips, 20 Lay's	180
Wheat Thins, 8 (0.5 oz)	135
Gatorade, 8 oz (240 ml)	110
Endurolytes (electrolytes), 1 capsule	100
Powerade, 8 oz (240 ml)	70
Beer, 12 oz (360 ml) can	15
Coke, 12 oz (360 ml) can	10
Orange juice, 8 oz (240 ml)	5
Potential loss in a 2 hr workout	**1,000-2,000**

Data from food labels, July 2007.

Active people who exercise for more than four hours and athletes who sweat excessively should be sure to consume extra salt. But for the ordinary exerciser, salt depletion is unlikely, even though this electrolyte is lost in the highest concentration. The concentration of sodium in your blood actually increases during exercise because you lose proportionately more water than sodium. Hence, your first need is to replace the fluid. You can replace sodium via the food you eat by sprinkling salt on your recovery meal or choosing salty items such as olives, pickles, crackers, or soup. Notice, however, that popular recovery foods such as yogurt, bagels, pizza, and spaghetti have more sodium than you may realize (see table 10.2).

If you are tempted to replace sodium losses with commercially prepared fluid-replacement beverages, note that most of these special sports drinks are sodium poor. Commercial fluid-replacement drinks are designed to be taken during intense exercise. They are very dilute, which helps them empty faster from the stomach. They are not the best recovery foods in terms of electrolyte content, carbohydrate, and overall nutritional value unless you drink large volumes.

Recovery Vitamins

After exhaustive exercise, many people believe that extra vitamins are needed to replace what was depleted during exercise. To date, there is no research to support that belief. Vitamins are not used up during exercise; they are recycled, like spark plugs in a car.

Some people believe that vitamins can help repair the oxidative damage that occurs during exercise and is thought to hinder muscle repair and enhance cancer risk. Hence, they take antioxidant vitamins (C, E, beta-carotene). A study of ultrarunners who took 1,500 milligrams of vitamin C for the week before a race suggests that they had higher blood levels of vitamin C compared with a group of peers who took no vitamin C, but this did not translate into benefits in terms of oxidative or immune changes. (The recommended intake of vitamin C is 75 to 90 mg, so this was an extremely high dose) (Nieman et al. 2002).

Another study of runners who took 1,000 milligrams of vitamin C and 1,000 IU of vitamin E for four weeks before a very hard 13-mile (21 km) run found no reduction in the indicators of muscle damage (Dawson et al. 2002). Research supports the concept that the body can handle the stresses of exercise. That's why eating well on a daily basis is undoubtedly a wise investment in optimal recovery; supplements are not the answer. See chapter 11 for more information on vitamins.

Taking Time to Recover

Although proper nutrition can optimize recovery, even active people who eat well can become chronically fatigued for a variety of reasons, including excessive training, inadequate rest, or too little sleep. If you have a strenuous and prolonged training schedule in addition to other commitments and responsibilities, you may find yourself with too little time for proper eating, sleeping, and self-care.

Overtraining symptoms can vary. Some physical symptoms include loss of appetite, losing weight (without trying), insomnia, frequent colds or respiratory infections, and muscle or joint pains that seem to have no cause (Sherman and Maglischo 1991). Mental symptoms included irritability and anxiety, either of which may be accompanied by depression. Unusually poor performance in training or competition and lack of improvement even when you're maintaining diligent training can also indicate overtraining. If you are experiencing two or more of any of these symptoms, be aware that your training could be doing more harm than good.

Rather than overtrain to the point of chronic fatigue, you should take steps to prevent it. Eat a proper sports diet that provides adequate carbohydrate and protein, allow recovery time between bouts of intense exercise, and plan your schedule so that you get enough sleep at night. You should also try to minimize stress in your life and curtail disruptive activities that might drain your physical and mental energy reserves.

Rest days with little or no exercise are an important part of your training program. Yet, some people feel guilty if they don't train every day. They fear becoming unfit, fat, and lazy if they miss a day of training. That scenario is unlikely. These compulsive exercisers overlook the important physiological fact that rest is essential for top performance. Rest enhances the recovery process, reduces risk of injury, and invests in future performance. To replace depleted glycogen stores completely, the muscles may need up to two days of rest with no exercise and a high-carbohydrate diet. True athletes plan days with no exercise. Compulsive exercisers, in comparison, push themselves relentlessly and often pay the price of poorer performance and overuse injuries.

The same athletes who avoid rest after an event also tend to overtrain while preparing for an event. Many athletes train for two or three hours per day, thinking that such a regimen will help them improve. That sort of training program, however, is unlikely to enhance performance. Research has shown that swimmers performed just as well after one

90-minute training session per day as they did with double workouts
of two 90-minute sessions (Costill et al. 1991). *Quality* training is better
than *quantity* training. Do not underestimate the power of rest.

CHAPTER 11 —

Supplements, Performance Enhancers, and Engineered Sports Foods

Once upon a time, athletes enjoyed a well-balanced diet based on natural sports foods—bananas, orange juice, yogurt, pasta, spinach, chicken. Today, many athletes fuel themselves from a shopping cart filled with engineered bars, powders, potions, and supplements. They graze on carbohydrate, protein, amino acids, and vitamin pills, with little mention of enjoyable meals shared with family and friends.

There's no denying the sports food and supplement industry is booming. Competitors are fighting for a niche, and advertisements for their products lead us to believe that engineered nutrition is a better way to optimize health and performance. (Doubtful.) Although there is a time and a place for engineered nutrition, commercial products should be used knowledgeably, at the right times for the right reasons. Commercial products advertise promises of enhanced performance and nutritional excellence, but please don't miss this important point: Natural foods contain components that interact in highly complex ways to synergistically benefit your overall health.

Eating food as close to its natural form as possible is by far the best bet for improving health, preventing disease, optimizing healing, and thus enhancing performance. Vegetables, fruit, whole grains, lean meats, low-fat dairy foods, nuts, and legumes are all rich in a combination of the important vitamins, minerals, fiber, protein, fat, carbohydrate, antioxidants, and phytochemicals that athletes need on a daily basis to stay in the game. The purpose of this chapter is to help you wade through the plethora of confusing information and understand the appropriate situations for choosing engineered sports foods, vitamin supplements, and energy enhancers.

Vitamin and Mineral Supplements

What are vitamins and minerals? Vitamins are metabolic catalysts that regulate biochemical reactions within your body; they are found in the plants we eat and are created by the plants themselves. Minerals are natural substances that plants must absorb from the soil. If the soil is void of the needed minerals, the plant fails to thrive or yields small fruits or vegetables that have a poor appearance. (Depleted soil does not yield depleted plants; this is a concept promoted by supplement salespeople.)

Your body cannot manufacture vitamins or minerals, which is why you must obtain them through your diet. By eating a variety of wholesome foods, you can consume the right balance of vitamins and minerals needed for optimal health and performance. To date, 14 vitamins and 15 minerals have been discovered, each with a specific function. Here are a few examples:

- Calcium maintains the rigid structure of bones.
- Sodium helps control water balance.
- Iron transports oxygen to the muscles.
- Thiamin helps convert glucose into energy.
- Vitamin D controls the way your body uses calcium.
- Vitamin A is part of an eye pigment that helps you see in dim light.

Many of my clients take vitamin supplements. If they don't, they feel guilty. They assume that active people need more vitamins and supplements to pave the way to better health and performance. This is not the case. Although you do need adequate vitamins and minerals to function optimally, no scientific evidence to date proves that extra vitamins and minerals offer a competitive edge. Despite claims to the contrary, vitamin supplements will not enhance performance, increase strength or endurance, provide energy, or build muscle in healthy, active people. Nor does exercise significantly increase your vitamin and mineral needs. Exercise does not burn vitamins, just as cars don't burn spark plugs.

Dietary Reference Intakes (DRIs)

To help you determine whether you are getting the right balance of nutrients, the government has established the dietary reference intakes (DRIs). The recommendations for vitamins and minerals exceed the average nutrition requirements of nearly all people, including athletes. The DRIs have several subgroupings:

- Recommended dietary allowance (RDA) is the amount per day that should decrease the risk of chronic disease.
- Adequate intake (AI) is used when an RDA cannot be determined for a particular nutrient.
- Tolerable upper intake level (UL) is the highest level of a daily nutrient intake that is likely to pose no health risks. Above this UL, there is potential for increased risk.

Another measurement of intake you've likely seen is the daily value (DV), which is a compilation of DRIs used for food labels. The DV is intended to help people get a perspective on their overall dietary needs.

Nutrient	Daily value (on food labels)	Recommended dietary allowance or adequate intake		Tolerable upper limit
		Women	Men	Women & Men
Vitamin A (IU/day)	5,000	2,333	3,000	10,000
Vitamin C (mg/day)	60	75	90	2,000
Vitamin D (IU/day)	400	200 (<age 50)	200	2,000
		400 (age 50-70)	400	
		600 (>age 70)	600	
Vitamin E (IU/day)	30	15	30	1,000
Vitamin K (μg/day)	80	90	120	ND
Thiamin (mg/day)	1.5	1.1	1.2	ND
Riboflavin (mg/day)	1.7	1.1	1.3	ND
Niacin (mg/day)	20	14	16	35
Vitamin B_6 (mg/day)	2	1.3	1.3	100
		1.5 (>age 50)	1.7	
Folate (μg/day)	400	400	400	1,000
		600 (if pregnant)		
Vitamin B_{12} (μg/day)	6	2.4	2.4	ND
Calcium (mg/day)	1,000	1,000	1,000	2,500
		1,200 (>age 50)	1,200	
Iron (mg/day)	18	18	8	45*
		8 (postmenopause)		
Zinc (mg/day)	15	8	11	40

ND = not determined
*The upper limit does not apply to people who are taking an iron supplement as a short-term medical treatment for iron-deficiency anemia.

Source: Food and Nutrition Board, Institute of Medicine. Dietary Reference Intakes. Landover, MD: National Academy Press. 1998, 2000.

(continued)

Dietary Reference Intakes (DRIs), continued

You can get the recommended intake of most nutrients (except possibly iron) by eating 1,500 calories of a variety of foods. This amount will not only prevent nutrition deficiencies but also reduce the risk of chronic diseases such as osteoporosis, cancer, and heart disease.

According to the International Olympic Committee (IOC 2004), the best way to get all the needed vitamins, minerals, and protein is to eat a variety of foods from all the food groups. Although taking a general multivitamin is unlikely to be harmful, the IOC recommends against taking high doses of vitamin C, vitamin E, beta-carotene, selenium, and manganese because they might have negative effects on the body's immune system.

Keep in mind that the more you exercise, the more you eat. Compared with inactive people with smaller appetites, most athletes consume more calories and therefore more vitamins and minerals. Deficiencies are more likely to occur in a sedentary person who eats very little, such as an elderly grandparent, than in an active person who eats hefty portions.

Vitamin and mineral deficiencies do not develop overnight but over the course of months or years, such as can happen in a person with anorexia or someone who eats an inadequate vegetarian diet. Your body actually stores some vitamins in stockpiles (A, D, E, and K—the fat-soluble vitamins) and others in smaller amounts (B and C—the water-soluble vitamins). Most healthy people have enough vitamin C stored in the liver to last six weeks. One day of suboptimal eating will not result in a nutritionally depleted body.

Paul, a triathlete, had heard that exercise increases harmful free radicals (particles that can cause oxidative damage and cancer). He was told to take supplements of cancer-protective antioxidants, including vitamins C and E, beta-carotene, and selenium. Little did he realize that high doses of antioxidants can sometimes turn into prooxidants. This is another reason the best way to get antioxidants is from food, because food contains them in the right amounts (as well as other nutrients the body needs).

By eating a variety of wholesome fruits, vegetables, whole grains, lean meats, and low-fat dairy foods, you can consume the vitamins and minerals you need. As a bonus, many of today's foods (including energy bars and breakfast cereals) are highly fortified, so many active people actually consume far more vitamins and minerals than they realize, further negating the need to take supplemental pills. For the most part, the people who take vitamins are health conscious, eat well, and do not need a supplement.

Consumer Beware

Vitamin and herbal supplements abide by a set of government regulations different from prescription drugs and other medications. The government has very little control over their purity, potency, safety, or effectiveness, and the supplement industry is able to hype their products with little need to prove their claims. *High potency* and *all-natural* tend to be promotional buzzwords.

The Food and Drug Administration is currently establishing a new set of rules. It is hoped that by 2010, dietary supplements will be produced in a quality manner, will not contain contaminants or impurities (such as natural toxins, bacteria, pesticides, lead, or other substances), will be accurately labeled, and will contain the amount stated on the label. But the manufacturers still don't need to show that the product is safe or prove that it works.

Are Supplements Health Insurance?

Although taking a simple multivitamin is unlikely to hurt your health, does taking vitamin supplements improve your health if you already have a good diet? In a review of carefully controlled research studies on the impact of vitamin supplements on cancer, heart disease, cataracts, or age-related macular degeneration and hypertension, the National Institutes of Health concluded that "the evidence is insufficient to prove the presence or absence of benefits from use of multi-vitamin or mineral supplements to prevent cancer and chronic disease" (Huang et al. 2006, National Institutes of Health 2007).

The latest results of carefully conducted clinical research suggest that many supplements are not as effective as hyped:

- Multivitamins have not been shown to offer a clear health benefit.
- Antioxidants (vitamins A, E, C, and beta-carotene) do not protect against heart disease (Marchioli et al. 2001). Recent studies have shown no benefits but, in fact, possible earlier death with high doses. (Bjelakovic et al. 2007).
- Antioxidants for athletes have shown potential harm and no benefits. The consensus to date is that daily high-dose antioxidant vitamin supplementation is unlikely to be of real practical benefit (Davison, Gleeson and Phillips 2007).
- Chromium does not help people lose body fat.
- B vitamins do not reduce the risk of heart disease, stroke, and memory loss.
- Zinc does not prevent colds.

Taking a multivitamin and mineral supplement does not compensate for a high-fat, low-fiber, junk food diet. Nor should it allow you to become overconfident in your nutrient intake to the extent you can rationalize eating suboptimally. The information in chapters 1 and 2 can help you make smart food choices that offer the nutrients you need. If you choose to take a vitamin supplement, look first at your daily foods to see if you are already consuming these vitamins through highly fortified foods, such as breakfast cereals.

Supplementing in Special Situations

Taking a simple multivitamin and mineral pill can be a good idea for certain individuals who are at risk of developing nutrition deficiencies. You should indeed consider taking a multivitamin and mineral pill if you fall into any of the following categories:

- **Restricting calories.** Dieters who eat less than 1,200 calories daily may miss some important nutrients.

- **Allergic to certain foods.** People who can't eat certain types of foods, such as fruits or wheat, need to compensate with alternative vitamin sources to avoid deficiencies in some nutrients.

- **Lactose intolerant.** The inability to digest the milk sugar found in dairy products is a common occurrence among African American and Hispanic people. Avoiding dairy foods can result in a diet deficient in riboflavin, vitamin D, and the mineral calcium.

- **An indoor athlete.** If you spend little time in the sun or consistently use sunscreen when you are outdoors, you might be short on vitamin D, the so-called sunshine vitamin. Milk fortified with vitamin D is among the best sources of this vitamin. If you cannot or will not drink milk, taking a calcium pill with vitamin D might be a smart idea, as well as 15 minutes of regular activity in the sunshine without sunscreen.

- **Contemplating pregnancy.** To help prevent certain types of birth defects, women who are thinking about becoming pregnant should be sure to have a diet rich in folic acid, and they should take a multivitamin with 400 micrograms of folacin.

- **Pregnant.** Expectant mothers require additional vitamins and iron, but they should consult with their physicians before taking a supplement. See chapter 12 for more about athletes and pregnancy.

Vitamin D

When the sun's ultraviolet rays shine on the skin, they activate the precursor to vitamin D. If you get very little sun or always use sunscreen (which blocks the production of vitamin D), you might have low levels of this vitamin. Enjoying 15 minutes of sunshine without sunscreen a few times a week can increase vitamin D levels without increasing the risk of skin cancer.

Vitamin D helps the body absorb calcium from the intestines; that's why it's important for bone health. Vitamin D may also be involved in preventing and treating high blood pressure; heart disease; diabetes; cancer of the breast, prostate, and colon; fibromyalgia; multiple sclerosis; and rheumatoid arthritis.

The current daily value (DV) for vitamin D is 400 international units (IU), but some nutrition experts believe the recommended intake should be increased to at least 1,000 IU per day. (Lappe et al. 2007). A light-skinned person can make 20,000 to 30,000 IU of vitamin D in 30 minutes of sunbathing with no sunscreen (CSPI 2006). Most daily multivitamin pills offer 400 IU; calcium pills have 200 to 400 IU. When reading the supplement label, note that D_3 (cholecalciferol) is preferable and more potent than D_2 (ergocalciferol). You can increase your intake of vitamin D by consuming the following foods:

Food sources	Vitamin D (IU)
Salmon, pink, 3 oz (90 g) canned	500
Tuna, light, 1/2 can (3 oz; 90 g)	200
Shrimp, 4 oz (125 g) raw	160
Milk, 8 oz (240 ml)	100
Orange juice, fortified, 8 oz (240 ml)	100
Soy milk, fortified, 8 oz (240 ml)	40-120
Yogurt, fortified, 6-8 oz (175-230 g)	40-80
Cereal, fortified (10% DV), 1 oz (30 g)	40
Egg, 1 large	25

- **Vegan.** Total vegetarians (people who abstain from eating any animal foods) may become deficient in vitamin B_{12}, vitamin D, and riboflavin. Those who eat a poorly balanced vegetarian diet can also become deficient in protein, iron, and zinc.

- **Elderly.** Poor nutrition is common among frail, elderly people who eat few calories. The fewer the calories, the higher the risk of vitamin and mineral deficiencies.

Deciding Whether to Supplement

Confused? If you are currently taking supplements and are not knowledge-able about vitamins or minerals, I recommend that you consult with a registered dietitian (RD), preferably a RD, CSSD (board certified specialist in sports dietetics). This nutrition professional will be able to evaluate your diet and tell you not only what nutrients you are missing but also how to choose foods that offer what you need. To find an RD, use the referral network at www.eatright.org and see the Registered Dietitians entry in appendix A for other resources

If you simply like the idea of taking a one-a-day type of vitamin pill for peace of mind and health insurance, here are some guidelines that can help you zero in on the best bets:

- Choose a supplement with the vitamins and minerals close to 100 percent of the daily values (DVs). Don't expect to find 100 percent of the DV for calcium and magnesium listed on a label; these minerals are too bulky to put in one pill.

- Don't buy supplements that contain excessive doses of vitamins and minerals, particularly minerals. High doses of one mineral can offset the benefits of another. For example, too much zinc can interfere with the absorption of copper.

- Buy and use a supplement before its expiration date. Store it in a cool, dry place.

- Ignore claims about natural vitamins; they tend to be blends of natural and synthetic vitamins and offer no benefits. Vitamin E is more potent in its natural form, but the difference is inconsequential.

- Chelated supplements offer no advantages, and neither do those made without sugar or starch or those with the highest price tag.

- Look for USP on the label. This indicates the manufacturer followed standards established by the U.S. Pharmacopeia.

- Choose nationally known brands; this may improve the likelihood of actually getting what you believe you are buying.

- To optimize absorption, take a supplement with or after a meal.

Above all, think food first. As I have said before, and will say again, no vitamin pill will compensate for hit-or-miss eating. If you eat wisely and well, you can get the nutrients you need from the foods you enjoy. Your overall dietary pattern is what's health protective, not isolated vitamins. Your best bet is to eat your vitamins from a variety of foods. For example, here's how to get some key antioxidants:

- For vitamin C, eat oranges and other citrus fruits, strawberries, kiwi, broccoli, peppers, tomatoes, and leafy greens.

- For vitamin E, consume sunflower seeds, almonds, peanut butter, wheat germ, and avocados.

- For beta-carotene, munch on carrots, sweet potatoes, broccoli, tomatoes, kale, cantaloupe, and apricots.
- For selenium, eat seafood, lean meat, chicken, whole grains, and low-fat dairy.

Performance Enhancers

Just as whole grains, fruits, vegetables, lean protein, and low-fat dairy foods can provide the vitamins and minerals you need for optimal health, they can also supply the protein you need to build muscles, carbohydrate to fuel performance, and healthful fat to provide energy to excel at your sport. Yet, many athletes fail to be responsible with proper fueling; they look for a quick fix from supplements, pills, and potions.

One of my clients, an aspiring baseball pitcher, skipped breakfast, failed to properly fuel himself before and after exercise, and then gobbled late-night fried rice and egg rolls from a Chinese restaurant. He came to me with abundant questions about supplements, asking about muscle builders, energy boosters, immune system enhancers, and bone and joint protectors. I reminded him that no quick fix can compensate for a lousy diet. We talked about how many of the popular performance enhancers have been overrated. Some advertise false claims; others fail to list the "magic ingredients" on the label. (And no one is watching very carefully.)

Some supplements might even be contaminated. If you are a serious athlete who undergoes drug testing, be aware that contaminated nutritional supplements have caused athletes to fail drug tests (van der Merwe and Grobbelaar 2005). See the Supplements entry in appendix A for a list of Web sites you can visit for more in-depth information and cutting-edge research.

A brief overview of what's known to date about a few of the popular sports supplements follows in this section. With new research and new products appearing on a weekly basis, you need to do your own research and draw your own conclusions. Again, please refer to the Supplements entry in Appendix A for the latest information. Whatever you do, remember that no supplement will compensate for a suboptimal sports diet. Be responsible, take mealtimes as seriously as you take your training, and observe the benefits associated with good nutrition.

Muscle Builders

To build muscle, you need to lift weights. With hard gym work and an appropriate sports diet eaten at the right times, you can feel good about enhancing your musculature the natural way. If, however, you decide to

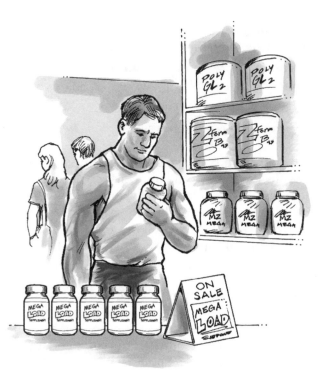

seek out muscle building supplements, here is some information on the most common types:

Creatine. A naturally occurring compound found in muscles (meat), creatine is an important source of fuel for sprints and bouts of high-intensity exercise lasting up to 10 seconds. This includes weightlifting; interval or sprint training with repeated short bouts of explosive efforts; and team or racket sports with intermittent work patterns, such as soccer, football, basketball, tennis, and squash. The typical diet of meat eaters contains about 2 grams of creatine per day; vegetarians have lower body stores of creatine.

Many athletes who take creatine report increases in lean body mass, perhaps because they are better able to recover during strength training; this allows more weightlifting repetitions. A study with 31 experienced bodybuilders who took a protein-carbohydrate supplement with or without creatine at midmorning, after their afternoon workout, and before bed (for a total of about 450 calories) suggests the protein-carbohydrate-creatine group gained more muscle mass and strength than those who consumed just protein and carbohydrate (Cribb, Williams, and Hayes 2007).

Not all athletes experience enhanced performance with creatine, however. The response is variable, with 20 to 30 percent of athletes failing to see any changes in performance. In a study with 21 subjects, 4 were classified as nonresponders (Kilduff et al. 2002).

In research studies, the subjects commonly take 3 grams of creatine per day, or they consume 20 grams of creatine in a loading dose for three to five days, then take 3 grams per day. Creatine holds water, so loading the body with creatine results in gaining water weight. This added weight might be counterproductive for weight-conscious athletes, such as sprinters.

Many health professionals agree that only fully developed athletes should take creatine. Young athletes need to learn to improve performance by training hard and developing sports skills. Although creatine is unlikely to cause medical problems, it might influence the mental desire to look for shortcuts to success.

DHEA (dehydroepiandrosterone). A precursor to testosterone, DHEA is considered a prohormone and touted to be a "fountain of youth" because it diminishes with age. Yet, there is no evidence that DHEA increases muscle mass or performance. In 1998, a small study of DHEA suggested that men (not women) experienced greater muscle strength (Morales et al. 1998). But seven studies later, DHEA has come up empty; a recent two-year study showed no benefits in men or women in their 60s and 70s (Nair et al. 2006).

HGH (human growth hormone). HGH regulates growth during childhood and metabolism during adulthood. The rumor is that HGH helps slow the aging process. The reality is that HGH can cause adverse side effects, such as swelling, painful joints, and, in men, enlarged breasts (Liu et al. 2007).

HMB (beta-hydroxy beta-methylbutyrate). HMB is a by-product of the essential amino acid leucine. HMB has been shown to quickly reverse muscle damage in rats, and it improves performance in race horses. In chronically ill, hospitalized patients, HMB helps prevent muscle wasting. In athletes, HMB is claimed to reduce muscle protein breakdown and improve recovery.

To date, the research is inconclusive, with only possible benefits for untrained people who start a weightlifting program. HMB had only possible minor effects on strength in well-trained athletes (Burke 2007). A small study from Poland indicated some gain when HMB was used alone and better results when it was combined with creatine (Jówko et al. 2001). Stay tuned.

Energy Boosters

The best energy booster is breakfast, followed by lunch, preexercise snacks, and adequate fluids. Please honor the information in chapters 1 though 6 before you seek alternative options such as the following:

Arginine. The amino acid arginine is a precursor to nitric oxide, which is discussed later in this list.

Caffeine. Caffeine is a known ergogenic aid that increases alertness, decreases reaction time, and makes effort seem easier. Many athletes enjoy a caffeine boost before, during, and after exercise. For information on caffeine, see chapters 3 and 8.

Coenzyme Q10. CoQ10 is produced by the body and is used by cells to produce energy. It is especially concentrated in heart cells. Patients with certain types of heart disease may have low CoQ10 levels, and if supplemented, may have greater exercise capacity. But several studies suggest that CoQ10 has a negative effect on athletes and can increase oxidative damage (Burke 2007).

Ginseng. Widely used in Asian cultures to reduce fatigue, ginseng is reputed to be an adaptogen that can improve recovery and help your body adapt to stress. The majority of research with athletes has failed to find benefits from ginseng supplements. A major problem is that ginseng supplements are unregulated, with varying and unknown concentrations and possible contaminants.

Glucuronolactone. Glucuronolactone is metabolized from glucose and is reported to increase feelings of well-being, reduce sleepiness, and enhance reaction time (Reyner and Horne 2002). It is found in some energy drinks (along with caffeine and taurine), in concentrations ranging from 200 to 2,400 milligrams per liter. It is found in wine (20 mg per L) and only a small number of foods. The safety of high doses has not been established.

Guarana. A "natural" stimulant, similar to caffeine, guarana is claimed to increase energy, enhance physical performance, and promote weight loss. One gram (1,000 mg) of guarana equates to about 40 milligrams of caffeine. It is often used in so-called energy drinks (Finnegan 2003).

Nitric oxide. Nitric oxide is a vasodilator that opens up the blood vessels and supposedly increases blood flow to the muscles. This is good for patients with cardiovascular disease but has yet to be proven as advantageous for athletes.

Sodium bicarbonate. Sodium bicarbonate is known to buffer the lactic acid that accumulates in the blood. Although consuming large doses of sodium bicarbonate (also known as baking soda) can improve performance in high-intensity exercise that lasts for 60 to 180 seconds, it also is known to cause nausea and diarrhea.

Synephrine. Also known as bitter orange or citrus aurantium, synephrine is used in "ephedra-free" supplements. (Ephedra is a weight-loss supplement that is now banned by the FDA.) Although it may contribute to greater alertness, it also raises blood pressure and has the potential to induce strokes and other cardiac abnormalities, particularly if taken with caffeinated beverages (Haller, Benowitz, and Peyton 2005).

Taurine. Named after the Greek word *taurus*, meaning bull, taurine is an amino acid found in high concentrations in the brain, heart, and muscles. In combination with caffeine, taurine is reputed to enhance concentration and reaction time, but more research is needed to determine if the effect is due more to the caffeine than to the taurine.

Taurine is found in protein-rich foods such as meat and seafood, and the body can make taurine from other amino acids. The typical daily intake is generally less than 200 milligrams, even in people eating a diet high in meat (Laidlaw, Grosvenor, and Kopple 1990). A can of Red Bull contains 1 gram (1,000 mg) of taurine. The safety of high doses of taurine both alone and in combination with caffeine has yet to be established.

Immunity Boosters

Almost all nutrients are linked to the immune system and play an important role in maintaining an optimal immune response. That's one reason you want to eat well on a daily basis. Immune system enhancers are found in a variety of foods, including apples, oats, broccoli, tea, spices . . . the list goes on! Taking extra nutrients will not boost the immune response above normal levels, but if you are training rigorously, you'll want to counter immune suppression by consuming carbohydrate before, during, and after exercise.

People who have low immunity tend to have a low food intake and are rapidly losing body weight—a syndrome more commonly seen in frail elderly or people experiencing a famine than robust athletes (unless they are in severe calorie deficit). For patients with HIV/AIDS, infections, and failing health, "immuno-nutrition" is being intensely researched. But whether the findings will translate to enhanced recovery for athletes is yet to be determined. Until then, optimize your immune system by avoiding overtraining, eating adequate carbohydrate, and sleeping well. The following is a list of a few immunity boosters popular among athletes.

Bovine colostrum. Bovine colostrum is a protein-rich, immunity-enhancing substance found in a mother cow's milk in the first few days after giving birth. Limited research suggests that bovine colostrum might boost immune function in athletes who do intense exercise (Shing et al. 2007). It did not prevent postrace colds in marathoners (Akerstrom and Pedersen 2007). More research is needed.

Carbohydrate. Consuming carbohydrate before, during, and after exercise is the best way for athletes to enhance immune function. Being adequately fueled with a steady stream of carbohydrate reduces the stress response. See chapters 9 and 10 for information about proper fueling tactics.

Echinacea. An herbal remedy, echinacea supposedly prevents or shortens the duration of colds (Turner et al. 2005). In a study of 437 people who were exposed to the common cold virus, taking echinacea before or after exposure did not affect the rates of infection or the severity of the symptoms.

Glutamine. Glutamine is an amino acid that provides an important source of fuel for immune cells. It is involved in healing wounds, boosting the immune system, fighting infection, and decreasing illness. During physical stress (cancer, surgery), glutamine levels drop. Glutamine supplements have been used with success in very sick patients with HIV/AIDS and cancer, but research on whether glutamine supplements can help healthy athletes when they are intensely training is weak and inconclusive. Most protein-rich foods are rich in glutamine, including beef, chicken, fish, beans, whey, and dairy.

Vitamin C. An antioxidant, vitamin C is abundant in fruits and vegetables. It is involved in boosting the immune response and reducing the potential cellular damage caused by free oxygen radicals. If you overtrain and do prolonged exercise, you can lower your immune response. Taking high doses of vitamin C, however, is unlikely to enhance your immune response. The exception might be for athletes doing a sudden increase in training (Burke 2007). The better choice is to consume carbohydrate during exercise (Davison and Gleeson 2005). If you insist on taking vitamin C, 500 milligrams is more than enough.

Vitamin E. In low doses, vitamin E plays an important role in the maintenance of immune function. In a study of 38 Hawaii Ironman triathletes who took high doses (800 IU) of this antioxidant for two months before the triathlon, the vitamin E unexpectedly *promoted* inflammation during exercise (Nieman et al. 2004). Although some antioxidant protection can be good, more may not be better. In fact, vitamin E can become a potentially health-eroding prooxidant. The bottom line: If you choose to take vitamin E, do so in moderation; 500 IU is more than enough. Because your body adapts to exercise by producing more antioxidants, an appropriate time to take an antioxidant supplement might be just before initiating an unusually high amount of exercise. See Chapter 10 for more information.

Bone and Joint Protectors

Runners, basketball players, baseball catchers, and others who put undue stress on their bodies often worry about their aching joints. Can they take anything to invest in bone and joint health? Here are two popular options:

Chondroitin. Chondroitin gives cartilage elasticity by helping it retain water. A review of 20 trials with 3,846 patients with osteoarthritis of the knee suggests that the benefit of chondroitin is minimal or nonexistant. To date, there is no evidence that chondroitin helps athletes prevent cartilage damage. Yet, many active people swear it helps them. Given a very low risk of harm, these chondroitin users can continue to take it if they believe it is effective (Reichenbach et al. 2007).

Glucosamine. Glucosamine is a key component used in the maintenance and regeneration of healthy cartilage in joints. Although it has not been conclusively proven to prevent joint deterioration, studies have shown that glucosamine sulfate (500 mg, three times a day) may help ease moderate to severe arthritis pain (but not mild pain). It is often taken in combination with chondroitin (Clegg et al. 2006).

Of 20 joint supplements marketed to people (and their pets) to ease arthritis pain, 40 percent failed to contain what their labels promised. One brand had only half the labeled chondroitin (possibly because chondroitin is expensive). Other brands had none, 8 percent, or chondroitin in a form that didn't break down quickly enough and was excreted (ConsumerLab.com 2007). It is hoped that legislation (which must be implemented by 2010) will correct this fraud. Until then, buyer beware.

Commercial Sports Foods and Fluids

The sports fuel industry has rapidly grown, starting in the 1970s with the introduction of Gatorade, continuing into the 1980s with the debut of PowerBar, and expanding in the 1990s with gels such as Gu. Since then, a multitude of companies have jumped on the bandwagon to create niche fuels for every possible dietary need—gluten free, vegan, kosher, lactose free, fructose free, you name it—and every possible time to eat (before, during, and after exercise).

If you feel confused and overwhelmed by the wide selection of commercial sports fuels to choose from, you are not alone. Athletes and casual exercisers alike inevitably ask me, "What's the best energy bar? Gel? Sports drink?" They are worried about consuming "the best ratio of carbohydrate to protein." The simple answer is you need to learn which products are best for your body by experimenting with them during training. The best choice for one person may be nauseating for another.

In general, commercial sports foods tend to be more about convenience than necessity. They can make fueling easier, take away the guesswork, and offer more benefits than you'd get from drinking plain water. But if you are on a budget, take note: A daily liter of postexercise sports drink at $1.59 adds up to about $50 a month for sugar water. The Homemade Sports Drink recipe on page 397 can save you a bundle of money!

Certainly, there is a time and place for engineered sports fuels, particularly if you are a high-level endurance cyclist, marathoner, triathlete, or adventure athlete who exercises intensely and is limited by a sensitive intestinal tract. But all active people should maintain a foundation of wholesome foods in their day-to-day diets, with engineered choices used to support their exercise programs. In other words, don't have a sports drink at lunch (instead of orange juice) or eat Jelly Belly Sport Beans (instead of fruit) for an afternoon snack. Be sure you toss a few apple cores and banana peels into the trash along with the engineered sports food wrappers. (When making your food choices, please consider the negative environmental impact of plastic sports drink bottles, gel packets, and energy bar wrappers.)

Many athletes are easily swayed by advertisements to take their sports diet "to the next level" with commercial products. Engineered foods, supplements, and energy boosters seem to offer the magic solution when life is too busy, performance is lagging, meals are hit or miss, and sleep is inadequate. But these products sometimes offer nutrients in an unnatural balance that will hinder performance. For example, we know that athletes can absorb more carbohydrate when it comes from a variety of sources, not just one source, such as the glucose found in a commercial sports drink (Wallis et al. 2005, Jentjens et al. 2006). We know that fat is important for refueling the intramuscular fat stores that are depleted during endurance exercise (van Loon et al. 2003), but many commercial products offer carbohydrate and protein but no fat. We need more research to prove that standard foods do as good a job as engineered products, if not better.

To help you untangle the jungle of "fuel tools," appendix C on page 443 provides a comprehensive (but incomplete) list of various types of sports fuels and fluids. (It is just a list and not an endorsement of the products.) Perhaps this list will help you see how the industry markets to seemingly every possible niche. Try not to be swayed by a product's name; the name might be more powerful than the sports food itself!

CHAPTER 12

Age-Specific Nutritional Needs

Whether you are the parent of an aspiring athlete, a teenager wanting to excel in high school sports with an eye to becoming a Division I college athlete, a female runner contemplating pregnancy, a masters runner, or a member of the Golden Sneakers Walking Club, you likely have some age-specific nutrition questions. This chapter offers some answers to the questions that casual exercisers and competitive athletes have throughout the life cycle.

Nutrition and Pregnancy

Many active women have sweet dreams about becoming a mom. Others have nightmares about the effect pregnancy will have on their bodies. Competitive athletes, in particular, worry about gaining too much weight. Remember that pregnancy and obesity are very different! The approximately 25 to 35 pounds (11 to 16 kg) gained during pregnancy can be accounted for by the weight of the baby (8 lb); placenta (2 to 3 lb); amniotic fluid (2 to 3 lb); uterus (2 to 5 lb); breast tissue (2 to 3 lb); blood supply (4 lb), and fat stores for delivery and breastfeeding (5 to 9 lb). Athletic women who are underweight at the start of pregnancy commonly gain more weight; overweight women may gain less.

Nutrition Before Pregnancy

If you are contemplating motherhood, you shouldn't wait until you are pregnant to start eating well. Every day, mothers-to-be should fortify their bodies with the nutrients needed for the current and future well-being of their bodies and of their unborn children. In particular, a prepregnancy sports diet should be rich in folate (see table 12.1), a B vitamin that helps prevent brain damage in the fetus at the time of conception and can reduce the risk of some types of birth defects. Folate is the natural form of this B vitamin found in food. Folic acid is the synthetic form found in supplements or enriched foods. The recommended intake is 400 micrograms of folate or folic acid per day.

Table 12.1   Sources of Folate or Folic Acid

Food	Amount	Folate or folic acid (μg)
Natural foods		
Spinach	1 cup cooked	260
Lentils	1/2 cup cooked	180
Asparagus	6 spears	130
Avocado	1/2 medium	80
Broccoli	1 cup cooked	80
Romaine lettuce	1 cup shredded	80
Chickpeas	1/2 cup canned	80
Kidney beans	1/2 cup canned	65
Orange	1 medium	50
Peas, green	2 tbsp	30
Peanut butter	2 tbsp	30
Egg	1 large	20
Fortified and enriched foods		
PowerBar	1	400
Cheerios	1 cup	200
Oatmeal, instant	1 packet	80
Flour, enriched	1/2 cup	80
Bread, whole wheat	2 slices	60

Information from J. Pennington, 1998, *Bowes & Church's Food Values of Portions Commonly Used*, 17th ed. (Philadelphia: Lippincott) and food labels.

Nutrition During Pregnancy

Each athletic woman experiences a pregnancy unique to her. Some feel fine, eat well, exercise regularly, and breeze through the nine months of pregnancy. Others experience fatigue, nausea, low-back pain, and other discomforts. Some gain more weight than anticipated. Others gain according to the standard guidelines. Eat according to your appetite, and trust that regularly scheduled meals and snacks will contribute to the weight gain appropriate for your body, the enjoyment of a comfortable exercise program, and the development of a healthy baby.

Your best bet for nutrition during pregnancy is to follow the nutrition guidelines in the first two chapters of this book as well as to read some of the pregnancy books suggested in appendix A. Your diet should focus on folic acid (see table 12.1 for sources), calcium-rich foods, dark green or colorful vegetables, fresh fruits such as oranges and other citrus fruits, whole grains, and foods rich in iron and protein. Athletes who enter pregnancy with low iron stores are at high risk for anemia. Pregnancy is already tiring enough!

For about two-thirds of women, tastes change during pregnancy. You may develop strong aversions to meat, vegetables, or coffee. If you can hold down nothing but a few crackers, rest assured that your baby will still manage to grow on the nutrients you've stored up from your prepregnancy diet. If your intake is very limited because of nausea that lasts for more than three months, you might want to consult with a registered dietitian who can suggest ways to balance your diet.

If you experience unusual cravings, such as for salt, fat, or red meat, it's possible that nature is telling you that those foods have nutrients you need. Food cravings, in moderation, tend to be harmless, so listen to your body and respond appropriately. Try to resolve your cravings for sweets with the most healthful choices, such as frozen yogurt instead of ice cream or raisins and dried fruits instead of candy. The reality of the situation may be that there's only one food that will do the trick: the food you crave! Eating a healthful prepregnancy diet ensures that you start off well nourished so your body can survive the strange cravings and morning sickness.

Nutrition After Pregnancy

If you are a new mother who worries that you'll never lose the weight gained during pregnancy, be patient and remember that life has seasons. The first year after pregnancy may not be the season to be as lean or as athletic as desired. Pregnancy lasts for 9 months, and many women need an additional 9 to 12 months to return to their prepregnancy physiques (see figure 12.1). Don't try to crash diet now.

Your better bet is to focus on eating healthfully and trusting that healthy eating will contribute to the return of your appropriate weight. But this process often gets confounded because motherhood brings its own set of nutrition challenges and frustrations. When your baby cries, your life stops, and so do many healthful eating habits. Fatigue, stressful life changes, family adjustments, and lack of energy to shop for and cook food can also take their toll on the quality of your diet. You may also lack the mental energy you need to reduce your weight and maintain your exercise program.

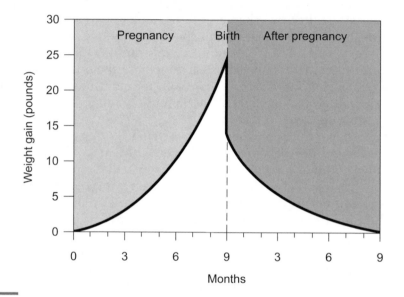

Figure 12.1 Pregnant women usually gain 25 to 35 pounds during pregnancy and may need 9 or more months to return to their prepregnancy weight after delivery.

The stresses and frustrations that accompany motherhood can interfere with your desired weight-loss plans and may even contribute to weight gain. If you are now home all day with readily available food, you may comfort yourself with candy, cookies, and other special treats. Physical exhaustion, lack of time, and child-care responsibilities may thwart your intentions to exercise. If this is the case, you might want to pay a babysitter so that you can have some time to exercise. This may help you feel better physically as well as feel better about yourself.

If you fear that you'll end up overweight for the rest of your life, take note of a survey of new moms. The women, who were all runners, reported that most returned to running five weeks after delivery and were at their prepregnancy weights in five months (Lutter and Cushman 1982). Yes, there can be a lean life after pregnancy, as verified by the many mothers you see around you who are lean. For now, love yourself from the inside out, enjoy your baby, be proud of your accomplishment, and be gentle on yourself.

Family Nutrition

Many of my active clients are health- and weight-conscious parents who are frustrated by their children's eating practices. As Janine, a triathlete and parent of two girls (11 and 14 years old) vented, "I wish I could get my kids to eat better and exercise more. They love junk food, spend hours chatting to their friends via computer, and weigh more than they should. Mealtimes are becoming World War III." Janine tried hard to teach her children about the importance of nutrition and health, but her messages fell on deaf ears.

I recommended that Janine not focus on "good" versus "bad" foods, but rather teach her children to enjoy food and appreciate how it helps a body do the wonderful things it can do. It is normal for children to want junk food, but it is also pretty normal for them to want good-for-you foods too. Balance—not restriction—is a key message. Otherwise, kids sneak-eat.

Despite popular belief, kids (and their parents) do not need to eat a perfect diet to have a good diet. Most children can meet their nutrient needs within 1,200 to 1,500 calories of a variety of wholesome foods. Hence, there is space for some treats, in moderation. (Active children can actually have trouble getting adequate calories if parents strictly limit treats.) One way to reduce your child's intake of not-so-good foods is to offer a healthful "second lunch" after school and before sports. Enjoying a peanut butter on crackers, an English muffin pizza, cereal with milk, a fruit smoothie, or a sandwich is preferable to the standard routine of munching on candy bars, cookies, and chips. A healthful second lunch is particularly important for kids who eat poorly at school. To help put an end to food wars, I highly recommend Ellyn Satter's *Secrets of Feeding a Healthy Family*.

Children's Growing Bodies

Paul, a fitness runner and the father of a 12-year-old swimmer, felt dismayed every time he saw his daughter in a bathing suit. "Sarah is pudgy, even though we try to keep her active." I reminded Paul that every child's body is different; some are petite, some are larger, and some are in the middle. That is normal and OK. Although Paul was unhappy about his child's physique, I warned him to express his concern from the point of health, not beauty. Conveying the message "you are not good enough" can be the root of future problems. Sarah was undoubtedly more than aware of her excess body fat; helping her accept and appreciate her body would be an important step for him to take.

Although dieting is standard among swimmers and participants in other sports that emphasize leanness (figure skaters, dancers, gymnasts, runners), the pressure to acquire the "perfect" body can lead to trouble if the dieter has a poor self-image and low self-esteem. All too often, diets are about feelings of being imperfect or inadequate rather than weight alone. Dieting increases the risk of developing a full-blown eating disorder.

As a parent, Paul needs to downplay body size as an important currency of worth and teach Sarah to love herself from the inside out. I advised Paul to never comment about the size of large children; Sarah could conclude she must be thin to be valued and loved. This is particularly important for young girls during puberty who are coping with body changes while struggling to be the best at their sports. Their efforts to control weight may lead to unhealthy dieting, frustration, guilt, despair, and failure.

Helping Your Overfat Child

Paul felt at a loss about how to help Sarah lose weight. I told him that childhood weight issues are complex and a topic of debate among parents and pediatricians alike. We know that restricting a child's food intake does not work. Rather, restricting kids' food tends to result in sneak eating, binge eating, guilt, shame—the same stuff that adults encounter when they "blow their diets." But this time, the parents become the food police—an undesirable family dynamic.

Despite Paul's best intentions to prevent creeping obesity, I warned Paul against putting Sarah on a diet, depriving her of French fries, or banning candy. Dietary restrictions don't work—not for adults and not for kids. If diets did work, then the majority of people who have dieted would all be lean, and the obesity epidemic would not exist.

Diets for children cause more problems than they solve. They disrupt a child's natural ability to eat when hungry and stop when content. Instead, the child overcompensates and stuffs himself through "last-chance eating." You know, "It's my last chance to have birthday cake, so I'd better eat a lot now because when I get home, I'm restricted to celery sticks and rice cakes." I suggested that Paul delicately ask Sarah if she is comfortable with her body. If she admitted discontent and expressed a desire to learn how to eat better, he could then arrange for a consultation with a registered dietitian who specializes in pediatric weight control.

If you, like Paul, are the parent of a chubby child, you should know that children commonly grow "out" before they grow "up." That is, they often gain body fat before embarking on a growth spurt. Talk to your pediatrician to determine if the problem is real. You can also assess your child's weight with growth charts available at www.cdc.gov/growthcharts.

You might be rightly concerned about your child's weight; we're seeing more and more medical problems linked to childhood diabetes, high cholesterol, and high blood pressure. But your concerns about your child's weight might reflect your own anxiety about having an "imperfect" kid. Yes, you say you want to spare your child the grief of being fat—but be sure to also examine your own issues. If you yourself are very weight conscious and put a high value on how you look, you may be feeling blemished if your child is overfat. Often, a child's weight problem is really the parent's issue. You may want a "perfect child."

Be sure to love your overfat child from the inside out—and not judge her from the outside in. Little comments such as "That dress is pretty, honey, but it would look even better if you'd just lose a little weight" can be interpreted by your child as "I'm not good enough." Self-esteem takes a nosedive and contributes to anorexic thinking, such as "thinner is better," and dieting can go awry (see chapter 16 for information on eating disorders).

So, what can you do to help fat kids slim down? Instead of maligning them and trying to get them thin by restricting food, get them healthier by helping them see the benefits of being more active. This could mean encouraging them to watch less TV, planning enjoyable family activities (unlike boot camp), and perhaps even creating a walking school bus with the neighborhood kids. As a family, you might want to sign up for a charitable walking or running event. As part of a society, make your voice heard about the need for safe sidewalks, health clubs that welcome overfat kids, and swimming pools that allow children (and adults, for that matter) to wear T-shirts and shorts instead of embarrassing bathing suits.

Foodwise, provide your kids with wholesome, nourishing foods as well as semiregular "junk foods." (Otherwise, they will go out and get them). Encourage your children to eat breakfast. Plan structured meals and snacks; take dinnertime seriously. Your job is to determine the what, where, and when of eating; the child's job is to determine how much and whether to eat. (Don't force your child to finish his peas or stop him from having second helpings.) If you interfere with a child's natural ability to regulate food, you can cause a lifetime of struggles. Trust your children to eat when hungry and stop when content—and to have plenty of energy to enjoy an active lifestyle.

Nutrition for Older Athletes

One hundred years ago, life expectancy was 42 years. Today, most of us will live twice as long. Without question, staying active is the key to maintaining your health, both physical and mental. With age, we gain not only wrinkles and gray hair but also wisdom, an appreciation for our mortality, and the desire to protect our good health. You may know that maintaining fitness into the golden years reduces the inflammation that can lead to heart disease, but you might not know that staying fit likely reduces the risk of Alzheimer's disease by 50 percent (Etnier et al. 2007).

If you are a masters athlete who has the desire to remain active for years to come, you may wonder if your nutrition needs differ from those of younger athletes. To date, research suggests that older athletes have no significantly different nutrition needs other than to optimize their sports diet so they'll have every possible edge over the younger folks. Your biggest nutrition concern should be to routinely eat quality calories from nutrient-dense, health-protective foods in order to reduce the risk of heart disease, cancer, osteoporosis, and other debilitating diseases of aging.

The last thing you want is to end up like Mickey Mantle, who once said, "If I'd known I was going to live this long, I would have taken better care of myself." It's never too late to start eating well, exercising appropriately, and adding life to your years. Here are a few specific tips to help older athletes (and aging athletes—that is, all of us) create a winning food plan that's appropriate for every sport, including the sport of living life to its fullest.

Protein. As people age, their protein needs slightly increase—but not enough to have a separate protein recommendation for masters athletes. Just don't skimp on protein-rich foods. Be sure to eat protein with at least two meals per day to build, repair, and protect your muscles. Protein-rich fish—in particular salmon, tuna, and other oily fishes—offer health-protective fat that reduces the risk of heart disease, cancer, and rheumatoid arthritis. Target 8 ounces of oily fish per week (two servings).

Whether you are young or old, if you want to get the most from your workouts, plan to refuel soon after you finish. In a 12-week training study of 74-year-old men, the subjects who refueled with carbohydrate and protein immediately after each exercise session developed significantly bigger and stronger muscles than the control group, who delayed refueling for two hours after their workouts (Esmarck et al. 2001).

Fat. Healthful plant and fish oils have a health-protective anti-inflammatory effect. Given that diseases of aging, such as heart disease and diabetes, are thought to be triggered by inflammation, consuming plant and fish oils that reduce inflammation is a wise choice. See chapter 2 for information on healthy fats.

Calcium. Even though your bones have stopped growing, they are still alive and need to be kept strong with resistance exercise and daily calcium. This advice applies to men as well as women. By selecting a calcium-rich food at each meal (including soy or lactose-free milk products), you'll invest in bone health. Having strong muscles attached to the bones is also essential, so be sure to do strengthening exercises such as lifting weights at least twice a week.

Fiber. Eat enough fiber-rich foods to have regular bowel movements; this not only enhances sports comfort but also invests in good health. The fiber in oatmeal, for example, reduces cholesterol and risk of heart disease.

Vitamins. The best all-natural sources of vitamins are colorful fruits and vegetables; eat a rainbow of produce. By keeping active and exercising, you can eat more calories—and more vitamin-rich fruits and veggies. These wholesome foods offer compounds that work synergistically and are more powerful than vitamin pills.

Supplementing antioxidant vitamins such as C and E is popular among masters athletes, but research has yet to support this practice. The body responds to extra exercise by making extra antioxidants.

Fluids. The older you get, the less sensitive your thirst mechanism becomes. That is, you may need fluids but may not feel thirsty. To reduce the risk of chronic hypohydration, drink enough so that you urinate every three to four hours. See chapter 8 for more information on how to stay well hydrated.

The bottom line: Eat wisely, drink plenty of fluids, exercise regularly, lift weights, refuel rapidly, and enjoy feeling young. Let wholesome food and enjoyable exercise be your winning edge!

Women, Weight, and Menopause

Even elite athletes gain a little weight with age, and nonelite folks have been known to gain a lot. The trick to weight management is to stay active and eat quality calories that invest in good health. Yet, many women fear midlife weight gain. As Mary, an avid tennis player complained, "No matter what I do, I can't seem to stop gaining weight." She was frustrated about her expanding waist and frightened about runaway weight gain. She fearfully asked, "Are women doomed to gain weight in midlife?"

The answer is no. Women do not always gain weight during menopause. Yes, women aged 45 to 50 commonly get fatter and thicker around the middle as fat settles in and around the abdominal area. But these changes are due more to lack of exercise and a surplus of calories than to a reduction of hormones (Wing et al. 1991). (Young athletes with amenorrhea and reduced hormones do not get fat.) In a three-year study of more than 3,000 women (initial age 42 to 52 years), the average weight gain was 4.6 pounds (2.1 kg). The weight gain occurred in all women, regardless of their menopause status (Sternfeld et al. 2004). If weight gain is not caused by the hormonal shifts of menopause, what does cause it? Let's explore a few of the culprits.

Menopause occurs during a time when a woman's lifestyle becomes less active. If her children have grown up and left home, she may find herself sitting more in front of a TV or computer screen than running up and down stairs, carrying endless loads of laundry. A less-active lifestyle not only reduces calorie needs but also results in a decline in muscle mass; when women (and men) age, they tend to lose muscle mass unless they do regular strength training. Muscle drives the metabolic rate, so less muscle means a lower metabolic rate and fewer calories burned.

Another problem is that sleep patterns commonly change in midlife, often due to night sweats and a husband who snores. Many women end up feeling exhausted most of the time. Exhaustion and sleep deprivation can easily drain motivation to routinely exercise, and this perpetuates more muscle loss and extends the drop in metabolism.

Sleep deprivation itself is also associated with weight gain. Adults who sleep less than seven hours per night tend to be heavier than their well-rested counterparts. When you are sleep deprived, your appetite grows. The hormone that curbs your appetite (leptin) is reduced, and the hormone that increases your appetite (grehlin) become more active (Taheri et al. 2004). Hence, you can have a hard time differentiating between being hungry or tired. In either case, cookies and chocolate can be very tempting.

Menopause may also coincide with career success, including business meals at nice restaurants, extra wine, plush vacations, and cruises. That means more calories and less exercise. By midlife, most women are tired of dieting and depriving themselves of tempting foods; they may have been dieting since puberty. The "No, thank you" that prevailed at previous birthday parties now becomes "Yes, please."

The best way to prevent weight gain is to exercise and maintain an active lifestyle. Research suggests that women who exercise do not gain the weight and waist of their nonexercising peers (Sternfeld et al. 2004). The optimal exercise program includes both aerobic exercise (to enhance cardiovascular fitness) and strengthening exercise (to preserve muscles and bone density). The book *Strong Women Stay Slim* by Miriam Nelson is a good resource for helping women develop a health-protective exercise program.

Despite popular belief, taking hormones to counter the symptoms of menopause does not contribute to weight gain. If anything, hormone replacement therapy may help curb midlife weight gain (DiCarlo et al. 2004).

If you have gained undesired fat, do not diet. If you have been dieting for 35 to 40 years of your adult life, you should have learned by now that dieting does not work. Rather, you need to learn how to eat healthfully.

This means fueling your body with enough breakfast, lunch, and afternoon snack to curb your appetite and energize your exercise program. Then, eat a lighter dinner. Think *small calorie deficit.* Consuming 100 fewer calories after dinner (theoretically) translates into losing 10 pounds (4.5 kg) of fat per year.

To find peace with food and your body, meet with a registered dietitian (RD) who specializes in sports nutrition. This professional can develop a personalized food plan that fits your needs. To find a local RD, go to www.eatright.org or www.SCANdpg.org. In addition, ask yourself, "Am I really overweight?" Maybe there is just more of you to love. Your body may not be quite as perfect as it once was at the height of your athletic career, but it can be good enough. I encourage you to focus on being fit and healthy rather than on being thin at any cost. No "perfect" weight will ever do the enormous job of creating midlife happiness.

PART III

Balancing Weight and Activity

CHAPTER 13

Assessing Your Body: Fat, Fit, or Fine?

When you look in the mirror or at people at the mall, you see that nature wants humans to have some body fat. In fact, the reference 24-year-old woman is about 27 percent fat, and the reference 24-year-old man is about 15 percent fat. Some of us have more fat than others—undesired bumps and bulges, spare tires around our waists, and fat on our thighs.

Society preaches that thinner is better, and consequently many of my clients yearn to have a fat-free image. Women strive to be sleek and slender. Men want to be muscular and trim. Although a certain amount of leanness is desirable for health and performance, obsessions about body fatness are unhealthy. One man did 1,000 sit-ups each day, hoping to get rid of the fat on his abdomen. A woman spent hours on the stair stepper, hoping to eliminate the fat on her thighs. Both came to me asking to have their body fat measured, and both were shocked to learn that they were leaner than they thought.

Scantily clad athletes commonly see themselves as being too fat, but rarely too thin. Measuring body fat can thus offer a helpful perspective about where a person is in the scheme of fatness. Body-fat measurement can be a positive tool that allows you to quantify loss of body fat or gain of muscle as you embark on your diet and exercise program. The purpose of this chapter is to talk about bodies, body fat, and body fatness; discuss the different methods of body-fat measurement; and offer perspectives about how fatness is less important than fitness. Even overfat people can be fit, healthy, and at peace with their bodies.

Body Fat: Why Do We Have It?

Although excess body fat is excess baggage that slows us down, we need a certain amount of fat for our bodies to function normally. Fat, or adipose tissue, is an essential part of our nerves, spinal cord, brain, and cell membranes. Internal fat pads the kidneys and other organs; external fat offers a layer of protection against cold weather. For the reference man, essential fat makes up about 4 percent of body weight, or 6 fat pounds for a 150-pound man (2.7 fat kg for a 68 kg man). In comparison, the reference woman has about 12 percent essential fat, or 15 fat pounds for a 125-pound woman (6.8 fat kg for a 57 kg woman). Table 13.1 further describes the various levels of body fatness.

Table 13.1   Defining Body Fatness by Percentage of Fat

Classification	Image	Males	Females
Very low fat	Skinny	7-10	14-17
Low fat	Trim	10-13	17-20
Average fat	Normal	13-17	20-27
Above normal fat	Plump	17-25	27-31
Very high fat	Fat	>25	>31
Essential fat		3-5	11-13

Adapted, by permission, from B. Getchell, 1982, *Being fit: A personal guide* (New York, NY: John Wiley and Sons, Inc.), 90.

Women store essential fat in their hips, thighs, and breasts. This fat is readily available to nourish a healthy baby if a woman becomes pregnant. If you are a woman fighting the battle of the bulging thighs, you may be fighting a losing battle. The activity of the enzymes that store fat in women's thighs and hips is very high compared with the enzyme activity in other fat storage areas in women and compared with fat storage in the hips and thighs of men. Moreover, the activity of the enzymes that release the fat is low, making it difficult to lose fat in these areas. The easiest time for women to lose fat in this area is during the last trimester of pregnancy and while breastfeeding. At those times, the activity of the fat-storing enzymes drops, and the activity of the fat-releasing enzymes increases. Nature, again, is protective of a woman's ability to care for her offspring.

Body Fat and Exercise

Myths and misconceptions are abundant surrounding the role of exercise in weight management. Here's a true or false quiz to test your knowledge about body fat and exercise.

If you start an exercise program, you'll lose body fat.

False. To lose body fat, you need to create a calorie deficit for the entire day. That is, you need to burn off more calories than you consume. Exercise can contribute to the calorie deficit, but exercise is often overrated as a way to reduce body fat. Exercise is better used as a tool to help prevent weight gain and to maintain weight loss. Exercise helps relieve stress (which can reduce stress eating), helps you feel good about yourself, boosts your metabolism, and often increases the desire to feed yourself healthfully.

Many people do lose weight by adding exercise. That happens because they start a total health campaign that includes not only adding activity but also subtracting some calories. After they work out, they tend to feel great, they've relieved stress, and they have less desire to unwind after a hectic day by munching through a bag of chips as they might have done before starting the exercise program.

But some of my clients complain to me that they have lost no weight despite hours of working out. That often happens because they are rewarding themselves afterward with generous amounts of calories that replace all they burned off. They may have exercised for 30 minutes and burned off 300 calories, but then they consumed 300 calories of "recovery food" in 3 minutes. Despite popular belief, appetite tends to keep up with your exercise load (except in extreme conditions). The more you exercise, the hungrier you will eventually become, and the more likely it is that you will eat enough to replace the calories you burned off. Nature does a wonderful job of protecting your body from wasting away, particularly if you are already lean with little excess fat to lose (Woo, Garrow, and Pi-Sunyer 1982; Woo and Pi-Sunyer 1985).

Another factor that influences the effectiveness of exercise as a means to lose weight relates to the toll of exercise on your total daily activity. Some avid exercisers put all their effort into exercising hard for one or two hours per day but then do little spontaneous activity the rest of the day (Thompson et al. 1995). For example, a group of moderately obese college-age students who participated in a 16-month aerobic exercise program had similar daily energy expenditures before starting and at the end of the program. The students seem to have become more sedentary at other times of the day (Bailey, Jacobsen, and Donnelly 2002). This pattern is common among both casual and serious exercisers, many of whom claim to maintain weight despite their hard workouts.

If you do want to use exercise to promote weight loss, think about doing exercise that builds muscle. Unlike aerobic exercise that burns calories primarily during the exercise session but very few thereafter, strength training builds muscles that boost your metabolism throughout the entire day and night. Muscle tissue actively burns calories. The more muscle mass you have, the more calories you burn.

To lose body fat, do low-intensity, fat-burning exercise.

False. To lose fat, you need to create a calorie deficit for the day. You can do this by adding exercise of any type, eating less, or combining the two. Just be sure that by the end of the day you have eaten fewer calories than you needed. That way, you'll dip into the stored body fat and burn it for energy.

Some people think that the key to body-fat loss is doing fat-burning exercise, or low-intensity exercise that uses more fat than muscle glycogen for fuel. Wrong. Studies have shown that burning fat during exercise does not affect loss of body fat (Zelasko 1995). But because you can sustain low-intensity exercise for longer than you can sustain high-intensity workouts, you can easily burn off more calories in, let's say, 60 minutes of jogging (600 calories) than in 10 minutes of fast running (150 calories).

High-intensity exercise may actually contribute to a lower percentage of body fat (Yoshioka et al. 2001). Research on 1,366 women and 1,257 men suggests that those who did high-intensity exercise tended to have less body fat than those who did lower-intensity fat-burning exercise (Tremblay et al. 1990). The big concern about doing high-intensity exercise relates to the higher risk of injury. If you choose to exercise harder, be sure to exercise wisely—warm up, stretch, and don't do too much, too soon. Keep in mind that you may not enjoy high-intensity activity as much and end up exercising less as a result.

Men are more likely to lose weight with exercise than are women.

True. In terms of evolution, nature wants women to have fat and be fertile; men are supposed to be lean hunters. Given that extreme amounts of exercise can be interpreted as a famine (because of the high calorie deficit), nature seems to work hard to protect women's body-fat stores. In one study of previously sedentary normal-weight men and women who participated in an 18-month marathon training program, the men reported increasing their food intake by about 500 calories per day and the women reported increasing by only 60 calories, despite having added 50 miles per week of running. The men lost about 5 pounds (2.4 kilograms) of fat; the women lost less than 2 pounds (1 kilogram) of fat, despite reporting (with questionable accuracy) a larger calorie deficit (Janssen, Graef, and Saris 1989). Similarly, other studies suggest that normal-weight women fail to lose significant amounts of fat when they add exercise.

In a study of previously sedentary overweight males and females (average age 22 to 24 years) who did fitness exercise five times a week for 16 months with no dietary restrictions, the men lost 12 pounds (5.4 kilograms), and body fat dropped from 27 to 22 percent. They failed to eat enough to compensate for the extra calories burned. The women, however, had no significant weight or body-fat changes; their appetites kept up with their calorie expenditures (Kirk, Donnelly, and Jacobsen 2002). As one of my female clients whined, "I've been running for 10 years, and I still haven't lost one pound." She's not the only one!

To reduce the fat around the stomach and hips, you should incorporate sit-ups into your exercise program.

False. Spot reducing sounds like a great idea. But the truth is that vigorous exercise won't reduce the fat cells in one localized area of your body. When you lose fat, you lose it everywhere, not just from the part of your body you are working most vigorously. Moreover, you need to create a calorie deficit for the entire day to reduce body fat. Muscle movement itself does not result in loss of body fat. For example, the man who did 1,000 sit-ups every day trying to burn off the fat in his abdomen certainly built strong abdominal muscles, but he failed to create a calorie deficit and lose abdominal fat.

If you become injured and are unable to exercise for a week, your muscles will turn into fat.

False. Muscle does not turn into fat, nor does fat turn into muscle. Muscle and fat are separate entities and not interchangeable. Perhaps you've noticed a fat layer on roast beef or pork chops. A similar fat layer occurs in humans. The fat tissue is a layer of fat-filled cells that covers the muscles. Muscle is the protein-rich tissue that performs exercise. When you exercise, you build up muscle tissue. When you consume fewer calories than you expend, you reduce the fat layer.

If you are unable to exercise because of injury or illness, your muscles actually shrink in size. For example, Joe, a skier, broke his leg and was shocked to see how scrawny his leg muscles looked when the cast was removed five weeks later. Once Joe started exercising again, he rebuilt the muscle to its original size.

If you overeat while you are ill or injured (as often happens with inactive athletes who are bored, depressed, and hopeful that chocolate-chip cookies will cure all ailments), you will become fatter. I often counsel wounded football players who gain 10 to 20 pounds (4.5 to 9.0 kilograms) after an injury. They continue to eat lumberjack portions although they need fewer calories. The extra fat takes up more space than the muscle, and the players become flabby.

Feeling frustrated and disappointed when you are injured is normal. Share your feelings with others who understand. Think positive, and visualize your injury getting better every day. Find the positive aspect. Time off from exercise can mean more time for friends, family, and other hobbies.

When injured, some very thin athletes do migrate to their natural weight (i.e., the weight they would naturally maintain without rigorous exercise and restricted calories). For example, a 13-year-old gymnast perceived herself as "getting fat" while she recuperated from a knee injury. She was simply catching up and attaining the physique that was appropriate for her age and genetics.

Cellulite is a special kind of fat that appears after a person has repeatedly gained and lost weight.

False. Cellulite is fat that has a bumpy orange-peel appearance and often appears on the hips, thighs, and buttocks. The fat is deposited in pockets just below the surface of the skin. Although much is written about cellulite, little is understood about it. Some medical professionals believe that the dimpled appearance of cellulite may result from restrictions of the connective tissue that separates fat cells into compartments. If you overeat and fill the fat cells, the compartmental restrictions may cause the fat to bulge.

Cellulite is more of a problem for women than for men because women have thinner skin and their fat compartments are larger and more rounded. Also, women tend to deposit fat in their hips, thighs, and buttocks, areas in which cellulite appears easily. In contrast, men tend to deposit fat around their waists. A genetic predisposition toward cellulite may exist. If a mother has cellulite, the daughter is likely to acquire it as well. Cellulite generally appears as a person ages because the skin loses its elasticity and becomes thinner.

Did you pass the quiz? If you are exercising primarily to lose weight, I encourage you to separate exercise and weight. Yes, you should exercise for health, fitness, stress relief, and, most important, enjoyment. I discourage you from exercising to burn calories. Under those conditions, exercise feels like punishment for having excess body fat. You'll likely quit your exercise program sooner or later because disagreeable exercise is not fun.

Your job is to find an exercise program that has purpose and meaning so that you will enjoy incorporating some type of exercise into your daily schedule for the rest of your life. Consider these examples:

- Jim bought a dog and is now walking the dog 3 miles (about 5 kilometers) per day.
- David enjoys gardening in the summer and walking in the woods in the winter.
- Gretchen, a busy executive, takes a 30-minute walk at lunch to relieve stress and process her feelings.
- Sherri commutes to work by bicycle.
- Kevin joined a marathon training program.

Although exercise without a calorie deficit fails to result in weight loss, we do know that exercise is important for maintaining weight loss and improving health. People who burn off 1,000 to 2,000 calories per week tend to be leaner and healthier than sedentary people. Again, find an exercise program that has purpose and meaning.

Body Image

Jessica, a competitive high school swimmer, was sensitive about her bulky body and described herself as "feeling fat." As I measured her body fat, she anxiously awaited the decisive moment. "You are actually very lean, Jessica," I said. "You simply have a lot of muscle and a big bone structure. You have very little excess fat."

Visual appearance and body weight are deceptive for athletes who tend to compare themselves with their teammates. We come in all different sizes and shapes, most of which are genetically determined. Although you can change your body to a certain extent by losing fat or building muscle, you can't do a complete makeover. Even if you lose the excess baggage, sometimes you still won't end up with the body you want.

If you are a woman who has large thighs (like all the women in your family), or if you are a man who hates your "love handles" (which all the men in your family have), you need to be realistic in your expectations.

You can trim the fat on your thighs or around your waist a bit by creating a calorie deficit, but you are unlikely to get it to vanish. Rather than obsess about your body flaw, I recommend that you let go of your dissatisfaction with your body, accept yourself for the sincere and caring person you are, appreciate your body for all the wonderful things it does for you, and focus on the relationships in life that really matter. You can waste a lot of mental energy fretting about undesired body fat.

Again, we come in sizes and shapes unique to our genetic makeup. Just as some of us have thick hair, others have thin hair. Some of us have blue eyes, and others have brown eyes. No one seems to care about hair thickness or eye color, but the media have made us all care about body fatness. As a result, too many self-conscious people feel inadequate because of repeated failures at transforming themselves into a shape they aren't meant to be.

To put into perspective how irrelevant body shape or size is, think about a person who has been most influential in your life. Does that person's weight modify your relationship with him or her in any way? Likely not. I suspect that there are few (if any) people in your life for whom your feelings are based solely on their appearance.

Remember that your value as a partner, colleague, or lover does not depend on your physical appearance. Your beauty comes from the inside. Your concern about how you look can be a mask for how you feel about yourself. People who obsess about their imperfect bodies commonly have low self-esteem. Somehow, they believe they are not good enough.

Are You Imagining the Wrong Body?

Because of today's appearance consciousness, you undoubtedly hold an image of what you are supposed to look like. Yet few people naturally possess their desired physique. Most of us are ordinary mortals, complete with bumps, bulges, fat, and fleshiness. Women, in particular, have a natural roundness and softness that tends to become rounder and softer with aging.

In general, about one-third of all Americans are truly dissatisfied with their appearance, women more than men. A woman will most commonly complain about her thighs, abdomen, breasts, and buttocks. A man expresses dissatisfaction with his abdomen, upper body, and balding scalp. Sometimes the problem is imaginary (such as when the anorexic skater complains about her fat thighs); sometimes it is real and ranges from a mild complaint about love handles that hang over the running shorts to a major preoccupation with flabby thighs that results in relentless dieting and exercise.

Even lean athletes, men and women alike, are not immune from the epidemic of body dissatisfaction, despite their fitness. Many perceive themselves as having unacceptable bodies, and this perception can lead to the development of eating disorders. The best predictor of who will develop an eating disorder relates to who struggles most with body image.

What you look like on the outside should have little to do with how you feel on the inside. But in reality, many people think like this:

1. I have a defect (fat thighs) that makes me different from others.
2. Other people notice this difference.
3. My looks affect how these people see me—as repulsive and undesirable.
4. I'm bad, inadequate, and not good enough.

This type of thinking is common among young dancers who develop hips and thighs as they blossom from girls into women, runners who feel pressure to be thinner, exercise leaders who think every student scrutinizes their bulges, and numerous other people who think they have imperfect bodies.

Men and Distorted Body Images

Since the creation of the Barbie doll, women have become increasingly obsessed about their looks. Today, men are also becoming more obsessed and feeling pressure to acquire a lean and muscular look. The G.I. Joe doll is one example of why the obsession is becoming more common. In 1964, if G.I. Joe were an actual man, he would have a 44-inch (112 centimeter) chest and 12-inch (30 centimeter) biceps. Today, if the G.I. Joe Extreme doll were an actual man, he would have a 55-inch (140 centimeter) chest and 27-inch (69 centimeter) biceps. His biceps would be almost the same size as his waist.

We should not be surprised, then, that body dysmorphic disorder (BDD)—preoccupation with an imagined defect in appearance or an excessive concern for a slight physical defect—is on the rise, even in men. Men with BDD feel socially anxious, believing that everyone around them is seeing their flaws and judging their appearance. Muscle dysmorphia, a subtype of BDD, affects men who are obsessed with thoughts that they are too small and do not have enough muscle mass. Many of these men spend extraordinary hours at the gym and take dangerous steroids and other drugs to bulk up. As one man commented, "Why should I be Clark Kent when I can be Superman?" (Olivardia 2002).

Learn to Love Your Body

If you are dissatisfied with your body, you might think the solution is to lose weight, pump iron, or do thousands of sit-ups. This "outside" approach to correcting body dissatisfaction tends to be inadequate. Concern about what you look like is really a mask for how you feel about yourself, your self-esteem. Given that about 25 percent of your self-esteem is tied to how you look, you can't feel good about yourself unless you like your body and feel confident about your appearance. Weight issues are often self-esteem issues.

The best approach to resolving your body-shape issues is to learn to love the body you have. As I mentioned before, much of what you look like, your size and shape, is genetically determined. You can slightly redesign the house that nature gave you, but you can't totally remodel it, at least without paying a high price of restrictive dieting and compulsive exercising.

If you are struggling with your body image, you need to think back to identify when you first got the message that something was wrong with your body. Perhaps it was a parent who lovingly remarked that you looked good in an outfit for a special occasion—but you'd look even better if only you'd lose a few pounds. Maybe it was the siblings who teased you about your flabby thighs. Then, you need to take the following steps to be at peace with your body and learn to like yourself:

- Rename your disliked body part (i.e., rename "ugly jelly belly" a more loving "round tummy").
- Identify the parts of your body that you like.
- Give yourself credit for your attractive body parts with positive talk.

If you find yourself obsessing about the look of your body, give yourself permission to live your life in a healthier way. The Declaration of Independence from Weight Obsessions (figure 13.1) provides a positive way to start accepting your body as it is. Please, do not dwell on the negative, but instead love all the good things your body does for you. It rides bikes, lifts weights at the gym, goes canoeing, and lets you have fun. How could you enjoy sports without your body? Remember that healthy bodies can come in many different sizes and shapes. You can even be fat and fit.

To start improving your relationship with your body, close your eyes and imagine that you have your desired body. Visualize the confident carriage, verbal expression, and body language you would use. Open your eyes and assume those characteristics. With practice, you'll come to

> ### Figure 13.1   Declaration of Independence From a Weight-Obsessed World
>
> I declare, from this day forward, I will choose to live my life by the following tenets. In doing so, I declare myself free and independent from the pressures and constraints of a weight-obsessed world.
>
> - I will accept my body in its natural size and shape.
> - I will celebrate all that my body can do for me each day.
> - I will treat my body with respect, give it enough rest, fuel it with a variety of foods, exercise it moderately, and listen to what it needs.
> - I will choose to resist our society's pressures to judge myself and other people on physical characteristics like body weight, shape, or size. I will respect people based on their depth of character and the impact of their accomplishments.
> - I will refuse to deny my body of valuable nutrients by dieting or using weight-loss products.
> - I will avoid categorizing foods as either "good" or "bad." I will not associate guilt or shame with eating certain foods. Instead, I will nourish my body with a balance of foods, listening and responding to what it needs.
> - I will not use food to mask my emotional needs.
> - I will not avoid participating in activities that I enjoy (e.g., swimming, dancing, enjoying a meal) simply because I am self-conscious about the way my body looks. I will recognize that I have the right to enjoy any activities regardless of my body shape or size.
> - I will believe that my self-esteem and identity come from within!
>
> Courtesy of the National Eating Disorders Association. www.nationaleatingdisorders.org

learn that appearance is only skin deep and that your real worth is the love, care, and concern that you offer your family and friends. You'll be able to muster the courage to face intimidating situations. You can even put on that bathing suit and feel at peace!

Don't Play the Numbers Game

Some people give too much power to the number on the bathroom scale. Jean, a dedicated exerciser, resorted to keeping her scale in the trunk of her car because it too easily ruined her day. Paul, a marathoner, said, "One morning I got so mad at the scale. It told me I'd gained 3 pounds, and I'd been starving myself for half a week. I angrily jumped up and down on it until it broke. That's the last time I've weighed myself!" Paul can laugh now when he recalls that story, but he wasn't laughing at the time.

If you worry about your weight, I advise against weighing yourself daily. You'll likely refer to yourself as being good when the pounds drop and bad when they go up. Nonsense. You are the same lovable person, regardless of a pound or two either way.

A scale measures not only fat but also muscle gain, water, food, intestinal contents, the coffee you drank just before weighing yourself, and so on. The scale often gives irrelevant information. For example, if you increase your exercise program, decrease your food intake, build up muscle, and lose fat, the scale may indicate that your weight has remained the same. You will feel thinner, look thinner, and your clothes will be looser, but you will not gain any psychological rewards if you depend on the scale.

Some athletes play games with the scales and fool only themselves. For example, runners, racquetball players, and other athletes who perspire heavily often prefer to weigh themselves after a hard workout. During exercise, they may have lost 5 pounds (2.3 kilograms)—5 pounds of sweat, not fat.

The only time to weigh yourself (if you insist) is first thing in the morning. Get up, empty your bladder and bowels, and then step on the scale before you eat or drink anything. You'll be weighing your body, pure and simple. If you weigh yourself at the end of the day, you'll also be weighing your dinner, beverages, and other foods in your intestines.

Also remember that weight is more than a matter of willpower. Weight, like height, has a genetic component. When it comes to height, you have likely accepted the fact that you can't force yourself to grow 6 inches (15 centimeters). But when it comes to weight, you may demand that your body lose an inappropriate number of pounds.

Certainly, if you are overfat, you can reduce to an appropriate level of body fatness. Weighing yourself weekly on the scale can provide positive reinforcement. But if you are already a lean athlete who is struggling to drop those final 5 pounds below an appropriate weight, you may feel like a failure and question your self-worth: "Why can't I do something as simple as lose 5 pounds?"

Some athletes are in a difficult situation when it comes to meeting the weight demands of their sports. Wrestlers, gymnasts, ballet dancers, and figure skaters participate in a sports system that does not accommodate athletes as designed by nature. This circumstance raises ethical concerns. Should genetically stocky people be discouraged from ballet, figure skating, gymnastics, and other sports that favor thinness? Should rowers be encouraged to drop 15 pounds (7 kilograms) to reach a lower weight class? How can the governing bodies of such sports accommodate the fact that health is more important than weight? These are tough questions.

How Much Should I Weigh?

Although only nature knows the best weight for your body, the following guidelines offer a method to estimate the midpoint of a healthy weight range (plus or minus 10 percent, depending on whether you have large or small bones). This rule-of-thumb guide does not apply to everybody—especially muscular bodybuilders.

- Women: 100 pounds for the first 5 feet of height, 5 pounds per inch thereafter (45 kilograms for the first 152 centimeters, 0.9 kilogram per centimeter thereafter).
- Men: 106 pounds for the first 5 feet of height, 6 pounds per inch thereafter (48 kilograms for the first 152 centimeters, 1.07 kilograms per centimeter thereafter).

For example, a woman who is 5 feet, 6 inches (168 centimeters) could appropriately weigh 100 + 30 = 130 pounds (45 + 14 = 59 kilograms), with a range of 117 to 143 pounds (53 to 65 kilograms). A man who is 5 feet, 10 inches (178 centimeters) could appropriately weigh 106 + 60 = 166 pounds (48 + 27 = 75 kilograms), with a range of 149 to 183 (68 to 83 kilograms).

Although athletes commonly want to be leaner than the average person, heed this message: If you are striving to weigh significantly less than the weight estimated by this guideline, think again. Pay attention to the genetic design for your body, and don't struggle to get too light. The best weight goal is to be fit and healthy rather than sleek and skinny.

If you are significantly overweight, your initial target should be to lose just 5 to 10 percent of your current weight. If you weigh 200 pounds (91 kilograms), losing just 10 to 20 pounds (5 to 10 kilograms) is enough to improve your health status and significantly reduce your risk of heart disease, diabetes, and high blood pressure. Although you may want to lose more fat for cosmetic reasons, you should know that losing the initial few pounds is a meaningful accomplishment.

Body Mass Index

The body mass index (BMI), a ratio of body weight to height, is often used as a screening tool to identify people who are overfat (BMI greater than 25) or obese (BMI greater than 30). In the general population, people with a high BMI are considered to have excess body fat and to be at risk of developing heart disease, diabetes, and other medical concerns. Yet, BMI is a poor method to screen for overfatness in athletes because it accounts for body mass, not body fat. Hulky football players, weight-lifters, and other power athletes who have lots of muscle mass easily get ranked as "obese"; this is generally far from the truth. In a study of 28 collegiate hockey players, the average BMI was 26 (overweight), but the average body fat was a lean 13 percent. Among 149 male wrestlers and basketball, hockey, and football players, 67 percent had a BMI that misclassified them as being overweight when their body-fat levels were actually normal (Ode et al. 2007).

In my counseling practice, I use BMI to determine who is too thin. If you have normal musculature, an appropriate BMI is 18.5 to 24.9. When an athlete's BMI is less than 18.5, I need to rule out the possibility of anorexia. To determine if you fit this underweight category, search the Web for "body mass index calculator" and you'll find a variety of tools to assess your BMI.

Body-Fat Measurements

When I counsel athletes who have a poor concept of an appropriate weight, I measure their body fat rather than rely on scales and height and weight charts. The fat measurement helps put in perspective the proportion of an athlete's body that is muscle, bone, essential fat, and excess fat. A scale provides a meaningless number because it doesn't indicate the composition of the pounds. Although some pounds are desirable muscle weight, others are less desirable fat weight. Obviously, the muscle weight contributes to top athletic performance in most sports. The fat weight is the bigger concern because excess fat can slow you down.

Believe me, judging from the tension that radiates from the body of a weight-conscious athlete, I believe that getting your body fat measured ranks high on the list of anxiety-provoking life experiences. This number unveils the truth. Hulky football players are often humbled to learn that 20 percent of their brawn is flab. Weight-conscious gymnasts are often thrilled to learn that they are leaner than they thought they were.

If you want to have your body fat measured, you'll certainly want to have it done correctly by a qualified health professional to eliminate any possibility of being told that you are fatter than you really are. Inaccurate readings can send people into a tizzy. If you later want to be remeasured, try to have it done by the same person using the same technique to ensure greater consistency.

When it comes to measuring body fat, no simple, inexpensive method is 100 percent accurate. Common methods, such as underwater weighing, air displacement, calipers, and electrical impedance, all have potential inaccuracies. The following information evaluates these options to help you decide the best way to estimate your ideal weight should you want to quantify the fats of life.

Keep in mind that body-fat measurements should include a conversation about an appropriate weight for your body. If you are far leaner than other members of your genetic family but still have a higher percentage of fat than you desire, you may already be lean for your body. For example, a 5-foot, 6-inch (168 centimeter) walker lost 50 pounds (23 kilograms), from 200 to 150 (91 to 68 kilograms) and wanted to reach a seemingly appropriate weight goal of 130 pounds (59 kilograms). Because she couldn't seem to lose beyond 150 pounds without severely restricting her intake, I measured her body fat. She was 28 percent fat, at the higher end of average but far leaner than anyone else in her family. I suggested that she be at peace with this healthier weight and remember that she was currently thin for her body.

Underwater Weighing

Underwater weighing traditionally has been considered the most accurate method for determining body fat. With underwater weighing, the subject exhales all the air in his or her lungs and then is weighed while submerged in a tank of water. Despite popular belief, this technique does not measure body fat. Instead, it measures body density, which translates mathematically into percent fat. During the translation, however, significant error can creep into the picture. The equations for translating density into fat are most appropriate for the standard male. This excludes many thin runners and muscular bodybuilders. The same equations can be inappropriately used for girls on the high school swim team, 50-year-old marathoners, and professional football players.

Body density differs among all types of athletes, and age, gender, and race affect it. Children and senior citizens differ from each other in body density. The anorexic ballerina with osteoporotic, low-density bones is far different from the standard male and may receive an inaccurate estimate of body-fat percentage unless the difference in density is accounted for using a population-specific equation.

Errors with underwater weighing also stem from the inexperience of the person being weighed. If you've never been submerged into a weighing tank, you are likely to be nervous and may not completely exhale all the air in your lungs before going under the water. This will affect the density reading. Exercise physiologists have estimated that as little as 2 cups (a half liter) of air can affect body-fat measurements by as much as 3 to 5 percent. Intestinal gas can also disrupt the accuracy, as can poorly calibrated equipment. Many portable underwater weighing systems (the kinds that show up at road races, health fairs, and runners' expos) may lack the precision of a weighing system used in a research laboratory.

Bod Pod

The Bod Pod uses a method similar to underwater weighing, except that the body displaces air instead of water. The Bod Pod is a podlike chamber with a top that swings open and a seat inside. The person sits inside, scantily clad. (Standard clothing takes up space and alters the reading, so the person should wear spandex clothing and a bathing cap). The technician closes the top of the Bod Pod and then takes air-pressure measurements that determine body volume from air displacement. These measurements are then translated into percent body fat, using a principle similar to underwater weighing. The accuracy is similar to that of underwater weighing; they agree within 1 percent (Fields, Goran, and McCrory 2002). Because the Bod Pod is quick, comfortable, easy, and less stressful than the underwater weighing method, it has become popular in health clubs, athletic departments at universities, and research settings.

Skinfold Calipers

Skinfold calipers are more convenient and less sensational than other methods of body fat measurement. The calipers are large pinchers that measure the thickness of the fat layer on specific body sites. Skinfold calipers are the most accurate of affordable ways for consumers to measure body fat (Peterson et al. 2007). However, health professionals well trained in the technique are the most qualified to use this method. Active people often obtain their measurements from students or novice technicians who may be using imprecise or poorly calibrated calipers at crowded health fairs or fitness events. A hasty measurement an inch above or below the established pinch point can add 5 to 15 millimeters of fat to the measurement. Those little millimeters can translate inaccurately into a high body-fat reading.

Even accurate measurements commonly translate into erroneous information because of inappropriate conversion equations. To be most accurate, the measurements from a runner, wrestler, bodybuilder, or gymnast should be plugged into sport-specific conversion equations. Such equations are seldom used for the average athlete.

The accuracy of body-fat measurements using calipers depends on the precision of the technician, the accuracy of the caliper, and the appropriateness of the conversion equations. Repeated measurements by different technicians using different calipers and different equations can yield widely different results.

Skinfold caliper measurements are best used to measure changes in body fatness. I often record on a monthly basis the measurements of people losing a significant amount of weight through regular exercise. By comparing the numbers (either as measurements in millimeters or converted into percent fat), the dieters can monitor changes. People recovering from anorexia may appreciate periodic skinfold measurements as a way to see that they are rebuilding muscle, not just gaining fat. This use of calipers may not give a 100 percent accurate picture, but it shows trends, particularly when the same technician measures the person each time, using the same calipers and same conversion equations.

Bioelectrical Impedance

Bioelectrical impedance analysis (BIA) measures body composition using a computerized system that sends an imperceptible electrical current through the body. The amount of water in the body affects the opposition to the flow of the current (impedance). Because water is found only in fat-free tissue, the current flow can be translated into percent body fat. As a result, it's relatively accurate if you are hydrated appropriately, but for sweaty athletes it is often less accurate than skinfold calipers.

Measuring body composition by bioelectrical impedance is a simple procedure that takes just minutes to perform. The whole-body machine (with electrodes attached to the wrists and ankles) is portable, easy to use, and popular at road races and health fairs. Other models that assess regional body composition come in the form of scales (leg to leg, such as the Tanita scale) and the handheld Omron model (arm to arm). Consumers who buy bioelectrical impedance scales should know that leg-to-leg measurements tend to be more accurate than hand-to-hand measurements.

Although it is a popular method, estimating body fatness by electrical impedance can be problematic, particularly among athletes. Because of the nature of the conversion equations, the body fatness of lean athletes is sometimes overestimated, and the fatness of overweight people is sometimes underestimated. If you measure yourself after you exercise, you'll likely have a lower percentage of fat compared with the preexercise measurement because hydration affects the reading (Demura et al. 2002). You will get an inaccurate reading if you are dehydrated (as often happens with wrestlers or in weight-class sports). Don't bother to be measured after hard exercise or after you've had any alcoholic beverages. As one of my clients reported, "I can be anywhere between 9 and 14 percent body fat, depending on when I use my Tanita scale."

Other factors that may affect the accuracy of the measurement include ethnic background, premenstrual bloat, food in the stomach, and carbohydrate-loaded muscles (water is stored along with the carbohydrate). The calculations are based on the assumption that the standard person is 73 percent water. Research has shown that young people tend to be 77 percent water and older folks 71 percent. If you are improperly positioned during the test (say, with part of your arms touching your body), you will also get an inaccurate reading. This error can easily happen in crowded exhibitions.

With the development of new sport-specific equations, accuracy is improving. Testing of the Omron handheld model indicates that it gives a reasonably accurate (within 3.5 percent) measurement 65 percent of the time with women and 70 percent of the time with men (Gibson, Heyward, and Mermier 2000).

What's the Use?

Until researchers find the definitive method to measure body fat, here's my advice. Consider body-fat measurement as a comparative tool to reflect changes in your body as you lose fat, gain muscle, shape up, and slim down. Don't expect more accuracy than is possible. The standard error is plus or minus 3 percent. Hence, if you are measured at 15 percent, you might be 12 percent or 18 percent. That doesn't take into account another 3 percent biological error because of individual variations in body fatness.

Just as weighing yourself on different scales results in different pound values, having your body fat measured by different people using different methods also results in different body-fat numbers. In a study done on 57 white male college students, their body fat ranged from 12.5 percent to 18.5 percent, depending on the method. This demonstrates the significant variability that occurs even under scientific conditions (Stout et al. 1994).

Your best bet is to see how the measurements change over time. Have the same person measure you at regular intervals to help you assess trends in your body-fat changes. But the measurements likely tell you nothing you didn't already know from looking at yourself in the mirror or from the fit of your clothing.

Words of Wisdom

I strongly recommend that instead of entrusting your fate to an unreliable number, you listen to your body. Each person has a set-point weight at which the body tends to hover. You may slightly overeat one day and slightly undereat the next, but your weight will stay more or less the same. If you drop below this natural weight, your body will start to talk to you. You may fight a nagging hunger, become obsessed with food, and feel chronically fatigued. On the other hand, if you are above your set point, you will feel uncomfortable and flabby.

My experience in counseling athletes of all ages and weights indicates that you likely do know your comfortable weight zone. As Tricia, a 5-foot, 2-inch masters swimmer, acknowledged, "I can diet down to 110 pounds, an appropriate weight for the average person of my height. But I don't stay there. My body is most comfortable between 117 and 120. That's heavier than most people my height, but that's what's normal for me and where I fit in with the rest of my family. Everyone is heavyset."

She had learned through years of unsuccessful dieting that she would never be able to fit her ideal image of perfectly thin. She has now accepted her build and recognizes that she can healthfully participate in sports regardless of the few extra pounds. Weight, after all, is more than a matter of willpower, and happiness is does not come from thinness.

CHAPTER 14

Adding Bulk, Not Fat

To listen to all the ads for diets and diet foods, one might think that the only people who struggle with weight concerns are those who want to lose body fat. Yet a significant number of people, primarily teenage boys and young men, and a few young women, struggle to gain weight. In a survey of 400 young men aged 13 to 18 (grades 7 to 12), 25 percent had deliberately tried to gain weight in the past 12 months (O'Dea and Rawstorne 2001). They wanted to bulk up by building bigger muscles so that they could be stronger, have a better body image, improve their sports performance, and better protect themselves in sports with physical contact such as football, soccer, rugby, hockey, boxing.

For those struggling to gain weight, eating can be a task, food a medicine, and the food bills an economic drain. Many skinny athletes devour doughnuts, cookies, ice cream, and fatty fried foods to help them pump in calories inexpensively (but unhealthfully). They often wonder about weight-gain drinks, thinking ordinary food is not good enough. That is not the case.

If you are feeling self-consciously thin, hate your skinny image, and seem to eat nonstop in hopes of putting a little meat on your bones, the information in this chapter, along with the protein information in chapter 7, can give you the knowledge you need to reach your goal healthfully.

Increasing Your Weight

Theoretically, to gain 1 pound (0.45 kg) of body weight per week, you'd need to consume an additional 500 calories per day above your typical intake. Some people are hard gainers and require more calories than other people do to add weight. In one landmark research study (Sims 1976), 200 prisoners with no family history of obesity volunteered to be gluttons. The goal was to gain 20 to 25 percent above their normal weights (about 30 to 40 pounds [14 to 18 kg]) by deliberately overeating. For more than half a year, the prisoners ate extravagantly and exercised minimally. Yet only 20 of the 200 prisoners managed to gain the weight. Of those, only 2 (who had an undetected family history of obesity or diabetes) gained the weight easily. One prisoner tried for 30 weeks to add 12 pounds (5 kg) to his 132-pound (60 kg) frame, but he couldn't get any fatter.

A varied response was also seen in another study of identical twins who were overfed by 1,000 calories for 100 days. Some twins gained only 9.5 pounds (4.3 kg), whereas others gained 29 pounds (13.2 kg). Each twin pair gained a similar amount of weight, suggesting strong genetic control (Bouchard 1990).

This discrepancy mystifies researchers. What happened to the excess calories that didn't turn into fat? Some say the body adjusts its metabolism to help maintain a predetermined genetic weight (Leibel, Rosenbaum, and Hirsch 1995). Others look at increases in fidgeting and greater activity in daily life (Levine, Eberhardt, and Jensen 1999).

If you are a hard gainer, take a good look at your genetic endowment. If other family members are thin, you probably have inherited a genetic predisposition to thinness. You can alter your physique to a certain extent with diet, weight training, and maturing, but you shouldn't expect miracles. Marathoner Bill Rodgers will never look like bodybuilder Charles Atlas, no matter how much eating and weightlifting he does.

Among my clients, I've observed that hard gainers are good fidgeters. They twiddle their fingers, swing their legs back and forth while sitting, and seem unable to sit still. All this involuntary movement burns calories. In comparison, the people who complain about their inability to lose weight generally sit calmly. I tell the fidgeters to mellow out. Chronic fidgeting can burn an extra 300 to 700 calories per day.

Extra Protein to Build Muscles?

Most people who want to bulk up believe that the best way to gain weight is to lift weights (true) and eat a very high protein diet (false). Although you do want to eat adequate protein, your body doesn't store excess protein as bulging muscles. The pound of steak just doesn't convert into bigger biceps. You need extra calories, and those calories should come primarily from extra carbohydrate rather than extra protein. Carbohydrate fuels your muscles so they can perform intense muscle-building exercise. By overloading the muscle not with protein but with weightlifting and other resistance exercise, the muscle fibers increase in size.

You are most likely to gain weight if you consistently eat larger-than-normal meals. I often counsel skinny athletes who swear they eat huge amounts of food. Peter, a swimmer, swore that he ate at least twice what his friends did. But he ate only two meals per day. Because he swam both before and after school, he lacked time to enjoy a hearty breakfast and afternoon snack. He found time to eat only lunch and dinner. Granted, he did eat a lot at those meals, but that merely compensated for the lack of breakfast and snacks.

Peter gained 3 pounds (1.4 kg) within three weeks after he started to eat three meals per day and an additional snack on a consistent basis. "I now look at food as my weight-gain medicine and have chosen to become more responsible and plan ahead so I have food with me at the right times. There are days when I'm rushed and almost forget about gathering my breakfast on the go—two energy bars and two juice boxes on my way to school. I've learned to put a big note on my swim bag, and that helps me remember to pack my sports breakfast. I'm enjoying the benefits—more energy, less morning hunger, plus a few pounds extra weight."

Keith, a 6-foot, 4-inch high school basketball player, expressed a different complaint about his efforts to gain weight. He felt embarrassed whenever he ate with his friends because he'd eat twice what they did. A large pizza was no challenge. When I calculated his calorie needs, he began to understand why he wasn't gaining weight. He needed about 6,000 calories per day to maintain his weight, plus more to gain weight. The pizza was 1,800 calories. Two pizzas would have been more appropriate.

I told Keith to feed his body what it needed and stop comparing his food intake with that of his shorter friends. I suggested that he explain to any teasers that his body was like a limousine that needed more gas to go the distance.

Boosting Your Calories

The trick to gaining weight is to eat larger-than-normal portions consistently for three meals per day and one or two snacks. If you have a busy schedule, finding the time to eat can be the biggest challenge to boosting your calories. You might need to pack a stash of portable snacks in your gym bag if you do most of your eating outside the home. To take in the extra calories needed to gain weight, you should eat frequently throughout the day, if that fits your lifestyle. Plan to have food on hand for every eating opportunity, or try these tips: eat an extra snack, such as a bedtime peanut butter sandwich with a glass of milk, and eat higher-calorie foods.

If you eat foods that are compact and dense (e.g., granola instead of puffed rice), more calories can fit into your stomach with less volume. Keith became an avid food-label reader; he learned that 8 ounces (240 ml) of orange juice has 110 calories, while 8 ounces of cran-apple juice has 160 calories; a cup of (canned) green beans has 40 calories, a cup of (canned) corn, 140; a cup of Bran Flakes, 200 calories; a cup of granola, 780. He then chose more calorie-dense foods.

When you make your food selections, keep in mind that fat is the most concentrated form of calories. One teaspoon of fat (butter, oil, margarine, or mayonnaise) has 36 calories; the same amount of carbohydrate or protein has only 16 calories. Most protein-rich foods contain fat (such as the cream in cheese, the grease in hamburgers, and the oil in peanut butter) and therefore tend to be calorie dense. But some of the forms of fat in such foods are bad for your health: the saturated fat in cheese, beef, butter, and bacon.

Try to limit your intake of bad fat and focus on healthful fat, such as peanut butter, walnuts, almonds, avocado, olive oil, and oily fish such as salmon and tuna. You should still eat a basic high-carbohydrate sports diet. Eating too much fatty food leaves your muscles underfueled.

Boost Those Calories!

These choices alone in one day will boost your calories by 890!

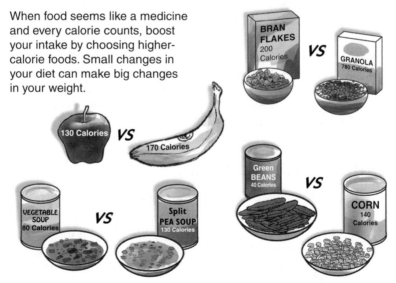

When food seems like a medicine and every calorie counts, boost your intake by choosing higher-calorie foods. Small changes in your diet can make big changes in your weight.

BRAN FLAKES 200 Calories **VS** GRANOLA 780 Calories

130 Calories **VS** 170 Calories

Green BEANS 40 Calories **VS** CORN 140 Calories

VEGETABLE SOUP 80 Calories **VS** Split PEA SOUP 130 Calories

The following foods and beverages can help you healthfully boost your calorie intake:

Cold cereal. Choose dense cereals (as opposed to flaked and puffed types), such as granola, Grape-Nuts, and Wheat Chex. Top with nuts, sunflower seeds, ground flaxseed, raisins, bananas, or other fruits.

Hot cereal. Cooking with milk instead of water adds calories and nutritional value. Add still more calories with mix-ins such as powdered milk, margarine, peanut butter, walnuts, sunflower seeds, wheat germ, ground flaxseed, and dried fruit.

Juices. Apple, cranberry, cran-apple, grape, pineapple, and most of the juice blends (such as mango-orange-banana) have more calories than do grapefruit, orange, or tomato juice. To increase the calorie value of orange juice, use frozen concentrate and add less water than the directions indicate—or simply drink a larger glassful.

Fruits. Bananas, pineapple, mangos, raisins, dates, dried apricots, and other dried fruits contain more calories than watery fruits such as grapefruit, plums, and peaches. Blend milk with fruit and enjoy fruit smoothies.

Milk. To boost the calorie value of milk, add 1/4 cup (30 g) of powdered milk to 1 cup (240 ml) of 2-percent milk. Or try malt powder, Ovaltine, Carnation Instant Breakfast, Nesquik, and other flavorings. Mix these up by the quart so they are waiting for you in the refrigerator. You can also make blender drinks such as milk shakes and fruit smoothies. Fixing these kinds of drinks is far less expensive than buying canned liquid meal supplements, which are typically just milk-based formulas with added vitamins. Plus, your homemade drinks taste much better. See chapter 24 for recipes.

Toast. Spread with generous amounts of peanut butter; soft, tub margarines (preferably made with canola oil); jam; or honey.

Sandwiches. Select hearty, dense breads (as opposed to fluffy types) such as sprouted wheat, honey bran, rye, and pumpernickel. The bigger and more thickly sliced, the better. Spread with a moderate amount of margarine or mayonnaise. Stuff with tuna, chicken, hummus, or other fillings. Peanut butter and jelly makes an inexpensive, healthful, and high-calorie choice.

Soups. Hearty lentil, split-pea, minestrone, and barley soups have more calories than brothy chicken and beef types, unless the broth is chock-full of veggies and meat. To make canned soups (such as tomato or chowder) more substantial, add evaporated milk in place of water or regular milk, or add extra powdered milk. Garnish with margarine, parmesan cheese, and croutons. If you wish to reduce your sodium intake, be sure to choose the reduced-sodium soups or homemade varieties.

Meats. Beef, pork, and lamb tend to have more calories than do chicken or fish, but they also tend to have more saturated fat. Eat them in moderation, and choose lean cuts. To boost calories, saute chicken or fish in canola or olive oil, and add wine sauces and bread-crumb toppings.

Beans, legumes. Lentils, split-pea soup, chili with beans, bean burritos, limas, and other dried beans are not only calorie dense but also packed with protein and carbohydrate. Hummus (made with chickpeas) is an easy snack, dip, or sandwich filling.

Vegetables. Peas, corn, carrots, winter squash, and beets have more calories than do green beans, broccoli, summer squash, and other watery veggies. Top with margarine, slivered almonds, and grated low-fat cheese. Add calories by stir-frying veggies in olive oil instead of steaming them.

Salads. What may start out being low-calorie lettuce can quickly become a substantial meal by adding cottage cheese, garbanzo beans (chickpeas), sunflower seeds, assorted vegetables, chopped walnuts, raisins, dried cranberries, tuna fish, lean meat, croutons, and a liberal dousing of salad dressing made with heart-healthy oil, preferably olive or canola.

Potatoes. Add soft, tub margarine and extra powdered milk to mashed potatoes. Although you might be tempted to add lots of butter and gravy for extra calories, think again. You'd also be adding saturated fat, which is unhealthful for your heart. Reduced-fat sour cream and low-fat gravies would be better alternatives.

Desserts. By selecting desserts with nutritional value, you can enjoy treats as well as nourish your body. Try oatmeal raisin cookies, fig bars, chocolate pudding, strawberry shortcake, low-fat frozen yogurt, apple crisp, or other fruit desserts. Blueberry muffins, cornbread with honey, banana bread, and other sweet breads and muffins can double as dessert. See the recipes in chapter 17 for ideas.

Snacks. Instead of a small snack, think "second lunch" and "second dinner." A second lunch at 3:00 p.m. or second dinner at 10:00 p.m. is an excellent way to boost your calorie intake. Pack an extra sandwich. At dinner, cook enough for a second meal. If you don't feel hungry, just think of the food as the weight-gain medicine you need to take.

If you aren't interested in or able to eat a whole second meal, at least enjoy some snacks. Healthful snack choices include fruit yogurt, low-fat cheese and crackers, peanuts, sunflower seeds, almonds, granola, pretzels, English muffins, multigrain bagels (with low-fat cream cheese and jelly), bran muffins, pizza, peanut butter on crackers, milk shakes, instant breakfast drinks, hot cocoa, fruit smoothies, bananas, dried fruits, trail mix, and even sandwiches.

Alcohol. Moderate amounts of beer and wine can stimulate your appetite and add extra calories, particularly when consumed with snacks such as peanuts and popcorn. Because alcohol offers little nutritional value, do not substitute it for juices, milk, or other wholesome beverages. Do not drink if you are underage, and never drink alcohol shortly before an event. It has a dehydrating effect, to say nothing of its potential to blunt reflexes, create problems with hypoglycemia, and hurt performance.

The sample menus in table 14.1 implement some of these suggestions. You can see how smart choices can accumulate into a hefty, carbohydrate-rich calorie intake that can help you meet your weight goals.

Table 14.1 Sample Weight Gain Menus

Menu plan 1	Approximate calories	Menu plan 2	Approximate calories
Breakfast			
16 oz (480 ml) orange juice	200	16 oz (480 ml) pineapple juice	280
6 pancakes	600	1 cup granola	500
1/4 cup syrup	200	1/4 cup raisins	120
1 pat margarine	50	16 oz (480 ml) low-fat milk	200
8 oz (240 ml) low-fat milk	100	1 large banana	130
Total	**1150**	**Total**	**1230**
Lunch			
4 slices hearty bread	400	1 7 in. (18 cm) pita pocket	240
6 oz (175 g) can tuna	200	6 oz (175 g) turkey breast	300
4 tbsp light mayo	200	2 tbsp light mayo	100
1 bowl lentil soup	250	16 oz (480 ml) apple juice	250
2 oatmeal cookies	100	1 medium muffin	300
16 oz (480 ml) low-fat milk	200	1 cup fruit yogurt	230
Total	**1350**	**Total**	**1420**
Second lunch			
2 slices hearty bread	200	1 large NY-style bagel	450
2 tbsp peanut butter	200	3 oz (90 g) light cheese	250
3 tbsp jelly	150	16 oz (480 ml) cran-grape juice	350
12 oz (360 ml) low-fat milk	150		
2 tbsp chocolate powder	100		
Total	**800**	**Total**	**1050**
Dinner			
1 medium cheese pizza	1,400	6 oz (170 g) chicken breast	300
16 oz (480 ml) lemonade	200	2 large potatoes	400
		2 pats margarine	100
		1 cup peas	100
		2 biscuits	300
		2 tbsp honey	100
		16 oz (480 ml) low-fat milk	200
Total	**1600**	**Total**	**1500**
Total calories for day	**4,900**	**Total calories for day**	**5,200**
60% carbohydrate (745 g)		65% carbohydrate (832 g)	
15% protein (193 g)		15% protein (180 g)	
25% fat (121 g)		20% fat (123 g)	

Weight-Gain Drinks

Weight-gain drinks (with enticing names such as Muscle Milk, N-Large, Muscle Juice, and Serious Mass) are high-calorie beverages (more than 500 calories per serving) that are more about convenience than necessity. A big jug of powder might cost as much as $55; the price for 1,000 calories ranges between $2.50 and $4.50, which is more than a few peanut butter and jelly sandwiches. The commercial weight-gain drinks do not offer any advantage you cannot get from eating real food (Godard, Williamson, and Trappe 2002) or by making your own weight-gain drink. But if you lack the time or inclination to make extra sandwiches and smoothies, weight-gain drinks can be a convenient way to consume adequate calories.

The ingredients in weight-gain drinks vary from brand to brand, but all brands supply plenty of protein to help build muscle and plenty of carbohydrate to help fuel muscle-building exercise plus the muscle-building process itself. The products are generally fortified with vitamins and minerals—and possibly other questionable ingredients as well. (Remember, the sports supplement industry is poorly regulated.) Weight-gain drinks tend to be low in (saturated) fat, which offers an advantage over boosting your calories with French fries, cheeseburgers, and ice cream.

As for what to look for in a weight-gain drink, the most important factor is taste. If you enjoy your calories, you'll have an easier time sticking to your weight-gain program. Each brand touts the type(s) of protein it has—whey, casein, egg, soy—and the type of carbohydrate—glucose, fructose, and glucose polymers (also called maltodextrins). Consuming a blend of protein and carbohydrate provides varying speeds of absorption, which creates a sustained release effect—similar to what you get with standard foods. Assuming your meals include a balance of protein- and carbohydrate-rich foods, you are likely already meeting your goals for those nutrients: 0.7 to 0.8 grams of protein per pound of body weight (1.5 to 1.7 g per kg); 3 to 5 grams of carbohydrate per pound of body weight (6 to 10 g per kg). Hence, you are using the weight-gain drinks for convenient, concentrated calories.

The type of carbohydrate, protein, or weight-gain drink you consume as a supplement to your sports diet will likely have an insignificant long-term impact on your ability to reach your weight goals. The biggest impact comes from your genetics, training intensity, timing of fueling, and ability to consistently consume additional calories.

If you are a collegiate athlete, be sure to follow the NCAA guidelines regarding acceptable weight-gain supplements. Like the NCAA, I believe that proper nutrition based on scientific principles, not commercial supplements, should lay the foundation for optimal performance. Generations of athletes have built muscles with hard work and real foods. You can, too.

Eating at the Right Times

If you are serious about gaining muscle weight, you need to have the right foods available at the right times so you can eat strategically and optimize muscular growth. The following actions will help you reach your goals:

- Fuel up before you strength-train with a carbohydrate–protein snack, such as a yogurt or bowl of cereal with milk. The snack will digest into readily available glucose for fuel and amino acids to protect muscles.

- Refuel immediately afterward with more protein to heal and rebuild muscles and more carbohydrate to refuel depleted glycogen stores.

- Eat frequently throughout the day. Eat at least every four hours: breakfast, lunch, a second lunch (if you train in the afternoon, split this meal into pre- and postexercise snacks), dinner, and an evening snack as desired. This even distribution of calories ensures that the muscles have a steady supply of glucose for fuel and amino acids for growth. When the amino acid levels in the blood are above normal, the muscles take up more of these building blocks; this enhances muscle growth. If you go for long periods without eating, your body will break down muscles for fuel; this happens to dieters and is counterproductive to reaching your goals.

You might be wondering how much of a difference meal timing really makes. The answer is quite a bit. A study of recreational male bodybuilders who consumed about 270 calories of carbohydrate–protein supplement immediately before and after midday exercise, as compared with taking the same supplement in the morning and evening (away from the workout), indicates significantly greater muscular growth at the end of a 10-week program—about 6 pounds versus 3.3 pounds (2.8 kg versus 1.5 kg) of muscle. That's almost twice as much gain! The bodybuilders who fueled before and after training were also able to bench press 27 more pounds (12.2 more kg) by the end of the study, as compared with only 20 more pounds (9 more kg) for the group who fueled in the morning and evening (Cribb and Hayes 2006). Clearly, when you eat makes a difference.

Eating several protein-containing meals and snacks is preferable to eating one big dinner at the end of the day. A simple way to ensure that a source of high-quality protein is readily available is to drink milk with meals and eat yogurt for snacks. Other examples of carbohydrate–protein combinations include chocolate milk, cereal with milk, a turkey sandwich, a fruit smoothie, an apple with cheese, a canned liquid meal (such as Boost or Slim-Fast), or any number of commercial sports foods. The muscle-building supplement used in the previously noted study included about 32 grams of whey protein, 34 grams of sugar (glucose) for fuel, and 5.5 grams of creatine, known to enhance muscle mass and strength during resistance exercise (Cribb and Hayes 2006).

Balancing Your Weight-Gain Diet

The best and simplest weight-gain diet follows a pumped-up version of the fundamental guidelines for healthy eating as described in chapter 1. I suggest that you keep food records for a few days to assess your typical intake, then figure out where you could plug in more calories. Steve, a volleyball player, described to me what he typically ate, and together we listed ways he could consume more, without much effort, at certain times of the day. The following chart shows what Steve typically ate as well as some suggestions for how he could work more calories into his daily intake:

Typical intake	Calorie booster	Added calories
Breakfast		
1 bagel	Another bagel	+300
2 tbsp peanut butter	Another 2 tbsp peanut butter	+200
8 oz (240 ml) orange juice	Another 8 oz (240 ml) orange juice	+100
Lunch		
1 sandwich	Another 1/2 sandwich	+200
8 oz (240 ml) milk	Another 8 oz (240 ml) milk	+100
1 cookie	Another cookie	+100
Snack		
Nothing	Granola bar	+200
	Cran-apple juice	+200
Dinner		
Lasagna	Apple	+100
Salad		
Bread		
Milk		

By adding more to his meals and snack, he could potentially pump his intake by 1,500 calories. Granted, that is a lot of additional food. He might not eat all of that every day, but at least he knew how to get more calories with little fuss or effort. He just needed to be responsible and set aside enough time to eat the extra calories.

If you are into the mathematical approach to weight gain, follow this more complex plan: Your muscles become saturated with glycogen when fed about 3 to 5 grams of carbohydrate per pound (6 to 10 g per kg) of body weight, and your body uses less than 1 gram of protein per pound (2 g per kg) under growth conditions, so your primary dietary goal is to satisfy these requirements for carbohydrate and protein. Then you can choose the balance of the calories from a variety of (preferably healthful) sources of fat or carbohydrate.

For example, Alex, a high school football player, wanted to gain weight. He was 5 feet, 10 inches (178 cm), weighed 140 pounds (64 kg), and wanted to gain 15 to 20 pounds (7 to 9 kg). I calculated that he was maintaining his weight at about 3,000 calories per day, and I recommended that he eat about 20 percent more to gain weight and try to hit the following targets.

Caloric increase. First, we calculated what a 20 percent increase in calories would mean for his daily eating plan:

$$20\% \times 3{,}000 \text{ cal} = \text{about } 600 \text{ more cal} = 3{,}600 \text{ total cal} =$$
$$4 \text{ meals at } 900 \text{ cal each}$$

Carbohydrate. Then, we calculated his carbohydrate requirements by planning for him to consume 4 grams of carbohydrate per pound of body weight. Remember, the carbohydrate consumption target is about 3 to 5 grams per pound, or about 6 to 10 grams per kilogram. This recommendation results in about 55 to 65 percent of calories from grains, fruits, vegetables, and other forms of carbohydrate.

$$4 \text{ g carb} \times 140 \text{ lb} = 560 \text{ g carb}$$
$$560 \text{ g carb} \times 4 \text{ cal} = 2{,}240 \text{ cal carb}$$
$$2{,}240 \text{ cal carb} / 3{,}600 \text{ total cal} = 62\% \text{ cal carb}$$

Thus, Alex needed about 560 carbohydrate calories (140 g carb) in each of his four meals per day).

Protein. His protein target was 0.7 to 0.9 grams of protein per pound (1.5 to 2.0 g per kg), resulting in about 12 to 15 percent of calories from lean meats, beans, nuts, and low-fat dairy products.

$$0.8 \text{ g protein} \times 140 \text{ lb} = 112 \text{ g protein}$$
$$112 \text{ g protein} \times 4 \text{ calories} = 448 \text{ cal protein}$$
$$448 \text{ cal protein} / 3{,}600 \text{ total cal} = 12\% \text{ cal protein}$$

Therefore, Alex needed about 40 grams of protein at three meals per day (or he could spread his protein intake over four meals a day plus snacks).

Fat. The balance of Alex's daily calories should come primarily from the healthful fat in peanut butter, nuts, and olive and canola oil, which places Alex's fat consumption in the recommended range of 25 to 30 percent of total calories.

$$26\% \times 3,600 \text{ total calories} = 936 \text{ cal fat}$$
$$936 \text{ cal fat} / 9 \text{ cal} = 104 \text{ g fat}$$

This means that Alex could include about 26 grams of primarily healthful fat at each of his four meals.

I taught another client, Martin, how to read food labels to learn more about the composition of the foods he was eating. He was surprised to learn that he could get most of his protein requirement from one 6-ounce (175 g) can of tuna (40 grams of protein) at lunch, two chicken breasts at dinner (80 grams of protein), and 1 quart (1 L) of low-fat milk (40 grams of protein) throughout the day. He no longer felt compelled to eat egg-white omelets for breakfast and to buy expensive protein bars for snacks. Instead, he ate balanced carbohydrate-based meals, such as tuna on a hefty whole-grain sub roll and 16 ounces (480 ml) of low-fat chocolate milk at lunch, then chicken, two baked potatoes, a hefty salad, and more milk at dinner.

Patience Is a Virtue

By consuming the prescribed 500 to 1,000 additional calories per day, you should see some weight gain. Be sure to include muscle-building resistance exercise (weight workouts, push-ups) to promote muscular growth rather than just fat deposits. Consult with the trainer at your school, health club, or gym for a specific exercise program that suits your needs. You may also want to have your body fat routinely measured to make sure your weight gain is indeed mostly muscle, not fat. Untrained men might gain about 3 pounds (1.5 kg) of muscle per month initially. The rate of gain in well-trained athletes is slower.

If you don't gain weight, look at your family members to see if you inherited a naturally trim physique. If everyone is thin, accept your physique and concentrate on improving your athletic skills. Rather than drain your energy fretting about being too thin, capitalize on being light, swift, and agile. You will likely be able to surpass the heavier hulks that lack your speed.

Also keep in mind that most people gain weight with age. If you are still growing or are in your 20s, your turn to bulk up may still come. All too often, scrawny young athletes fatten up once they get out of school and start working. That's why I hesitate to encourage my clients to force-feed themselves. Doing so upsets the natural appetite regulatory mechanisms, and people lose the natural ability to stop eating when they are content.

Such was the case with Wes, a 30-year-old photographer and former football player. He reported with a sigh, "I was skinny all through high school. In college, my football coach insisted that I gain weight by eating extra buttered bread, piles of French fries, and mounds of ice cream. I developed quite a liking for these foods. I continued to eat them even after I'd reached my weight-gain goals. Voila—look at me now! I'm 60 pounds overweight and can barely walk, to say nothing of play football. I long for those days when I was lean and mean."

With a food plan that contained no fatty snacks or sugary soft drinks, Wes did lose weight over the course of a year. That fall, he coached an after-school football program. He advised the thin kids to be patient, eat healthfully, and develop smart, lifelong eating habits.

I offer you the same advice. To gain weight, you need to choose larger portions of healthful foods at meals and snacks, eat on a regular schedule—no skipped or skimpy meals—and be responsible. You need to work hard to eat your fill consistently. You also have to work hard at weightlifting and other muscle-building exercise.

Questions From Parents of Skinny Kids

If you are the parent of a skinny kid, you undoubtedly want to help your child add weight healthfully—without eating tons of ice cream, super-sized fast-food meals, and expensive (as well as questionable) nutrition supplements. The following are some answers to the questions parents commonly ask about how to support appropriate weight gain in growing kids.

Q: My 16-year-old son insists that I buy him protein powders and weight-gain drinks so he can bulk up. Are these necessary?

A: No. The single most important thing your son needs is extra calories to perform resistance exercise, which builds muscle. Most of these extra calories should come from carbohydrate (not protein supplements) because carbohydrate will fuel his muscles and give him the energy he needs for exercise. I recommend replacing water (apart from during exercise) with extra juice and low-fat milk as a simple way to boost calories. Note that even with no exercise, just eating extra calories stimulates a little muscle growth. Sedentary people gain about 1 pound of muscle with every 3 pounds of total weight that creeps on.

Q: My 12-year-old son is shorter than many of the girls his age. He feels embarrassed and asked me about protein supplements. Would they help him grow faster?

A: No amount of extra protein will speed the growth process. Boys generally grow fastest between the ages of 13 and 14. After this growth spurt, he will have enough male hormones to add muscle mass and start to grow a beard ("peach fuzz"). This growth spurt lasts longer in boys than in girls. After the growth spurt, boys continue to grow slowly until about age 20.

Q: My 13-year-old son wants to start lifting weights to bulk up for football. Should he?

A: A well-supervised weightlifting program (to prevent stress on immature bones and ligaments) with light weights can help your son grow stronger and help prevent injuries. But it will not contribute to bulkier muscles until he has enough male hormones to support muscular development. (This corresponds with the growth of adultlike pubic hair.) Boys generally bulk up after they have finished their growth spurts. Remind him that patience is a virtue!

Q: Is creatine a safe way to gain weight?

A: Creatine is a naturally occurring compound found in meat and fish. Creatine is also available in powder and pills. The muscles use creatine phosphate to generate energy for one to ten seconds of intense work (such as occurs in weightlifting, wrestling, ice hockey, and sprinting). In people who respond to creatine supplements, their muscles may perform better during these brief, all-out exercise bouts (Terjung et al. 2000). But not everyone responds.

Research to date suggests that creatine causes no physical harm if taken in the recommended doses. The initial weight gain commonly seen with creatine supplementation may be due to water gain, but in the long term, the gain can be attributed to muscle mass. To date, no sports medicine organization has recommended the use of creatine in individuals under the age of 18; its use has not been extensively tested in growing children.

Q: My 14-year-old son is uncomfortable with his scrawny physique. He's heard that creatine will help him gain weight and asked me to buy some for him. What should I tell him?

A: As a 14-year-old, your son is at an impressionable age. Taking a muscle-building, performance-enhancing substance establishes a risky attitude that could lead to the desire to take other dangerous substances down the road. Your job is to encourage him to do his best and discourage a win-at-all-cost attitude. Although you must be truthful about possible benefits from the use of creatine, you can also send a strong message that discourages the use of creatine in young bodies that are still growing.

Remind your son that there is no shortcut to excellent performance; it takes hard work. He will be proud when he achieves his weight goals "the old-fashioned way," with dedicated training and good nutrition. Tell him you think that using this substance is a poor choice for him. Remind him that the body he has at age 14 is not the body he will have when he is 15, 16, 17, or 18. He can look forward to lots of natural growth and development.

CHAPTER 15

Losing Weight Without Starving

Weight loss is far more complex than the simple recommendation to "just eat less and exercise more." Both serious athletes and fitness exercisers struggle to either lose weight or keep off the weight they have lost. Why is weight loss so difficult? Does the body adapt to a reduced calorie intake? Does dieting "ruin your metabolism"? Or do dieters just have poor compliance? The answer, to date, seems to be that most people have trouble with compliance; it's hard to eat less food (Heymsfield et al. 2007).

As a result of the abundance of yummy food that pervades our environments, flabby thighs and big butts (either real or perceived) haunt many active people. Hence, they work extra hard to burn calories and trim excess body fat. Although some of them successfully lose weight and attribute that loss to their exercise programs, others express frustration that they don't shed an ounce of fat despite consistent workouts. As Sarah, an avid runner and newspaper editor, complained, "I've been running for 10 years now, and I haven't lost a single pound. I must be doing something wrong." Her husband, Peter, had the opposite experience. "I started going to the gym a month ago. I've painlessly dropped 5 pounds." Yes, gender differences exist when it comes to exercise and weight loss.

The purpose of this chapter is to help you learn how to lose body fat by appropriately managing your food supply. You'll learn how to eat wisely, improve your health, have energy to enjoy exercise, and be able to lose excess body fat without feeling denied or deprived. Yes, despite popular belief, you can lose weight without dieting. Even if you are a bodybuilder, wrestler, lightweight rower, or other athlete who needs to make weight for your sport, the same rules that apply to fitness exercisers also apply to you.

Diets Don't Work

Because I'm a dietitian, most of my clients assume that I will put them on a diet. I don't. I teach them how to eat healthfully and appropriately. Athletes—and all people, for that matter—who go on a diet simply go off a diet. They have a high chance of not only regaining all the lost weight but also regaining proportionately more fat than muscle. That represents a lot of wasted (or is that waisted?) effort.

Dieting conjures up visions of rice cakes, salad with fat-free dressing, and Shredded Wheat with skim milk. Diets can actually contribute to a person's weight problem because they are associated with extreme hunger. The body rebels against hunger and the state of starvation by triggering binge eating, more commonly known as blowing the diet, and the dieter gains weight despite extreme efforts to lose weight.

A study of 4,746 teens indicates that those who dieted in the fourth grade ended up heavier in high school. Dieting was associated with weight gain (to the classification of "overweight"), disordered eating, and eating disorders (Neumark-Sztainer et al. 2006). Another study of 370 male athletes (boxers, weightlifters, wrestlers) who had to make weight for their sports suggests they were at higher risk of becoming obese later in life, as compared with a control group of nonathletes (Saarni et al. 2006). Dieting is simply the wrong way to try to lose weight.

To lose weight healthfully and to successfully keep it off without dieting, you must pay attention to the following:

- **How much you eat.** There is an appropriate portion of any food.
- **When you eat.** Enjoy big breakfasts rather than big dinners.
- **Why you eat.** Eat when your body needs fuel, not when you are simply bored, stressed, or lonely.

We can learn a lot about weight reduction from people who have lost weight and kept it off. According to the National Weight Control Registry (a sample of more than 5,000 people who have lost more than 30 pounds and have kept it off for more than a year), the tricks to losing weight and keeping it off include the following (Wing and Phelan 2005):

- Get enough sleep.

- Weigh yourself regularly (once a week).
- Eat breakfast.
- Choose a lower-fat (less than 25 percent fat) food plan.
- Eat consistently, and maintain the same eating patterns on weekends as on weekdays.
- Engage in regular (and often vigorous) exercise for about an hour a day.

Yet, there is not one weight-reduction food plan that fits everyone.

The upcoming section includes numerous food-management tips to help you achieve your weight-loss goals. But before attempting a weight-loss program, you might want to get your body fat measured (see chapter 13). By knowing what percentage of your weight is excess body fat, you'll have a valid perspective for setting an appropriate weight goal. All too often I counsel active people who weigh more than they desire, but their weight is primarily muscle with little excess fat. No wonder they struggle with trying to reduce.

Avoiding Weight Gain

The best way to deal with weight loss is to not gain the weight in the first place. That's where exercise helps. A seven-year survey of about 6,100 male and 2,200 female runners who participated in the National Runners' Health Study indicates those who ran more miles gained less weight (Williams 2007).

On average, the men and women who ran more than 30 miles (48 kilometers) per week gained half the weight of those who ran less than 15 miles (24 kilometers). And all the runners gained less weight than their sedentary peers.

The 25- to 34-year-old men gained about

- 1.4 pounds (0.6 kg) annually if they ran less than 15 miles per week,
- 0.8 pound (0.4 kg) annually if they ran between 15 and 30 miles per week, and
- 0.6 pound (0.3 kg) annually if they ran more than 30 miles per week.
- This trend is mirrored in women. Women between the ages of 18 and 25 gained about
- 2 pounds (0.9 kg) annually if they ran less than 15 miles per week,
- 1.4 pounds (0.6 kg) annually if they ran 15 to 30 miles per week, and
- 0.75 pound (0.4 kg) annually if they ran more than 30 miles per week.

Other benefits to running more miles each week included fewer inches gained around the waist in both men and women and fewer inches added to the hips in women.

Losing Weight by Eating More

If diets worked, then everyone who has ever gone on a diet would be thin. That's not what happens. Most dieters are heavy. The way to lose weight for the long haul is to learn how to eat—healthfully and appropriately. Chapters 1 and 2 offer guidelines for making healthful food choices. This chapter builds on that information to help you choose the right portions at the right times so that you can lose weight without feeling denied or deprived. I'll teach you nutrition skill power, which is more powerful than the willpower you might yearn for. Such was the case with Roberta, a 42-year-old computer programmer, mother of two teenagers, and fitness runner.

"If only I had more willpower, I could lose weight," Roberta complained. "I've been trying to lose these same 8 to 10 pounds for 12, yes 12, years. I'm the diet queen!" Feeling completely helpless, Roberta came to me as a last resort to help her achieve her weight goals.

When reviewing her dieting history, I noticed that Roberta needed a more realistic food plan. She would diet by trying to exist on coffee for breakfast, salad for lunch, yogurt for a snack, and fish with vegetables for dinner. Her intake was spartan, to say the least, and it included a limited variety of food. I asked, "When you are not dieting, what do you eat?" She quickly listed her favorite foods (what she fed her children): cereal for breakfast, peanut butter and jelly sandwich for lunch, spaghetti for dinner. Every time she went on her diet to lose weight, she denied herself these favorite foods. She went to extremes to keep cereal and peanut butter out of her sight so that she wouldn't eat them. She deemed them too much temptation for her weak willpower, so she had her kids hide them from her.

I encouraged Roberta to stop looking at food as being fattening and instead start fueling her body appropriately with satisfying meals. Eating good food, after all, is one of life's pleasures. Given that she had liked cereal, breads, and pasta since childhood, she was naive to think she could stop liking them. Instead of trying to keep these foods out of her life, I encouraged her to eat them more often. I pointed out that her standard diet foods (salad, yogurt, and fish) had no power over her because she gave herself permission to eat them whenever she wanted. I encouraged her to eat an adequate portion of cereal every day for breakfast (and even lunch, dinner, and snacks) to take the power away from that food.

If you, too, struggle with weight issues, you need to learn how to manage your favorite foods, not how to deny yourself of them. By enjoying appropriate portions of whatever you'd like to eat, as often as you'd like, you no longer need willpower to avoid them. Nutrition skill power, not willpower, enhances permanent weight loss without denial and deprivation.

One skill that enhances your ability to eat appropriate food portions is to eat mindfully (not mindlessly). That is, chew the food s-l-o-w-l-y, taste it, and savor each mouthful. By doing so, you'll need far less quantity to be satisfied, and you'll be content to eat a smaller portion. By mindfully eating your favorite foods, you will also defuse the urge to do last-chance eating. (You know, "Last chance to eat peanut butter before I go back on my diet. I'd better have another spoonful!") You can enjoy more peanut butter—even in a sandwich—when your body becomes hungry again. Nutrition skill power wins in the end.

A second skill that enhances weight loss is to eat "closer to the earth" and choose more whole foods: fruits, vegetables, unrefined grains, and other fiber-rich foods. Fiber can assist with weight loss by promoting satiety and delaying a return of hunger, which contributes to eating less in subsequent meals. Calorie for calorie, fiber-rich fruits, veggies, and whole grains are more satiating than sugary sodas, lollipops, and gummy bears. You still need to limit calories, but you can feel fuller on calories from wholesome foods.

By regularly choosing wholesome forms of carbohydrate, lean meats, and low-fat dairy, you'll not only lose weight but also reduce your risk of cancer, heart disease, and hypertension. The food plan that helps you manage your weight should be consistent with dietary guidelines for healthy eating. Don't go on a crazy diet only to regain the weight you lost because you failed to learn how to eat healthfully.

One Size Does Not Fit All

Time and again, I hear people complain, "I know what I should do to lose weight. I just don't do it." Lack of control over food has humbled these knowledgeable dieters. The truth is that successful weight reduction isn't as easy as it sounds, because one diet does not fit everyone. That's why professional advice, individually tailored to a person's lifestyle and food preferences, is far more effective than packaged programs or self-inflicted diets.

If you want to lose weight for the last time, I recommend that you get personalized professional guidance from a registered dietitian (RD), preferably one who is a board certified specialist in sports dietetics (CSSD). This health professional has fulfilled specific educational requirements, has passed a registration exam, and is a recognized member of the largest organization of nutrition professionals in the United States, the American Dietetic Association. Because some states lack specific standards defining who can rightfully call himself or herself a dietitian or nutritionist, you can protect yourself from frauds and nutrition gurus by seeking guidance from RDs. To find your local RD, use the referral networks at www.eatright. org and www.SCANdpg.org.

Counting Calories—Correctly

Most of my dieting clients are afraid to eat real meals. They believe that eating, let's say, a tuna sandwich makes people fat. Eating diet foods, such as rice cakes and carrots, feels safer. The problem is that self-created diets commonly allow too few calories and too limited a selection of (boring) foods. The dieter ends up becoming too hungry and craves calorie-dense foods (Gilhooly et al. 2007). As a result, he or she blows the diet and regains any lost weight, plus more.

I calculate for my clients an appropriate calorie budget so that they know how much is OK to eat to maintain or lose weight. Just as you know how much money you can spend when you shop, you might find it helpful to know how many calories you can spend when you eat. A calorie, or more correctly, a kilocalorie, is a measure of energy. It is the amount of heat needed to raise one liter of water by one degree Celsius. (If you need to convert kilocalories to kilojoules, you can do so by multiplying the number of calories by 4.1868.) To assess your calorie needs, you should meet with a registered dietitian. Alternatively, you can use a "calorie calculator" on the Web (see appendix A), or you can make a ballpark estimate of your calorie needs by using the following steps.

   1. **Estimate your resting metabolic rate**—the number of calories you need simply to breathe, pump blood, and be alive (see table 15.1)—by multiplying your healthy weight by 10 calories per pound (or 22 calories per kilogram). If you are significantly overweight, use an adjusted weight, a weight about halfway between your desired weight and your current weight. That is, if you weigh 160 pounds but at one time normally weighed 120 pounds, use 140 as your adjusted weight. For example,

Table 15.1   Resting Metabolic Rate

Organ	Calories per day*	Percentage of resting metabolic rate
Brain	365	21
Heart	180	10
Kidneys	120	7
Liver	560	32
Lungs	160	9
Other tissues	370	21

*Number of calories burned by a 150-pound (68 kilogram) man while resting in bed all day.

Roberta weighed about 130 pounds but could healthfully weigh about 120 pounds. Hence, she needed approximately 1,200 calories (120 ×10) simply to do nothing all day except exist.

2. Add more calories for daily activity apart from your purposeful exercise. If you are moderately active throughout the day, add about 50 percent of your resting metabolic rate (RMR). If you are sedentary, add 20 to 40 percent; if very active (in addition to your purposeful exercise), add 60 to 80 percent of your RMR. Roberta was moderately active throughout the day with her two kids and her job. She burned about 600 calories (50 percent × 1,200 calories) for activities of daily living. Her totals were as follows:

$$1,200 \text{ RMR} + 600 \text{ cal daily activity} = 1,800 \text{ cal per day}$$
$$(\text{without purposeful exercise})$$

3. Add more calories for purposeful exercise. For example, when Roberta went to the health club, she exercised aerobically for about 45 minutes and burned about 400 calories on the treadmill. Hence, this was her total calorie need:

$$1,200 \text{ cal RMR} + 600 \text{ cal daily activity} + 400 \text{ cal purposeful exercise} =$$
$$2,200 \text{ total cal/day}$$

Be honest and accurate in assessing your calorie needs. Athletes who exercise hard are often very sedentary as they rest and recover from their rigorous workouts. This affects their daily calorie needs. In one study, men and women (aged 54 to 76) who added one hour of brisk walking ended up eating the same number of calories per day and did not lose weight. They simply napped more and reduced by 62 percent their overall energy expenditure throughout the rest of the day (Goran and Poehlman 1992).

4. To lose weight, subtract 20 percent (or even less; small deficits add up and can be easier to sustain) **of your total calorie needs.** Roberta deserved to eat about 2,200 calories per day to maintain her weight. Subtracting 20 percent of 2,200 calories (20 percent × 2,200 = about 400 calories) left her with about 1,800 calories for her reducing diet.

In the past, Roberta had tried to reduce on 1,000 to 1,200 calories per day. She was skeptical about my proposed reducing plan of 1,800 calories. "If I can't lose weight on 1,000 calories, why would I lose weight on 1,800?" she questioned. I reminded her that when she cut back too much, she'd get too hungry and blow her diet. She also lost muscle, slowed her metabolism, and consumed too few of the nutrients she needed to protect her health and invest in top performance. I reminded her that slow and steady weight loss stays off; quick weight loss rapidly reappears.

A reasonable weight-loss target is 0.5 to 1 pound (0.25 to 0.5 kg) a week for a person who weighs less than 150 pounds (68 kg); 1 to 2 pounds a week is reasonable for heavier bodies.

The theory of "the less you eat, the more fat you will lose" contains little practical truth. Generally, the less you eat, the more you blow your diet and overeat because of extreme hunger. For example, if you knock off only 100 calories at the end of the day (the equivalent of two Oreo cookies or a spoonful of ice cream), you'll theoretically lose 10 pounds (4.5 kg) of fat a year, because 1 pound of fat equals 3,500 calories. If you eat 500 fewer calories per day than you normally do, you should lose 1 pound per week. Now think of the number of times you've tried to knock off 1,000 calories per day and have ended up gaining weight.

Remember, though, that weight loss is not always mathematical. Nature makes weight loss harder for people who try to get below their set-point weight (Leibel, Rosenbaum, and Hirsch 1995). If you have no excess fat to lose, nature will cause your body to conserve energy. I've had thin clients who claim they eat far less than they deserve yet maintain weight. They have cold hands and report they are "always freezing"—just one way nature conserves calories.

Once you've established your total daily calories, divide them evenly throughout the day. Some people like having six small meals: breakfast, snack, lunch, snack, dinner, snack. Others, like Roberta, find that four meals per day work well for them.

Roberta was initially skeptical about this four-meal plan; meals, after all, are "fattening." She complained, "I'm afraid I'll get fat from eating so much at breakfast and two lunches." I reminded her that the purpose of the daytime meals is to ruin her appetite for dinner. By eating more during the day, she would then be less hungry that evening, have more energy to exercise from 5:00 to 6:00 p.m., and be able to eat less (diet) at night.

If you hold the fear that meals are fattening, think again and remember these ideas:

- You won't gain weight from eating a substantial breakfast or lunch. You'll have more energy to exercise and burn calories. Even if you were to eat too much at those meals, you could compensate by eating less at night.

- If you skimp on daytime meals and develop a deep hunger, you'll be likely to overeat at night because of the strong physiological drive to eat.

- You'll end up eating fewer calories, even though the breakfast and lunch and second lunch may be larger than before. You'll simply trade in the evening blown-diet calories for wholesome foods earlier in the day.

• If you are not hungry at night, you can skimp at dinner and simply eat soup or salad. But don't have just soup or salad for lunch. It's not enough.

Become familiar with the calorie content of the foods you commonly eat, and then spend your calories wisely. That is, include at least three of the five food groups at each meal (see chapter 1) and two kinds of foods per snack. Too many dieters repetitively eat a single food, such as cottage cheese, for a meal. This practice limits their intake of the variety of vitamins, minerals, and other nutrients offered by a range of foods.

Roberta was an expert calorie counter. In fact, she expressed fear about becoming neurotic about counting calories. I reminded her to count calories loosely (0, 50, or 100) and to consider them a general guideline and helpful tool to determine how much (rather than how little) food she could appropriately eat.

More important, she needed to start listening to her body and learn what, for example, 600 calories feels like. She could then use that feeling for future reference. For example, she could tell the right amount to eat at a restaurant by listening to her body's message of being pleasantly fed. Calorie counting can be a helpful bridge to get you in touch with your body's ability to tell you how much is OK to eat so that you feel satisfied. You can and should quickly replace calorie counting with listening to your body's signals for hunger and satiety. Calorie counting should not become an obsession.

Ten Steps for Successful Fat Loss

Now that you know how many calories you can eat to lose body fat gradually, you need to learn how to eat those calories appropriately. Here are 10 steps for successful fat loss.

1. Write it down. Keep accurate food records of every morsel and drop for three days, if not more. Research suggests that people who keep food records tend to lose weight effectively. A handy place to keep food records is on the Internet. See Dietary Analysis and Nutrition Assessment in appendix A for Web sites that can help you not only record your food but also calculate calories.

Record why you eat. Are you hungry, stressed, or bored? Include the time and amount you exercise as well. Evaluate your patterns for potentially fattening habits such as skimping at breakfast, nibbling all day, overeating at night because you've become too hungry, entertaining yourself with food when you're bored, or rewarding yourself with chocolate when you're stressed.

Pay careful attention to your mood when eating. Roberta discovered that at times a hug and human comforting could have better nourished her than food did. She acknowledged that eating a tub of popcorn diverted her loneliness or anxiety and distracted her from her problems but did nothing to resolve the problem that triggered her eating.

If you eat for reasons other than to obtain fuel, you need to recognize that food should only be fuel. Like a drug, food should not be abused. Food becomes dangerously fattening when it is eaten for entertainment, comfort, or stress reduction. And no amount of any food will solve your problems.

2. **Frontload your calories.** If you eat lightly during the day and excessively at night, experiment with having a bigger breakfast and lunch and a lighter dinner. Roberta was surprised that I thought her diet breakfast of cereal with skim milk was too skimpy. She thought that diets were supposed to start at breakfast. I told her to start her diet at dinner. She needed more energy to get through her active day.

3. **Eat slowly.** Overweight people tend to eat faster than their normal-weight counterparts do. Because the brain needs about 20 minutes to receive the signal that you've eaten your fill, slow eating can save you many calories. No matter how much you consume during those 20 minutes, the satiety signal doesn't move any faster. Try to pace your eating time so that you eat less and avoid the discomfort that often occurs after rapid eating. For example, choose a broth-based soup for a first course before dinner at a restaurant. Hot soup takes time to eat and decreases the appetite for the entree. You'll be content to have a lighter meal.

Roberta had the bad habit of inhaling her meals in a matter of minutes. She'd eat nonstop, without enjoying the pleasures of the meal. I encouraged her to put her fork down frequently, taste the food, and eat it mindfully. You should pay attention to what you are eating. Remember, the best part about food is its taste. If you aren't taking time to enjoy the taste of food, you are missing one of the pleasures of life.

Because Roberta had eaten quickly for most of her life, I suggested that she practice slowly eating at least one meal per day and then build that up to two, then three meals. She discovered that lunchtime became more enjoyable once she gave herself permission to relax and enjoy both the meal and mealtime. She felt less tempted to eat dessert because the slowly savored lunch satisfied her appetite.

4. **Eat your favorite foods.** If you deny yourself permission to eat what you truly want to eat, you are likely to binge. But if you give yourself

permission to eat your desired foods in diet portions, you will be less likely to blow your reducing plan. If chocolate-glazed doughnuts are among your favorites, then have one once or twice a week. Simply determine how many calories are in the doughnut, and spend your calorie budget accordingly (many chain restaurants provide calorie information online). When eating this treat, remember to chew it slowly, savor the taste, and fully enjoy it. You'll free yourself from the temptation to devour a dozen doughnuts in one sitting.

Roberta's downfall was chocolate-chip cookies. "I can go for four days without a cookie fix, but then I inevitably end up eating two great big ones." I encouraged Roberta to have a cookie at lunch at least twice per week to prevent those unnecessary binges. When she did that, she discovered that she had less desire for cookies as treats because she did not feel denied or deprived. Eating bigger meals also helped abate the cookie cravings. By preventing herself from getting too hungry, she lost interest in sugary treats (see chapter 5).

5. Avoid temptation. Out of sight, out of mind, and out of mouth. If you spend a lot of free time in the kitchen, you might consider relocating to the den when you want to relax, where food is less likely to be available. At parties, socialize in the living room, away from the buffet table and away from the snacks. At the market, skip the aisle with the cookies.

Roberta used to take walks that went by the bakery. No wonder she'd succumb to temptation. I suggested that she walk down another street. This became the simple solution to what had been a major problem. She also learned to enter her house through the front door and go immediately upstairs to change her clothes and unwind from the day. Previously, she had entered the house through the kitchen door. She would then habitually open the refrigerator and graze for a few minutes while making that transition from working to being at home.

6. Keep a list of nonfood activities. When you are bored, lonely, tired, or nervous, you need to have some strategies in mind that have nothing to do with eating. You might want to call a friend, check your e-mail, take a bath, water the plants, listen to music by candlelight, surf the Web, work on a puzzle, go for a walk, take a nap, play with your kids, or meditate. Food is designed to be fuel, not entertainment, and not a reward for having survived another stressful day.

When Roberta felt tired and stressed, she would treat herself to food. I encouraged her to ask herself before indulging, "Am I hungry? Or am I tired and stressed? Does my body need this fuel?" If the answer was that she was tired, she talked herself into going to bed early. If the answer was that she was stressed, she learned to recognize that no amount of food would resolve the stress, so she shouldn't even start to eat. Making a phone call to her best friend or writing a page in her journal became her slimming alternatives.

When you overeat because you are stressed, you are only trying to be nice to yourself. Food alters your brain chemistry and may put you in a happier mood—for the moment, that is. In the end this inappropriate coping skill will leave you even more stressed and depressed from the weight gain. Learning how to manage stress without food is the obvious solution.

Instructors from the Mind/Body Medical Institute in Boston suggest taking three deep, slow breaths—breathe in peace, breathe out stress—to dissipate stress. Meditation can also be helpful. Calm your mind by sitting in a comfortable position and focusing on the word *ocean*. Slowly inhale on "O" and exhale on "cean." Soon the calm vision of ocean waves will help soothe your nerves . . . and perhaps save you some calories.

7. **Make a realistic eating plan.** You don't have to lose weight every day. Rather, every day you can choose to lose, maintain, or even gain weight. For example, if you face a hectic schedule and wonder how you will survive the stresses of the day, give yourself permission to fuel yourself fully and have a maintain-weight day. You'll need the energy to cope. If you are going to an elegant wedding and want to enjoy the full dinner, go right ahead. A gain-weight day from time to time is part of normal eating. Your body will simply be less hungry the next day, and you'll be able to compensate by eating a little less. (Note: Do not "save calories" for a big dinner by skimping on daytime food; doing so tends to backfire, and you'll inevitably end up seriously overeating in the evening.)

Roberta had always considered a diet to be a nonstop event that would last for weeks or months until she reached her target weight. I invited her to see weight reduction as being a daily choice that depends on the stress level of the day. I also recommended that she plan on a treat once a week. Just as people need a day off from work, dieters need a day off from dieting. Roberta acknowledged, "Knowing that I can enjoy going out to eat on Friday night helps me stay with my reducing program the rest of the week."

8. **Schedule appointments for exercise.** If you are a serious athlete who is trying to lose weight, you likely have a regular training program. But if you are a fitness exerciser who has trouble following a consistent exercise program, you might be helped by scheduling the time to exercise in your appointment book. You want to exercise regularly to tone muscles, relieve stress, and improve your health, but you should not overexercise. If you exercise too much, you will likely end up injured, tired, and irritable.

As I mentioned before, exercise should be for fun and fitness, not simply for burning off calories. Be sure that you enjoy yourself.

Roberta would sometimes punish herself with extra-hard workouts—more time on the stair stepper or longer, faster walks to burn more calories. Although she did expend 500 to 600 calories per session, she'd end up so hungry that by the end of the day she would inevitably replace those calories, plus more. I encouraged her to stop using exercise as punishment for having extra body fat. She should exercise to improve her health and performance. Remember, exercise only contributes to weight loss if it culminates in a calorie deficit at the end of the day.

My clients commonly ask, "How much exercise is enough?" Enough for what? Enough to lose weight? You can lose weight without exercising; you just need to eat fewer calories. Enough for overall health and fitness? The American College of Sports Medicine (ACSM 1998) recommends accumulating at least 30 minutes of moderate physical activity most days of the week (about 150 calories per day, or 1,000 calories per week). The classic Harvard Alumni Health Study found that the lowest death rates from cardiovascular disease occurred among those who burned more than 1,000 calories per week (Sesso, Pfaffenbarger, and Lee 2000). The Institute of Medicine recommends 60 minutes each day of moderate physical activity (2,000 calories per week) to prevent weight gain and optimize health (Couzin 2002).

9. **Make sleep a priority.** Getting too little sleep can make you feel hungrier. When you are tired, the signals to your brain to stop eating are very quiet, and the signals to eat more are very loud. Roberta often found herself tired and hungry at the end of her long day. She learned to go to bed earlier and reminded herself she needed to "snooze to lose." She knew if she started eating, she would have great difficulty stopping.

10. **Think fit and healthy.** Every morning before you get out of bed, visualize yourself being fitter and leaner. This picture will help you start the day with a positive attitude. If you tell yourself that you are eating more healthfully and are successfully losing weight, you will do so more easily. Positive self-talk is important for your well-being.

Roberta constantly reminded herself that she'd rather be healthier and leaner than allow herself to overeat. She took smaller portions. She made a daily eating plan and stuck to it. On her way home after work, she visualized herself eating a pleasant (but smaller) dinner, chewing the food slowly, savoring the taste, relaxing after dinner with a book rather than cookies, and successfully following her food plan. By practicing this scene before she arrived home, she discovered that she was better able to carry through with her good intentions.

Roberta also reminded herself that when she ate well, she felt better and exercised better. She also felt better about herself. After years of unsuccessful dieting, she liked feeling successful, perhaps even more than feeling thinner.

Fad Dieting

Every dieter wants to lose weight quickly, and a fad diet that promises instant success is appealing. Unfortunately, fad diets tend to work for only a short time because the dieter gets tired of being denied and deprived of favorite foods. In a year-long study of 311 women (average age 40 years) who were instructed to read a popular diet book (such as Atkins, Zone, or Ornish), none of the women lost much weight, and almost all started gaining it back after 6 months. By the end of 12 months, they had lost and kept off only 3.5 to 11 pounds (1.6 to 5 kg); that averages less than a pound a month (Gardner et al. 2007). The bottom line: Instead of hopping from one fad diet plan to another, you need to learn how to eat appropriate portions of the foods you like. You need to learn how to manage food—not how to eliminate foods by going on a diet.

I have clients who abandon my weight-reduction advice, which is based on balance and moderation; they want to lose weight faster—and easier. A year or two later, they inevitably end up back in my office, heavier than when they first came. Here is a brief summary of some of the tempting fad diets that have failed to work for them, and likely for you, too.

Zone Diet. This 40-30-30 plan prescribes 40 percent of calories from carbohydrate, 30 percent from protein, and 30 percent from fat, the philosophy being that eating less carbohydrate will reduce insulin and consequently fat storage. The truth is, excess calories (of any type), not excess carbohydrate, promote fat storage. (If carbohydrate is fattening, why aren't the people in rice-eating countries fat—such as natives of Japan and China?)

The Zone Diet was the fad response to high-carbohydrate, low-fat diets that failed to achieve weight-loss promises. The seeming success of the Zone Diet demonstrates that a strong intake of protein and fat can enhance weight reduction because these types of foods are more satisfying than fat-free foods. When you feel less hungry, you can more easily eat fewer calories and thereby lose weight.

The bad news is that athletes generally need more than 40 percent carbohydrate to fuel their muscles for top performance. You cannot expect to do repeated days of hard exercise without having carbohydrate as the foundation of each meal. If you are a casual exerciser, you may be able to exercise well enough with a reduced carbohydrate intake. But do you really want to live your life calculating 40-30-30 meals? As one dieter said, "I didn't know if my meal would equate to 40-30-30, so I just didn't eat it." No wonder he lost weight.

Atkins Diet. Based on high-protein, high-fat foods, this diet eliminates carbohydrate to the extent that the body goes into ketosis. Ketosis is an abnormal condition in which the carbohydrate-depleted body resorts to fueling the brain with ketones (a fuel created when protein is burned for energy). Ketosis kills the appetite, which makes it easier to lose weight. But take heed: People who are in ketosis have bad-smelling breath as well as poorly fueled muscles and suboptimal workouts.

Like the Zone Diet, this plan labels insulin and carbohydrate as fattening, but that is not the case. And although this high-protein plan promotes the concept that you can eat all you want, just how many chicken breasts and cans of tuna can you eat for days in a row? The lack of variety contributes to food boredom and reduced calorie intake . . . to say nothing of reduced phytochemicals, fiber, and other health-protective food components because of the lack of fruits and vegetables.

South Beach Diet. Many people swear by this modified Atkins-type diet, which simply eliminates rice, pasta, breads, and other starches but (thankfully) includes fruits and vegetables. If you are a recreational exerciser, you may be able to get enough carbohydrate from fruits and vegetables for fitness workouts from the South Beach Diet. But the question arises: Do you never want to eat pasta or bagels for the rest of your life?

The goal of losing weight is to learn how to eat smaller portions of the foods that you always have (and always will) like. Diets that deny favorite foods have a very limited life. Plus, the dieter ends up feeling guilty if he or she "cheats" and has a bagel. In my value system, food is not a moral issue, and eating is not cheating. Is living with guilt and self-anger for having eaten a bagel conducive to optimal health? I doubt it.

Low glycemic index diet. The theory is that foods with a high glycemic index are fattening because they create a rapid rise in blood sugar, stimulate the body to secrete more insulin, and thereby (supposedly) promote fat storage. For athletes and active people, this is not the case because fit people have a reduced insulin response. Each person's response to a carbohydrate-containing food is variable, so the glycemic index is almost meaningless (see chapter 6).

Ultra Slim-Fast plan. By drinking this canned beverage at breakfast and lunch and then eating a normal dinner, the pounds supposedly drop off. Clearly, a 180-calorie can of Slim-Fast offers fewer calories than does a standard meal, but the reality is that you work *very* hard to eat less dinner when your body is starving for more calories. That is, the Ultra Slim Fast Diet doesn't work; *you* do.

A better bet than a 180-calorie starvation meal is to eat at least 500 calories at breakfast and lunch, if not more. Adequate daytime meals provide needed fuel so your body does not shut down, conserve energy, and leave you feeling lifeless and unable to enjoy an afternoon workout. If you insist on Slim-Fast, have it for dinner (along with a generous serving of vegetables), but not for breakfast and lunch.

Double-duty exercise program. Doubling your workouts to burn more calories and melt away body fat may sound like a good idea. But what often happens is that the more you exercise, the more you'll want to eat. You may burn an extra 400 calories but then succumb to eating 500. Or, if you are able to restrict your caloric intake, your body will conserve energy in response to this perceived "famine" caused by the huge calorie deficit. In addition, you can easily end up injured, exhausted, and sick with a cold or the flu. Exercise should be for enjoyment, not punishment.

Fat-burning thermogenic program. Thermogenic weight-loss supplements are indeed popular. The primary ingredient in any of the thermogenic products is ephedrine, ephedra, or ma huang. These are powerful stimulants—so powerful that they not only boost the metabolic rate and contribute to (short-term) weight loss but also kill people. At least 70 deaths and 1,400 adverse events have been linked to ephedrine-containing products. Weight loss is not worth dying for. My advice is to stay away from these products.

Portion-plate program. A simple yet effective non-fad-diet approach is to use portion-controlled plates, bowls, and glassware. A study of (inactive) overweight people indicates that those who used special dishes with markings for the recommended portion of protein, starch, and vegetables lost more weight than those who got verbal instructions about proper portions (Pedersen, Kang, and Kline 2007). For many active people, the standard portions will be too skimpy, so you may need to plan for double portions, depending on how much you exercise.

Weight-Loss Myths and Truths

Weight reduction is more complex than adding exercise and eliminating dietary fat. Confusion abounds among athletes, exercisers, and obesity researchers themselves about the best way to lose body fat. The one-diet-fits-all approach to losing weight is not appropriate; different people have different histories. Some overweight people are genetically heavy; others are genetically lean. Some are men; others are women. Some are recently overfat; others have been fighting the battle of the bulge for years. Some have taken comfort in food since childhood; others have recently turned to food to smother tough emotions.

Despite these factors that contribute to the complexities of weight loss, people are forever searching for a simple method to shed excess body fat. This section addresses some of the weight-reduction myths and misconceptions among athletes and fitness exercisers alike.

Myth: **Carbohydrate is fattening.**

Truth: No! As I explained in chapter 6, excess calories are fattening. Calories come from carbohydrate (4 calories per gram), protein (4 calories per gram), alcohol (7 calories per gram), and fat (9 calories per gram). Excess calories from fat are the main dietary demons. Your body can easily store excess dietary fat as body fat, whereas you are more likely to burn off excess calories of carbohydrate. Butter, margarine, oil, mayonnaise, salad dressing, and grease are obvious sources of fat. Fat is also hidden in meats, cheeses, peanut butter, nuts, and other protein foods. Although some forms of fat are healthier than others, all fat is equally fattening.

Excess calories from alcohol also quickly add up and can easily inflate your body fat stores, as can the calories from the high-fat munchies that commonly accompany alcohol. But calories from carbohydrate are excellent for muscle fuel. Your body preferentially burns them for energy rather than stores them as fat.

Myth: **High-protein, low-carbohydrate diets are the best choice if you want to lose weight.**

Truth: If you want to lose weight, your best bet is to eat smaller portions at dinner and create a calorie deficit for the day. The fundamental type of calories eaten, either protein or carbohydrate, seems to have less importance. In one eight-week study, subjects who ate 1,600 calories of either a high-protein diet (30 percent protein, 40 percent carbohydrate) or a high-carbohydrate diet (15 percent protein, 55 percent carbohydrate) lost the same amount of weight (Luscombe et al. 2002). In another study comparing diets with varying amounts of carbohydrate, protein, and fat, the subjects lost similar amounts of weight. The bottom line is that all calories count!

A high-protein, low-carbohydrate diet seemingly works because of several factors:

1. **Dieters lose water weight.** Carbohydrate holds water in the muscles. For each ounce of carbohydrate you store as glycogen, your body simultaneously stores 3 ounces of water. When you deplete carbohydrate during exercise, your body releases the water. You experience a significant loss of weight that's mostly water, not fat.

2. **People eliminate many calories when they eliminate carbohydrate.** For example, you might eliminate not only the baked potato (200 calories) but also two pats of butter (100 calories) on top of the potato, and this creates a calorie deficit.

3. **Because it lingers longer in the stomach, protein (and fat) tends to be more satiating than carbohydrate.** Having high-protein (and high-fat) eggs and bacon for breakfast stays with you longer than does a high-carbohydrate bagel with jam. By curbing hunger, you have fewer urges to eat and can more easily cut calories.

The overwhelming reason that high-protein, low-carbohydrate diets do not work is that dieters fail to stay on them for a long time. They may lose weight, only to regain it. The trick to losing weight is to learn how to manage the food supply so that you won't regain the weight. Remember: You should never start a food program that you do not want to maintain for the rest of your life.

Myth: **If you eat fat, you will get fat.**

Truth: If you eat excess calories, you will get fat. Weight control relies on a calorie budget, not only on a fat-gram budget. Fat loss occurs when you burn off more calories than you eat. If you require 2,400 calories per day to maintain your weight but eat only 2,000 calories, you will lose body fat. The kind of calories you eat may be of less consequence. If you choose to spend 300 of your 2,000 calories on high-fat peanut butter instead of fat-free bagels, you can still lose body fat. Fatty foods that fit into your calorie budget are not inherently fattening (Alford, Blankenship, and Hagen 1990; McManus et al. 2001). Look at your friends. I'll bet you know several people who eat fat but are not. You can appropriately eat 25 to 30 percent of your calories from (primarily healthful) fat.

Some people eat large portions of fat-free foods thinking that *fat free* means *calorie free*. Bad idea! Excess calories, regardless of the source, will ultimately be stored as fat (Hill et al. 1992). Dieters who eat only fat-free foods fool only themselves. Sharon, a personal trainer, reported that she'd been known to eat a whole box of fat-free pretzels for a snack. Paul, a bodybuilder, routinely polished off a half gallon of fat-free frozen yogurt. And Nancy, a swimmer, used to eat at least six fat-free bagels per day. No wonder they all complained that they hadn't lost weight even though they avoided foods containing fat. They were eating too many calories.

The advice to lose body fat by eating no fat tends to work best for overweight people who eliminate fatty foods and lose weight because they eat fewer calories. For example, instead of having 700 calories of bacon, eggs, and buttered toast for breakfast, Elliott switched to 400 calories of cereal and banana as part of a conscious effort to lose 50 pounds (23 kg). He successfully dropped weight because of the continued calorie deficit.

In contrast, when already lean people eat a low-fat diet, they commonly feel driven to eat more calories of carbohydrate to compensate for the reduction in fat calories. Weight reduction becomes increasingly hard if you strive to be lighter than nature designed (Leibel, Rosenbaum, and Hirsch 1995). Paula, who wanted to lose 3 pounds (1.4 kg) but was already at her set-point weight, reported that she craved bread, pretzels, and other low-fat foods. I recommended that Paula include some fat in her diet so that she could eat a wider variety of food and enjoy better dietary balance (her extremely low-fat diet was lacking in protein, iron, and zinc), feel more satisfied (foods with fat provide a pleasant feeling of fullness), and be more at peace with food.

Her fat-free food plan created guilt feelings whenever she succumbed to eating a food with fat. For example, she declined a piece of birthday cake because it contained fat. She said that she would have felt too guilty if she had eaten some. I reminded Paula that other people enjoyed the cake and didn't get fat from eating it. Clearly, she was confusing appropriate eating with her desire to be in control. This desire to control fat had little to do with weight and more to do with rigidity and misinformation.

Myth: **Food eaten after 8:00 p.m. readily turns into body fat while you sleep.**

Truth: If you are hungry at night, you should honor hunger and eat, particularly if you have calories left in your calorie budget for the day. Many active people, because of their hectic work or training schedules, enjoy most of their calories at night. Other people, however, undereat by day only to blow their diets at night. They eat more than what their bodies require and consume excess calories.

The verdict is unclear as to whether night eating is inherently fattening. One survey of 1,800 women found no connection between weight and big evening meals (Kant, Ballard-Barbash, and Schatzkin 1995). But the night eaters did consume more fat, protein, and alcohol and less carbohydrate, vitamin C, vitamin B_6, and folic acid, indicative of a fast-food diet with too few fruits and vegetables. At night, people tend to eat fewer carrots and more cookies.

Gymnasts and runners who eat skimpily during the day tend to have more body fat than those who keep themselves better fueled. By minimizing the time they are in calorie deficit, they are less likely to conserve energy (Deutz et al. 2000). The bottom line for dieters is that you should fuel appropriately during the day and then eat less at night. You'll not only have more energy for training but also prevent yourself from becoming too hungry and overeating. Remember that when you get too hungry, you may no longer have the energy to care about how much you eat. You simply want to eat. That drive to eat is physiological and has little to do with willpower.

Myth: **Exercise kills your appetite.**

Truth: Exercise may temporarily kill your appetite, but hunger will catch up with you within one to two hours. Temperature control regulates appetite to some extent. Therefore, if you feel hot after a hard workout, you may experience a temporary drop in appetite. But if you are chilled, such as after swimming, you may feel ravenous.

The effect of exercise on appetite varies according to gender. Regularly exercising male rats tend to lose their appetite and drop weight, whereas female rats get a bigger appetite, eat more, and maintain weight (Staten 1991). Human studies suggest that exercise makes food more attractive to women (Pomerleau et al. 2004).

Postexercise appetite also varies according to body fatness. Studies of obese women who added moderate exercise to their sedentary lifestyles indicate they did not eat more, and hence they lost weight. Diet and exercise studies with men suggest that the fatter they were, the more weight they lost (in comparison with their thinner peers) because their meals didn't compensate for the calories burned during exercise (Westerterp et al. 1992).

Myth: **The more you exercise, the more weight you'll lose.**

Truth: Often, the more you exercise, the hungrier you get and the more you eat. For example, you may spend an hour on the stair stepper burning off 500 calories and then devour 12 Oreos (600 calories) in less than six minutes. After a hard workout, your body is hungry. Your soul may also be hungry for a reward. You now deserve a treat for having survived the workout, right?

The effects of exercise on weight loss are complex and unclear. Nature seems to replenish fat stores of lean athletes efficiently to prevent them from wasting away. Lean female athletes, in particular, struggle harder than do males to lose body fat and maintain an even leaner physique. This makes sense in terms of evolution. Nature wants women to be able to reproduce; men are supposed to be lean hunters. I tell my female clients to exercise to train and improve performance and to count calories to create a calorie deficit.

Myth: **If you train for an Ironman Triathlon, your body fat will melt away.**

Truth: Wishful thinking. I commonly hear marathoners, triathletes, and other highly competitive endurance athletes complain, "For all the exercise I do, I should be pencil thin." They fail to lose fat because they put all of their energy into exercising then tend to be sedentary the rest of the day as they recover from their tough workouts. A study of male endurance athletes who reported a seemingly low calorie intake found they did less spontaneous activity than their peers in the nonexercise parts of their day (Thompson et al. 1995). You need to eat according to your whole day's activity level, not according to how hard you trained that day.

Alternatively, athletes who complain they eat like a bird but fail to lose body fat may simply be underreporting their food intake. A survey of female marathoners indicates that fatter runners underreport their food intake more so than their leaner peers (Edwards et al. 1993). Remember, the calories you mindlessly eat while talking on the phone or eating on the run count just as much as calories from a meal.

Myth: **The fatter a person is, the fewer calories he or she should eat.**

Truth: This is plain wrong. Just as 18-wheel trucks need more fuel than do compact cars, large bodies need more calories than do smaller bodies. Contrary to popular belief, obese people rarely have slow metabolisms. Rather, they require significant amounts of food. A 250-pound (113 kg) person may need 3,000 to 4,000 calories per day to maintain weight. An appropriate reducing plan would be 2,400 to 3,200 calories. That's far more than the 800 to 1,000 calories offered by many quick weight-loss programs (that fail in the long run).

My obese clients repeatedly report that they don't have time for breakfast and commonly work through lunch. The fact is they choose to skip those meals. They believe they don't deserve to eat. They eat meagerly during the day, then succumb to excessive amounts of food at night. Of course, obese people do deserve to eat. As one of my obese clients said, "Nancy, you are the only person who has ever told me it's OK to eat."

Athletes with Weight Limits

If you are a jockey or light weight wrestler, boxer, or rower, you are probably not overweight. But you may have to cut weight to achieve a lower weight standard for your sport or else be denied permission to compete. Use the information here to help you lose weight healthfully. Contrary to popular belief, you do not need to starve yourself.

If you are worried that strict dieting as a teenager will stunt your growth, note that you will catch up after the competitive season. Many wrestlers are short in stature not because of malnutrition but because of genetics. They tend to have short parents. Small people often select a low-weight sport because they are more suited for it than they are for football or basketball.

The first step to attaining your weight class is to get a realistic picture of how much weight you need to lose by getting your body fat measured (see chapter 13). If you don't have access to calipers or another means of measuring your percent body fat, give yourself the less professional pinch test. If you can pinch more than half an inch of thickness over your shoulder blade or hips, you can safely lose a little more weight.

The absolute minimal weight includes 5 percent fat for men and 12 percent fat for women. The minimum weight recommended for wrestlers commonly includes about 7 percent body fat. If possible, do not try to achieve a weight that will result in your having to starve yourself to lose muscle or dehydrate yourself to lose water weight. Achieving an unrealistic weight is difficult and can hurt rather than enhance your health and performance.

Second, start to lose weight early in the season or, better yet, before the start of the season. That way you'll have the time to lose weight slowly (0.5 to 1.0 pound [0.25 to 0.5 kg] per week) and more enjoyably. Your goal is to achieve and stay at your lowest healthy body-fat level.

To lose weight, follow the calorie guidelines outlined on pages 270 to 272. No matter how much weight you have to lose, do not eat less than that required to sustain your resting metabolic rate. Most athletes need to eat at least 1,500 calories of a variety of wholesome foods every day to prevent vitamin, mineral, and protein deficiencies. Do not eliminate any food group. During the day or two before the event, choose low-fiber foods to reduce the weight of intestinal contents and restrict salty foods to reduce water weight.

Remember that water is not extra weight. Your body stores the precious water in a delicate balance. If you disrupt this balance, you will decrease your ability to exercise at your best. Using diuretics, rubber suits, saunas, whirlpools, or steam rooms to dehydrate yourself is dangerous. And when replacing sweat loss after training sessions, note that sports drinks, soft drinks, and juices all have calories. Ration them wisely when refueling after exercise, then drink water the rest of the day.

To lose weight rapidly before an event is counterproductive. If you do, depleted muscle glycogen and dehydration will take their toll. The odds are against the starved wrestler who crash diets to make weight as compared with the well-fueled wrestler who routinely maintains or stays within a few pounds of his competition weight during training.

In a study of wrestlers who quickly lost about 8 pounds (4.5 percent of their body weight), the wrestlers performed 3.5 percent worse on a six-minute arm-crank test designed to be similar to a wrestling competition. These results suggest that rapid weight loss by athletes before competition may be a detriment rather than a competitive advantage (Hickner et al. 1991). Yet, if the athlete follows an aggressive refueling program after the weigh-in, drops in performance can be minimized (Slater et al. 2007). Choose high-carbohydrate, salty foods and drink lots of fluids. For example, enjoy juice and pretzels. Be careful, though, to consume only the amount you can comfortably tolerate.

CHAPTER 16

Dieting Gone Awry: Eating Disorders and Food Obsessions

For most active people, the *e* in *eating* stands for enjoyment. But for some, the *e* stands for *evil*, and for them, food is the enemy. These food- and weight-obsessed exercisers spend their days trying not to eat. They worry constantly about what they'll eat, when and where they'll eat, how much weight they'll gain if they eat a normal meal with their friends, how many hours they will need to exercise to burn off those calories, how many meals they should skip if they overeat by a few morsels, and so on. The endless fretting about food, weight, exercise, and dieting consumes them. But some of these people fail to understand that their anxiety is abnormal. After all, doesn't everyone talk about food and diets all the time?

Why Eating Disorders Happen

Eating disorders such as anorexia and bulimia commonly occur in people with low self-esteem; they feel they are not "good enough." They believe that thinness will make them into better and almost perfect people. The truth is that a thinner body does not make a person better, just smaller. There is simply less of the person to love. The individual is the same person, just obsessed, withdrawn, and tired. And when someone severely restricts food, he or she loses muscle, strength, and stamina. This is not the way to become a star athlete.

The risk of developing an eating disorder seems to increase dramatically when an athlete with low self-esteem is physically beautiful, has traits of perfectionism, and tends to be hypercritical and anxious. Add to the scenario a mother who may have had (or still has) food and weight issues, and her daughter becomes a prime target for developing a full-blown eating disorder.

Athletes with eating disorders are less available to their friends. After all, when a person is constantly exercising and counting calories (calories eaten at meals, calories burned during exercise, calories saved by skipping lunch, calories about to be eaten at dinner, and so on) as well as counting fat grams and sit-ups, his or her brain has little energy left to manage bigger issues, such as life's problems and relationships. The anorexia or bulimia creates a smokescreen that masks the underlying issues.

What Is Anorexia?

People with anorexia nervosa tend to either consistently restrict food or restrict and then binge and purge. The American Psychiatric Association's definition of anorexia includes the following characteristics*:

- Intense fear of gaining weight or becoming fat, even though underweight
- Disturbance in the way a person experiences his or her body (i.e., claiming to feel fat even when emaciated), with an undue influence of body weight or shape on self-perception
- Weight loss to less than 85 percent of normal body weight or, if during a period of growth, failure to make expected weight gain leading to 85 percent of that expected
- Refusal to maintain body weight over a minimal normal weight for age and height
- Denial of the seriousness of the current weight loss
- Absence of at least three consecutive menstrual cycles

*Adapted from American Psychiatric Association, 1994, *Diagnostic and statistical manual of mental disorders*, 4th ed. (Arlington, VA: American Psychiatric Association), 251-252.

If you think that you or someone you know might have anorexia, look for these signs and symptoms:

Signs and Symptoms of Anorexia

- Significant weight loss
- Loss of menstrual periods
- Loss of hair
- Growth of fine body hair, noticeable on the face and arms
- Cold hands and feet and extreme sensitivity to cold temperature
- Layers of baggy clothing to hide thinness (and keep warm)
- Wearing sweaters in summer heat because of feeling cold all the time
- Light-headedness
- Inability to concentrate
- Low pulse rate
- Hyperactivity; compulsive exercise beyond normal training
- Recurrent overuse injuries and stress fractures
- Comments about being fat; distorted body image
- Expression of intense fear of becoming fat
- Nervousness at mealtimes; avoids eating with friends or in public
- Food rituals, such as cutting food into small pieces and playing with it
- Antisocial behavior; isolates from family and friends
- Excessive working or studying, compulsiveness, and rigidity
- Extreme emotions: tearful, uptight, oversensitive, restless

What Is Bulimia?

The person with the purging type of bulimia nervosa may purge by self-induced vomiting and by misusing laxatives, diuretics, or enemas. With the nonpurging type of bulimia, the person uses other inappropriate compensatory mechanisms to prevent weight gain after a binge, such as fasting or exercising excessively. The definition used by the American Psychiatric Association includes these aspects*:

- Recurrent episodes of binge eating, characterized by
  1. eating an unusually large amount of food in a discrete period of time (the amount eaten is larger than most people would eat during a similar time period and under similar circumstances) and
  2. feeling out of control during the eating episode (unable to stop eating or control what and how much is eaten)
- Compensating for the food binge to prevent weight gain, such as inducing vomiting; misusing laxatives, enemas, or other medications; fasting; or exercising excessively

- Binge eating and purging, on average, at least twice a week for three months
- Evaluating self-worth according to body shape and weight

*Adapted from American Psychiatric Association, 1994, *Diagnostic and statistical manual of mental disorders*, 4th ed. (Arlington, VA: American Psychiatric Association), 252-253.

If you think that you or someone you know might have bulimia, look for these signs and symptoms:

Signs and Symptoms of Bulimia

- Weakness, headaches, dizziness
- Frequent weight fluctuations because of alternating binges and fasts
- Swollen glands that give a chipmunklike appearance
- Difficulty swallowing and retaining food; damage to throat
- Frequent vomiting
- Damaged tooth enamel from exposure to gastric acid when vomiting
- Petty stealing of food or stealing of money to buy food for binges
- Strange behavior that surrounds secretive eating
- Disappearance after meals, often to the bathroom to "take a shower"
- Running water in the bathroom after meals to hide the sound of vomiting
- Extreme concern about body weight, shape, and physical appearance
- Ability to eat enormous meals without weight gain
- Compulsive exercise beyond normal training
- Depression
- Bloodshot eyes

Eating Disorders and Active People

Eating disorders among active people seem to be on the rise. The staff at health clubs commonly express concerns about some of their clients, as do coaches about their athletes, especially athletes in sports that emphasize weight, such as running, gymnastics, and wrestling. Research indicates that eating disorders are widespread among athletes in all sports. An estimated 15 to 30 percent of collegiate female athletes have some type of disordered eating pattern, be it anorexia, bulimia, laxative abuse, excessive exercise, crash diets, or other unhealthy weight-loss practices that place them at risk of developing a full-blown eating disorder (Beals and Manore 2002). Most people with eating disorders exercise compulsively, either to create a calorie deficit and be thinner or to burn off the calories consumed during a binge.

Approximately half of all dieters report abnormal eating binges. Many of these dieters abuse exercise as a means to help control their weight. Some call themselves athletes, when in reality they could be better named compulsive exercisers. Many live in fear of becoming fat, and they constantly restrict their food in hopes of losing weight. They live with chaotic eating patterns and body hatred.

I estimate that at least 40 to 50 percent of my clients are obsessed with food, and they represent only a minority of people who seek professional nutrition guidance. Most people who are obsessed with food struggle on their own for years before asking for help. They are embarrassed that they can't seem to resolve their food imbalances. One 65-year-old woman, a regular at the health club, confided that I was the first person in 50 years to whom she had talked about her bulimia.

For these people, food is not fuel. It is the fattening enemy that thwarts their desire to be perfectly thin. Their goal is thinness at any price, and that price is often guilt, shame, mental anguish, physical fatigue, injuries that fail to heal, anemia, weakened bones, stress fractures, and impaired athletic performance. These athletes perform suboptimally because they eat poorly. One high school runner failed to connect her inability to finish track workouts with her one-banana-a-day diet. She thought she fell asleep in classes because she had stayed up too late studying, not because she was underfed.

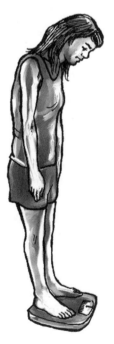

If you struggle with anorexia or bulimia, I recommend that you seek help from a professional counselor experienced with eating disorders and obtain nutrition guidance from a registered dietitian. (See Eating Disorders in appendix A for Web sites that offer referral networks.) Extreme eating disorders usually reflect an inability to cope with the day-to-day stresses of life.

For example, a woman in charge of fund-raising for a charitable organization smothered her stress with homemade chocolate-chip cookies, warm from the oven. This treat certainly diverted her attention from her problems, but it didn't resolve any of them. Afraid of gaining weight, she'd burn off the calories with a long workout that was pure punishment. She became injured from the excessive exercise, panicked at her inability to exercise, tried to eat next to nothing, became ravenous, binged, and then resorted to self-induced vomiting as a means of purging the calories because she could no longer exercise the way she desired. She came to me looking for help with food. I insisted that she also get psychological counseling to help her deal with stress and her feelings of being out of control.

Eating disorders plague all types of casual exercisers and competitive athletes, males and females alike, and perhaps even you or one of your friends. About 4 percent of female athletes struggle with anorexia, 39 percent with bulimia. Among male athletes, an estimated 1.5 percent struggle with anorexia, 14 percent with bulimia. These numbers (Beals and Manore 2000), if anything, are conservative because people who feel ashamed about their eating habits commonly give inaccurate self-reports.

These numbers also exclude the large group of people with subclinical eating disorders who do not fit the diagnosis of anorexia (because they have a seemingly normal weight) but have an abnormal relationship with food and spend too much time thinking about food and weight. They fritter away each day, trying to get thinner.

In-depth interviews of women with subclinical eating disorders delineate these characteristic eating behaviors:

- They restrict their calorie intake to lose weight and eat a repetitive diet, with little or no variety in the types and amounts of foods they consume.

- They follow strict dietary rules and experience guilt and self-anger if they break one of their rules.

- They limit their intake of "bad foods" and usually choose low-fat or fat-free foods.

- Almost all these women perceive themselves as being slightly to very overfat and are preoccupied with weight (Beals and Manore 2000).

Surprisingly, women with subclinical eating disorders tend to have higher body fat than normal eaters do, despite exercising more and reportedly eating less than their normal-eating counterparts. They also tend to consume less dietary fat than the normal eaters do. These findings challenge the two commonly held nutrition beliefs: (1) The more you exercise, the thinner you'll be, and (2) avoiding dietary fat helps you lose body fat.

The women seemingly adapt to the combination of intense exercise with high calorie expenditure and restricted calorie intake. The big deficit causes the body to shut down and conserve energy (similar to hibernation). As mentioned in chapter 13, this seems to be nature's survival technique to prevent women from becoming too thin to reproduce.

Research suggests that those women who maintain a stable weight actually do get the calories they need, but through chaotic binge eating (Wilmore et al. 1992). Yet, if you believe that your body is hibernating, and you think that you eat less than you "deserve" to eat given your exercise level, the solution in both cases is to increase your daytime calorie intake gradually to an appropriate level, stop living in calorie deficit, and curb binge eating. You can do this by adding about 100 calories to your daily intake for four days, then adding another 100 calories for the next four days, and so on until you approach your calorie requirements as outlined in chapter 15. A registered dietitian can be very helpful in this process.

Hunger: A Simple Request for Fuel

Being hungry all the time is not a personality quirk. Rather, hunger is the body's request for fuel. Hunger is a powerful physiological force that creates a strong desire to eat. Unfortunately, in our thin-is-in society, many active people fail to honor this simple request because they fear food as being fattening. The thought of eating elicits a sense of panic: "Oh, no, if I eat, I'll get fat. But if I stay hungry, I know I am not gaining weight." This is an unhealthy mind-set.

Athletes can eat without getting fat. Food, after all, is fuel. But problems arise when a person denies himself or herself food (as happens with a strict reducing diet), when hunger becomes the norm. The result is an abnormal physiological state known as starvation.

Starvation has been inflicted on many people, including people in developing countries suffering through famines, poverty-stricken people at the end of the month when they have no money for food, and victims of World War II concentration camps. Starvation is also common among exercisers who are intent on losing weight.

Hunger Scale

If you have spent years dieting and not eating when you are hungry, then blowing your diet and stuffing yourself until you need to loosen your belt, you may feel troubled by the struggle to regulate your food intake. The hunger scale can help you get back in touch with normal eating (i.e., eating like a child). Children eat when they are hungry and stop when they are content—and they rarely run out of energy.

1	5	10
Starved	Content	Stuffed
Light-headed	Pleasantly fed	Uncomfortable
Unable to concentrate	Satiated	Painfully full

Your job is to listen to your body and eat until you are satisfied and feel pleasantly fed—not stuffed, not hankering for more because you are still hungry. The trick to feeding yourself appropriately is to eat slowly and mindfully, paying attention to the pleasant feeling of satiety that is midway between starved and stuffed.

A question arises: What is the cost of starvation? What happens to the body and the mind when food is restricted and body weight is abnormally low? In 1950, Ancel Keys and his colleagues at the University of Minnesota studied the physiology of starvation (Keys et al. 1950; Garner 1998). They carefully monitored 36 young, healthy, psychologically normal men who for six months were allowed to eat only half their normal intake (an amount similar to that consumed on a strict reducing diet or with anorectic eating). For three months before this semistarvation diet, the researchers carefully studied each man's behaviors, personality, and eating patterns. After the semi-starvation diet, the men were then observed for three to nine months of refeeding.

As their body weight fell to 25 percent below baseline, the researchers learned that many of the symptoms that might have been thought to be specific to anorexia or bulimia were actually the result of starvation. The most striking change was a dramatic increase in preoccupation with food. The subjects thought about food all the time, just as hungry dieters and people with anorexia do. They talked about it, read about it, dreamed about it. They even collected recipes. They dramatically increased their consumption of coffee and tea, and they chewed gum excessively. They became depressed; had severe mood swings; and experienced irritability, anger, and anxiety. They became withdrawn, had little interest in sex, and lost their sense of humor. They had cold hands and feet, they felt weak and dizzy, and their hair fell out. Their basal metabolic rates (the amount of food needed to exist) dropped by 40 percent as their bodies adapted to conserve energy. Perhaps these changes sound familiar.

During the study, some of the men were unable to maintain control over food; they would binge eat if the opportunity presented itself. During the refeeding period, many of the men ate continuously—large meals followed by snacking. Several ate until they were uncomfortably full, became nauseated, and then vomited. These abnormal eating behaviors lasted for about five months. By eight months, most of the men regained their standard eating behaviors. On average, they initially regained 10 percent more than their original weights but then gradually lost that excess and returned close to their baseline weights.

So what can we learn from this starvation study?

- Preoccupation with food is a sign that your body is too hungry. Hunger creates a strong physiological drive to eat.
- Binge eating stems from starvation. If you worry about being unable to stop eating once you start, you have likely become too hungry.
- Weight is more than a matter of willpower. If you lose weight, your body will fight to return to a genetically normal level.
- Dieters who restrict to the point of semistarvation are likely to regain the weight they lost, plus more. If you have weight to lose, lose it slowly, not by starvation.

To prevent hunger, you might find it helpful to know how many calories your body requires to maintain or to lose weight. Then, the next time you get into a food tizzy, overeat, and wonder if you are borderline bulimic, you can compare your intake to your requirements. You'll likely see a huge discrepancy between what you have eaten and what your body needs. Hunger is powerful. Avoid becoming too hungry!

Thin at Any Cost

The restriction of food that accompanies the struggle to be perfectly thin creates health problems for casual exercisers and competitors alike. It can greatly reduce the intake of vitamins, minerals, protein, and carbohydrate, placing the athlete at risk of poor nutrition status. Food restrictions can also lead to health problems such as chronic fatigue, compromised immune function, poor or delayed healing, anemia, electrolyte imbalance, menstrual dysfunction, reduced bone density, and a four times higher risk of stress fracture (ACSM 2007).

I counsel many people with eating disorders and disordered eating; they fill the majority of my counseling hours. They come in believing that if only they were thinner, they'd be better athletes (and their overall lives would be better). I disagree. Their efforts to achieve their desired thinness reduce their energy and performance. They would be better athletes if they fed themselves better. Such was the case with Gretchen, an avid cyclist. She came to me complaining about her inability to lose 5 pounds (2.3 kilograms): "If only I could shed this extra fat, I'd be so much faster climbing hills." She was severely restricting her food intake. I pointed out how few calories she was eating compared with what her body required. Once she started to eat adequately, she discovered she could keep up with the other cyclists. Food works!

The following case studies are typical of the clients I treat. They may sound familiar and might help those of you who constantly struggle with food and exercise.

The Stair-Stepper Mistress

Alicia, a 41-year-old teacher, had never been concerned about her weight and had never dieted until her 39th birthday. But in the past two years, she had gained a few pounds because of the stress of a new job. Not liking the extra weight, she decided to join a health club. She forced herself through 60 minutes of stair stepping every morning before school, ate very little during the day, but would then devour any food in sight on arriving home from work. "I feel so guilty about the boxes of crackers, pretzels, and cookies I devour. After a binge, I won't eat dinner. Instead, I'll go back to the health club to burn off the excess calories. I'm exhausted all the time. I'm doing a poor job of teaching. I get easily irritated and feel like yelling at the students. I'm frustrated that I'm unable to do something as simple as lose a few pounds. I can't even eat normally now. I either starve or binge. I don't know if I should be seeing you or a therapist."

To help Alicia balance her food and exercise goals and to normalize her disordered eating patterns, I measured her percent body fat (a lean 18 percent) and calculated how many calories her body required each day. She needed about 1,200 calories for her resting metabolic rate, 600 calories for moderate daily activity, and 500 calories for purposeful exercise, adding up to about 2,300 total calories per day. Then I devised a meal plan to stabilize her eating.

Like many of my clients, she dieted too hard and unrealistically restricted her calories. She would burn off 500 calories at the health club but would not eat anything until lunch, when she limited herself to 250 calories of a frozen meal. No wonder she felt starved and stuffed herself with food the minute she arrived home after school. I advised her to stop dieting, start eating breakfast and lunch, and eat reasonably at night. She changed her habits and stopped binge eating after school.

Alicia followed my recommendations to eat 2,300 calories, divided into four even-sized meals: breakfast, first lunch, second lunch (after school), and dinner. When she returned two weeks later she reported with a big smile, "When I get home after school, I no longer act like a maniac in the kitchen, eating whatever I can get my hands on. I feel so much better and am even losing a little weight because I'm not binge eating. Having a substantial breakfast and lunch helps me feel better and gives me enough energy to have fun with my students. I'm less irritable—back to my old happy self. And, most important, I'm back in control of my food."

Alicia normalized her eating by stopping her dieting and starting to eat appropriate meals at breakfast and lunch. She simply needed a better food plan to correct her food binges, which stemmed from extreme hunger, not from an eating disorder. She'd thought that dieting would help her lose weight, but instead she learned that normal, healthful eating is really the better path to weight management.

The Exercise Addict

Bill, a regional sales manager for a computer company, was addicted to exercise. He'd get up at 5:15 a.m. and arrive at the front door of the health club when it opened at 6:00. He'd do a stationary cycling class from 6:00 to 7:00 and then lift weights from 7:00 to 8:00. At lunchtime, he'd do a step-aerobics class at his company's fitness facility. After work he'd swim laps for an hour at his local YMCA. Because he exercised at three different locations, few people knew how much time he spent exercising, except his wife and family. They constantly complained that he was never home.

Holidays brought even more complaints. "Why do you have to exercise on Christmas morning?" his eight-year-old daughter complained when Bill announced that he was going for his two-hour Merry Christmas run, his present to himself. His family knew he would be incredibly irritable if he didn't run, so they waited patiently for his return before opening gifts.

Without question, Bill was addicted to exercise. He'd feel irritable, anxious, guilty, and depressed if he was unable to do at least four hours of exercise a day. He needed to do increasingly more exercise to achieve the same physical and emotional highs. He'd exercise even when injured or sick. He had little energy for the rest of his life and was fearful that he would lose his job because of a steady decline in his work performance.

Bill's ability to exercise came to a halt when he experienced debilitating back pain. He could barely walk without severe anguish. While seeing the back doctor, he admitted he needed help. "I can no longer exercise the way I'd like to, and I'm petrified of getting fat. I'm trying not to eat because I cannot exercise, but I end up sneaking food—and stealing my daughter's M&M's." The doctor insisted that Bill make an appointment with me. To my eyes, Bill had a long way to go before anyone would consider him fat. He was 5 feet, 10 inches (178 centimeters) and weighed 130 pounds (59 kilograms), but I listened to his fears. I reminded him that people in the hospital do little or no exercise, and they still eat and don't get fat; in fact, they often lose weight.

I worked with Bill on normalizing his eating and exercise practices, suggested some reading material (such as *Hooked on Exercise* by Rebecca Prussin), and convinced him that meeting with a counselor would help keep his life from falling apart. With a doctor, therapist, and nutritionist on his treatment team, as well as a family therapist and the love of his wife and children, he evolved into a happier person. He learned to communicate his wants and needs so that he no longer felt the desire to run away from his problems. He came to understand that his underlying belief that he wasn't good enough was a misperception. He came to like and accept himself as the truly loving person he wanted to be.

How Much Exercise Is Enough?

Exercise should be a way to train and improve athletic performance, not a means of purging calories. If you are an exercise bulimic who spends too much time working out, note these recommendations from the 2005 *Dietary Guidelines for Americans* (www.health.gov/dietaryguidelines) as well as from the American Heart Association (Mosca et al. 2007).

For health, fitness, and reducing the risk of disease, adults should participate in the following most days of the week:

- A minimum of 30 minutes of moderate activity to prevent chronic disease
- 60 minutes of moderate-to-hard activity to manage body weight and prevent gradual weight gain in adulthood
- For people who have been obese, 60 to 90 minutes to keep from regaining lost weight

If you are an athlete training for a sport, you might spend more time than this. But consider getting help if you are a compulsive exerciser whose motivation is to burn off calories.

The Marathon Runner With Bulimia

Carol, a 29-year-old graduate student, had gained 12 pounds (5.4 kilograms) in the two years since she had started studying for her MBA. She tended to overeat when schoolwork became overwhelming and she felt as if she couldn't do all that was expected of her. "I binge at night and then vomit and go for a long run. I'm exhausted all the time and think of little else other than what, when, and how I'll binge. I've stopped socializing with my friends at mealtimes because I'm afraid I'll overeat and be unable to purge. Instead, I spend my time studying and training for a marathon. I'm hoping the added exercise will contribute to weight loss. But I'm a foodaholic. When I finish my run, I inevitably end up at the corner store, where I buy at least two big muffins and heaven only knows what else. I just can't seem to control my food intake."

After listening to Carol's story, I recognized that she seemed addicted not only to food but also to schoolwork and exercise. She constantly pushed herself to meet self-imposed deadlines, weight goals, and exercise demands. She always felt stressed and overextended. She lacked healthy balance in her life.

I asked if anyone in Carol's family had trouble with alcohol. She quietly admitted that her mother was an alcoholic. She seemed ashamed of this family secret. At least one-third of my clients with eating disorders grew up in families with some type of dysfunction, most commonly related to alcohol. The clients themselves may not be addicted to alcohol, but some are recovering alcoholics or drug abusers (Varner 1995). Alternatively, they express other addictive behaviors through overworking, overeating, overachieving, and overexercising. The traits and attitudes outlined in table 16.1 are characteristic of people who grew up in an alcoholic or otherwise dysfunctional family.

Table 16.1   Red-Flag Traits

Characteristic trait	Common expression of trait
Drive for perfection	"I've exercised for an hour every day for the past 2 years."
Desire for control	"I never eat after 7:00 p.m."
Compulsive behavior	"I work out for 2 hours every day, even if I have to get up at 4:00 a.m."
Feelings of inadequacy	"I could have biked even faster if I'd lost more weight."
Difficulty having fun	"Thanks for inviting me to the movie. I'll pass—I have to do my workout at the gym."
Trouble with relationships	"My spouse complains that I spend too much time exercising and not enough time with my family."

Carol displayed all these traits. She had a strong drive to be perfect and a desire for control. Since childhood she had tried to be perfect to compensate for her family's problems. Now, she was trying to eat the perfect diet, achieve the perfect weight, develop the perfect career, and maintain the perfect training schedule. She ran 10 miles (16 kilometers) every day, despite blizzards, illness, or fatigue. She lived on calorie-free coffee, diet soda, and fat-free foods, until ravenous hunger overwhelmed her good intentions. After a binge, she'd vomit to bring a feeling of control back to her life and compensate for her imperfect eating.

I helped Carol get a better perspective on an appropriate weight by measuring her percent body fat. By designing a meal plan, I helped her eat an appropriate diet. A referral to a coach at the local running club allowed her to train with an appropriate program. I also advised her to read some books about adult children of alcoholics (see appendix A), seek guidance from a suitable counselor, and perhaps join a support group such as Al-Anon or ACoA (Adult Children of Alcoholics).

"For the past two years, I have tried to avoid food, thinking it was fattening," she wrote in a follow-up letter. "I've come to learn that food wasn't the problem. My inability to handle stress was the problem. I'm now gentler on myself. I no longer strive to be the perfect student. For example, I took three days off from both school and running when I went on a ski weekend with my friends! I'm eating well and exercising healthfully rather than punishing myself with megamiles to burn off calories. I feel better and am at peace with myself and my body."

The Figure Skater With Anorexia

Emily, a 16-year-old student at a highly competitive figure skating program, was sent to me by her coach. Emily's mother made the appointment for her. Because she was chronically tired, Emily was compromising her ability to jump high and skate hard. Emily's first words to me were, "My coach and mother made me come here. They think I don't eat enough."

Emily weighed 92 pounds (42 kilograms). A year ago, she had weighed 110 pounds (50 kilograms), and at 5 feet, 3 inches (160 centimeters), she could have appropriately weighed 115 pounds (52 kilograms). She was limiting herself to 1,000 calories per day but required about 1,800 calories, if not more. Because she was eating so little food, she was consuming inadequate amounts of protein, calcium, iron, zinc, and numerous other vitamins and minerals that her body needed to be healthy.

Emily was so afraid that she'd get fat if she were to eat more, I had to constantly remind her that food is fuel and health. She was currently unhealthy. She had stopped menstruating (one sign of poor health), and her complexion was splotchy and grayish (a second sign). Emily needed to eat a wider variety of food than cottage cheese, egg whites, and apples to balance her diet and provide the nutrients in which she was deficient. She also needed to include more dietary fat.

I reminded Emily that she deserved to eat, even if she was not exercising. I asked her to take notice of all her friends who were nonexercisers. All ate, and most were lean. Eating more would not provide excess calories but fundamental fuel. We agreed on the following goals for a food plan that would optimize her health:

- Fuel her body appropriately by gradually increasing calories at meals and snacks.

- Rebuild her body to an appropriate weight to optimize her strength and health.

- Reduce the risk of stress fractures and future osteoporosis by eating enough to support regular menstrual periods.

- Attain peace with food and weight.

Emily agreed to increase her intake gradually, by 100 calories per week, adding more food at breakfast and lunch until she ate three 500-calorie meals that included at least three or four kinds of foods (such as cereal, milk, and fruit; pita bread, turkey, and yogurt; fish, rice, broccoli, and milk) as well as a snack with food from two food groups. These dietary improvements would help her have more energy to concentrate better at school and skate with enthusiasm. I suggested that she practice eating more healthfully, just as she practiced her skating, and that she focus on how much better she felt when she fueled herself better.

Over the course of weeks, Emily stopped rigidly controlling her food and started to eat more appropriately. My nutrition advice had provided helpful guidelines, but a key factor in her recovery was counseling. A psychologist skilled in handling eating disorders counseled her, as did a family therapist who met with Emily and her parents and sister. By communicating and resolving many of the family's issues, Emily was able to express her needs rather than withhold words and use food restriction to starve her feelings and be her silent cry for help.

Within three months, Emily started to menstruate, a good sign that she was adequately nourishing her body. She was feeling physically stronger, was happier with her family, and felt at peace with food and her body. She no longer felt that she had to be perfect to earn her parents' love, nor did she need to be perfectly thin, eat the perfect diet, and be the perfect student and figure skater. She learned to enjoy being human, like the rest of her family and friends. She let go of her fantasy that a perfect body would bring a perfect life. "I thought I'd be happier once I was thinner, but I was wrong. I've learned that happiness comes from loving myself from the inside out, not from the outside in."

Athletes and Amenorrhea

Athletes with eating disorders commonly stop menstruating (amenor- rhea). Athletes without eating disorders can also stop menstruating. This can happen, for example, if a woman steps up her exercise program with- out boosting her calorie intake. In either case, if you are an athlete who previously had regular menstrual periods but have stopped menstruating, don't ignore it. Although you may think amenorrhea is desirable because you no longer have to deal with the hassles of monthly menstrual periods, amenorrhea can lead to problems that interfere with your health and ability to perform your best. These problems include the following:

- A four-times-higher incidence of stress fractures that put you on the sidelines (Nativ 2000)
- Premature osteoporosis that can affect your bone health in the not-too-distant future
- An inability to conceive easily should you want to start a family

Amenorrhea Is Complex

If you believe you miss periods only because you are too thin and are exercising too much, you may be wrong. Studies have shown no body- fat differences between athletic women who menstruate regularly and those who don't (Sanborn et al. 2000). Many very thin athletes do have regular menses. Clearly, leanness and intense exercise are not the simple explanation to the complexities of amenorrhea.

But the question remains unanswered: Why are you amenorrheic when your peers, who have similar exercise programs and the same low percent body fat, are not? You are likely eating inadequate calories to support your training program and are experiencing nutritional amenorrhea.

Resolving the Problem

Current research suggests that amenorrhea is not caused by exercising too much, but by eating too little food. To resume menses, you need to eat enough calories to support not only your exercise program but also your body's ability to reproduce. To be able to menstruate, your body requires at least 13.5 calories per pound (30 calories per kilogram) of lean body mass (weight without any body fat) (Loucks 2004). By comparison, the average (nonathletic) woman maintains energy balance at about 20.5 calories per pound (45 calories per kilogram) of lean body mass.

An athletic woman who weighs 120 pounds and has 20 percent body fat, for example, has a lean body mass of 96 pounds (20% × 120 lb = 24 lb fat, which means she has 96 lb LBM). She needs to eat at least 1,300 calories (13.5 cal/lb × 96 lb LBM = 1,300 cal) that are not burned off, that are "available energy." If she burns 500 calories in exercise, she needs to consume at least 1,300 + 500 = 1,800 calories; this is still far too little to fully fuel her muscles and enjoy optimal performance.

A registered dietitian or sports nutritionist can help you improve your patterns of skimpy eating—a task that for some women is easier said than done. The following tips may also be of help:

1. **Throw away the bathroom scale.** Rather than strive to achieve a certain number on the scale, let your body weigh what it weighs. Rather than exert willpower to achieve a desired weight, let your body acquire its genetic weight. The information in chapters 13 and 15 can help you estimate a weight you can comfortably maintain without constantly dieting. Your physician or dietitian can also offer unbiased professional advice.

2. **Don't restrict calories by more than 20 percent.** If you have weight to lose, do not eat less than 1,200 calories (Woolsey 2001) per day or, more precisely, no less than 13.5 calories per pound of lean body mass (Loucks and Thuma 2003). By following a healthy reducing program, you'll not only have greater success with long-term weight loss but also have enough energy to enjoy participating and improving in your sports program.

3. **Practice eating as you did when you were a child.** If you are at an appropriate weight, focus on eating when you are hungry and stopping when you are content. If you are always hungry and constantly obsessing about food, you are undoubtedly trying to eat too few calories. Your body is complaining and requesting more food; hunger is simply a request for fuel. The information in chapter 15, plus advice from your doctor and dietitian, can help you determine an appropriate calorie intake.

   Amenorrheic women commonly eat in nontraditional ways, with chaotic eating patterns (Wilmore et al. 1992). They may eat little at breakfast and lunch, only to overeat at night, or they restrict themselves on Monday through Thursday and then overeat on the weekends. If your weight is stable, you have somehow consumed the number of calories you need, so you might as well eat them on a regular schedule of wholesome, well-balanced meals. A registered dietitian can help you develop an appropriate food plan if you are struggling on your own.

4. **Eat adequate protein.** In one study, 82 percent of the women with amenorrhea ate less than the recommended intake for protein (Nelson et al. 1986). Vegetarians, in particular, need to be sure to get adequate protein. Vegetarian women who consume adequate protein and calories tend to have regular menstrual periods (Barr 1999).

5. **Eat at least 20 percent of your calories from fat.** Some fat is absolutely essential for your health and well-being. Your body needs fat to build healthy cell membranes and to make hormonelike substances called prostaglandins. You want to boost your intake of good fat and carefully balance in the saturated ("bad") fat in red meats and other protein-rich foods. For most active women, eating 40 to 60 grams of fat per day would be an appropriate low-fat diet. This plan clearly allows salmon, peanut butter, nuts, olive oil, and other health-promoting fats, as well as smaller amounts of saturated fat as found in lean beef, low-fat cheese, and other nourishing foods that provide balance to a sports diet. If you just cannot bring yourself to add butter to bread or oil to salads, then
   o sprinkle sunflower seeds or slivered almonds on salads,
   o enjoy trail mix with nuts and raisins for snacks,
   o choose whole-wheat breads and cereals (they have more healthy fat),
   o eat fatty fish twice a week,
   o use olive or canola oil for cooking, and
   o skip the fat-free products (they are devoid of taste).

6. **Maintain a calcium-rich diet.** If you are amenorrheic, you should regularly consume three or four 8-ounce (250 milliliter) servings of low-fat milk or yogurt (or other calcium-rich foods) daily to protect your bones. Your bones benefit from the protective effect of exercise, but exercise does not compensate for lack of calcium. Although you may cringe at the thought of spending 300 to 400 calories on dairy foods, remember that milk is a wholesome food that contains many important nutrients. Women who consume three or more glasses of milk or yogurt tend to be leaner than those who do not (Pereira et al. 2002). If you are eating a diet that includes lots of bran cereal, fruits, and vegetables, you may have

an even higher need for calcium because the fiber may interfere with calcium absorption.

Many amenorrheic women worry about their bone health, and rightfully so. If the amenorrhea is associated with anorexia, you might be losing bone density at the rate of 2.5 percent a year (Miller et al. 2006). Multiply that by several years, and it's no wonder many of my clients have bones similar to those of 70-year-old women and problems with stress fractures. Teenagers, in particular, need to optimize their bone density because about 90 percent of bone density is gained by age 17. If you don't have dense bones as a teenager, you may never reach your peak bone mass and will have a higher risk of osteoporosis in later life (Weaver 2002).

You can recover much of the bone loss by eating well enough to rebuild muscles and gain weight, but not always all of it (Dominguez et al. 2007). A case study of a 31-year-old distance runner indicates she was able to bring her bone mineral density back to within normal values by eating better and rebuilding her body, despite a long history of anorexia and amenorrhea (Fredericson and Kent 2005). Not everyone is as lucky.

Many amenorrheic athletes have been advised to take the birth control pill to resume menses, and theoretically, this would help prevent bone loss. Research does not support that theory. Eating adequate calories to negate an "energy drain" and rebuilding muscles is the key to reversing bone loss. Adequate calories include adequate carbohydrate to replace depleted glycogen stores, adequate protein to build muscles, and enough fuel to maintain energy balance (Zanker and Cooke 2004; Nativ 2007).

Although female athletes fear that eating more and exercising less will hurt their performance, this is not the case. A 19-year-old amenorrheic runner reduced her training by one day per week, increased her daily food intake with one can of a 360-calorie liquid meal supplement, gained 6 pounds (2.7 kilograms) over about four months (from 106 to 112 pounds, or from 48 to 51 kilograms), and resumed menstruation. She set more personal records than she did during any prior season, broke two school records, and qualified for a national track meet (Dueck et al. 1996). What are you waiting for?

How to Help

Perhaps you have friends, family, or teammates who struggle with food, and you wonder what you can do to help resolve the problem. Seeing a

Healing Mantras and Affirmations

If you are determined to start eating better, you might find the task easier said than done. Here are some mantras that have helped my clients as they strive to fuel their bodies appropriately:

- My body is hungry; that means it has burned off what I fed it, and it now needs more fuel. Hunger is simply a request for fuel.
- This food is fundamental, not "extra," not "fattening."
- One meal is not going to change my life forever.
- Let me be more flexible. I can always go back to my old ways, if I need to.
- My body is stronger when I fuel better, and I become a better athlete.
- I don't need to have a perfect diet to have a good diet.
- I can be human, not perfect.
- Starving my body will not solve my problems.
- Being happy and healthy is more important than any number on the scale.
- I have a choice: Do I want to be a person with anorexia or a well-fueled athlete?
- Everything will work out OK. I just need to keep focused on the big picture—I need to be healthy.

loved one seemingly waste away can be sad and scary. Often it's hard to tell if the person is really struggling or just being a dedicated athlete. Even health professionals can have trouble distinguishing between the person who is lean and mean and the one who is battling anorexia.

An athlete with anorexia is generally a compulsive exerciser who trains frantically—out of fear of gaining weight—and never takes rest days. In comparison, a dedicated athlete trains hard with hopes of improving performance but also enjoys days with no exercise. Both push themselves to perfection—to be perfectly thin or to be the perfect athlete. Sometimes the two intertwine. Unfortunately, too many coaches, parents, friends, and teammates fail to confront the devastating stressfulness of this struggle for ultimate thinness. After all, how can anyone who is training hard and seems happy be sick?

If you suspect that your friend, training partner, child, or teammate has a problem with food, don't wait until medical problems prove you right. Speak up in an appropriate manner. Anorexia and bulimia are life-threatening conditions that shouldn't be overlooked. Here are 10 tips for approaching this delicate subject.

1. **Heed the signs.** You may notice that people with anorexia wear bulky clothes to hide their abnormal thinness or that their food consumption is abnormally restrictive and sparse in comparison to the energy they expend. Runners with anorexia, for example, may eat only a yogurt for dinner after having completed a strenuous 10-mile (16 kilometer) workout. Perhaps you'll never see them eating in public, at home, or with friends. They find some excuse for not joining others at meals. Or if they do, they may push the food around on the plate to fool you into thinking they're eating. You may also notice other compulsive behaviors, such as excessive studying or working.

   Bulimic behavior can be subtler. The athlete may eat a great deal of food and then rush to the bathroom. You may hear water running to cover up the sound of vomiting. The person may hide laxatives or even speak about a magic method of eating without gaining weight. She or he may have bloodshot eyes, swollen glands, and bruised fingers (from inducing vomiting).

2. **Express your concern carefully.** Approach these individuals gently but persistently, telling them you are worried about their health: "I'm concerned that your injuries are taking so long to heal." Talk about what you see: "I've noticed that you seem tired, and your race times are getting slower and slower." Give evidence for why you believe they are struggling to balance food and exercise, and ask if they want to talk about it.

   Individuals who are truly anorexic or bulimic commonly deny the problem, insisting they're perfectly fine. Continue to share your concerns about their lack of concentration, light-headedness, or chronic fatigue. These health issues are more likely to be stepping-stones for the athlete to accept help, given that she or he undoubtedly clings to food and exercise as attempts to gain control and stability.

3. **Do not discuss weight or eating habits.** The athlete takes great pride in being perfectly thin and may dismiss your concern as jealousy. Avoid any mention of starving and bingeing as the issue. Focus on life issues, not food issues.

4. **Suggest unhappiness as the reason for seeking help.** Point out how anxious, tired, or irritable the athlete has been lately. Emphasize that he or she doesn't have to be that way.

5. **Be supportive, and listen sympathetically.** Don't expect someone to admit right away that there's a problem. Give it time, and constantly remind your friend that you believe in him or her. Your support will make a difference in recovery.

6. **Offer a list of professional resources.** If someone you know has a full-blown or subclinical eating disorder, you may feel frustrated about your unsuccessful efforts to resolve the problem. You may think, "If only my friend would eat normally, everything would be OK." Likely not. Food is just the symptom. The problem is this person is unhappy. To help you understand more about these underlying issues, you might want to read *Surviving an Eating Disorder: A Survival Guide for Parents and Friends* by Michelle Siegel, Judith Brisman, and Margot Weinshel. This helpful resource can teach you what to say to your friend.

   Your job is to help your friend or loved one by taking her or him to get professional guidance. This might mean finding a registered dietitian in your area who specializes in sports nutrition and eating disorders. Remind your friend that no weight will ever be good enough to create happiness. Happiness comes from within, not from a number on the scale. And although the athlete may deny the problem to your face, she or he may admit despair at another moment. If you don't know of a mental-health counselor skilled in the treatment of eating disorders, the resources and national organizations listed in appendix A can help you find an expert where you live. You can also call your local sports medicine clinic and ask to speak to a physician or nutritionist, your university health center or eating disorders program, or your local medical center and ask to have an eating disorders assessment.

7. **Limit your expectations.** You alone can't solve the problem. It's more complex than food and exercise; it's a life problem. Share your concerns with others. Seek help from a trusted family member, medical professional, or health service. Don't try to deal with the problem alone, especially if you are making no headway and the athlete is becoming more self-destructive.

8. **Recognize that you may be overreacting.** Maybe there is no eating disorder. Maybe the athlete is appropriately thin for enhanced sports performance. But how can you decide? To clarify the situation, insist that he or she have a mental-health evaluation. If necessary, make the appointment, and take the athlete there yourself. Only then will you get an unbiased opinion of the degree of danger,

if any. The therapist may tell you to go home and stop worrying, or the therapist might detect misery and suicidal tendencies in the athlete and encourage immediate care.

9. **Seek advice from health care professionals about your concerns.** You may need to discuss your feelings with someone. Remember that you are not responsible for the other person's health. You can only try to help. Your power comes from using guidance counselors, registered dietitians, medical professionals, or eating disorders clinics.

10. **Be patient.** Recognize that the healing process can be long and arduous, with many relapses and setbacks, but your reward will be that you can make a critical difference in that person's life. People die from anorexia and bulimia.

Preventing Eating Disorders

Many people think, or feel pressured to believe, that by restricting their food intake to lose weight they will exercise better, look better, and enhance their overall performances. Ironically, dieting precedes the onset of obesity, disordered eating, and eating disorders. Dieting is a risky behavior; it can result in depleted muscles, amenorrhea, stress fractures, fainting, weakness, fatigue, impaired performance, and sooner or later, disordered eating or eating disorders. Clearly, dieting is not a solution to weight issues.

Eating disorders would fade if people could learn to love their bodies and feel good about themselves. You might want to stop reading glamour magazines; they can make you feel worse about yourself to the extent that you end up exercising to punish yourself for how you look and buying cosmetics and hair products to "fix" yourself.

As a society, we must

- dispel the myth that diets "work" and that thinness equates to happiness and success,
- discourage the notion that the thinnest athlete is the best athlete,
- love our bodies for what they are rather than hate them for what they are not,
- emphasize being fit and healthy as more appropriate goals than being skinny, and
- be careful about how we acknowledge weight loss.

When Your Friends Lose Weight, What Should You Say?

When someone has lost weight, the knee-jerk response is to exclaim, "Wow! You look great!" This praise is intended to be positive, but it implies that

1. the dieter looked horrible before,
2. physical size is more important than health, and
3. the person is somehow better or more valuable because of the weight loss.

Be it 2 pounds or 20 (1 kilogram or 10), the better way to acknowledge weight loss is to shift the focus away from physical weight change and focus instead on the praiseworthy aspect: the person's improved health status. Here are some recommended phrases to share with people who are losing or have lost weight:

- "It looks as if you've been working hard at losing weight." The dieter will be ever ready to talk about how proud she or he is of the hard work it took to lose weight. Listen to the story and be sure that the person is healthy.

- "You look smaller. . . . Is there less of you to love?" The message is that your friend is not *better* for having lost weight, just *smaller.*

- "You look pleased with your weight loss. How do you feel about it?" The person may feel healthier and more energetic, but you may also hear him or her express some frustration in not being quite thin enough yet.

- "You are looking fit. How are your workouts going? How is your energy level? How do you feel?" If your friend is losing weight appropriately, she or he will feel great.

- "You appear to be trading some of your excess fat for muscle." Acknowledge what you see, but don't suggest that dieting has made him or her a better person.

Regardless of the response, the goal is to help the dieter hold a solid appreciation of her or his value as a person. Beauty is in the sincere smile shared, the friendship offered, the positive qualities exhibited—not in being a size 2 instead of a size 12. People need to know they are loved from the inside out, not judged from the outside in. When dieters lose weight, they need to realize that there is simply less of them to love. They are not better or more likable. They are just smaller. With appropriate dieting, they are healthier, stronger, more energetic, and happy about these benefits of weight loss.

PART IV

Winning Recipes for Peak Performance

CHAPTER 17 ─────────────

Breads and Breakfasts

Fresh from the oven, breads are one of the favorite forms of carbohydrate for active people. Here are some baking tips to help you prepare the yummiest of breads.

- The secret for light and fluffy quick breads, muffins, and scones is to stir the flour lightly and for only 20 seconds. Ignore the lumps! If you beat the batter too much, the gluten (protein) in the flour will toughen the dough.

- Breads made entirely with whole-wheat flour tend to be heavy. In general, half white and half whole-wheat flour is an appropriate combination. Many of these recipes have been developed using this ratio. You can alter the ratio as you like. When substituting whole-wheat flour for white flour in other recipes, use 3/4 cup whole-wheat flour for 1 cup white flour.

- Most of these recipes have reduced sugar content. To reduce the sugar content of your own recipes, use one-third to one-half less sugar than indicated; the finished product will be just fine. If you want to exchange white sugar with honey, brown sugar, or molasses, use only 1/2 teaspoon baking powder per 2 cups flour, and add 1/2 teaspoon baking soda. This prevents an "off" taste.

- Most quick-bread recipes instruct you to sift together the baking powder and flour. This method produces the lightest breads and best results. In some recipes, I direct you to mix the baking powder with the wet ingredients and add the flour last. My method is easier, produces an acceptable product, and saves time.

- To prevent quick breads from sticking, use nonstick baking pans or cooking spray, or place a piece of waxed paper in the baking pan before pouring the batter. I've found that using waxed paper is foolproof. After the quick bread has baked, let it cool for five minutes, tip it out of the pan, then peel off the paper.

- To hasten cooking time, bake quick breads in an 8- by 8-inch square pan instead of a loaf pan. They bake in half the time. You can also bake muffins in a loaf or square pan, eliminating the hard-to-wash muffin tins.

Fresh from the stove top, oatmeal is not only a healthful addition to your sports diet but also an easy-to-digest preexercise breakfast. Many people like oatmeal before long runs, hard workouts at the gym, swim practices, or other workouts. The following oatmeal additions will add variety to your breakfasts:

- Dried apricot pieces, honey, and a dash of nutmeg
- Raisins and cinnamon
- Sliced banana (cooked with the oatmeal), brown sugar, and peanut butter
- Dried cranberries, honey, and chopped pecans
- Diced apple (cooked with the oatmeal) and maple syrup

Instead of adding sweetener to the oatmeal, some people choose to add a little salt and eat the oatmeal as a grain instead of a sweetened cereal. Because active people need some salt to replace what they lose in sweat, eating salted oatmeal is certainly an acceptable practice—plus most athletes find the oatmeal tastes a lot better.

RECIPE FINDER ─────────────────────────────────────

See also: Tofu burritos, Oatmeal cookies, Peanutty energy bars, Peanut butter banana roll-up, Diana's supersoy and phytochemical shake, Fruit smoothie, Protein shake, Rainbow fruit salad

Banana Bread

The key to success for this all-time favorite is using well-ripened bananas that are covered with brown speckles. Banana bread is a favorite for premarathon carbohydrate loading and for snacking during long-distance bike rides and hikes. Add some peanut butter and you'll have a delicious sandwich that'll keep you energized for a long time.

3 large well-ripened bananas

1 egg (or substitute) or 2 egg whites

2 tablespoons oil, preferably canola

1/3 cup (80 ml) milk

1/3 to 1/2 cup (66 to 100 ml) sugar

1 teaspoon salt

1 teaspoon baking soda

1/2 teaspoon baking powder

1 1/2 cups flour, preferably half whole wheat and half white

1. Preheat the oven to 350 °F (180 °C).
2. Mash bananas with a fork.
3. Add egg, oil, milk, sugar, salt, baking soda, and baking powder. Beat well.
4. Gently blend the flour into the banana mixture. Stir for 20 seconds or until moistened.
5. Pour into a 4- × 8-inch loaf pan that has been lightly oiled, treated with cooking spray, or lined with waxed paper.
6. Bake for 45 minutes or until a toothpick inserted near the middle comes out clean.
7. Let cool for 5 minutes before removing from the pan.

Yield: 12 slices

Nutrition Information   1,600 total calories; 135 calories per slice; 24 g carbohydrate; 3 g protein; 3 g fat

Blueberry Oatmeal Muffins

Blueberries and oatmeal are a tasty combination. Enjoy these muffins for breakfast or snacks. With any baked product, buttermilk offers a nice flaky texture. If you don't have any on hand, you can substitute 1 cup milk mixed with 1 teaspoon vinegar (let stand for a few minutes).

1 cup (80 g) uncooked oatmeal, instant or regular

1 cup (240 ml) buttermilk (or 1 cup milk + 1 teaspoon white vinegar)

1 egg (or substitute) or 2 egg whites

1/4 to 1/3 cup (50 to 66 g) sugar

1/4 to 1/3 cup (60 to 80 ml) oil, preferably canola

1 cup (140 g) flour

1 teaspoon baking powder

1/2 teaspoon baking soda

1 teaspoon salt

1 to 1 1/2 cups (145 to 215 g) blueberries, fresh or frozen

Optional: 1/4 teaspoon nutmeg or cinnamon

1. Preheat the oven to 400 °F (200 °C). Prepare 12 muffin cups with cooking spray or paper liners.
2. In a medium bowl, combine oatmeal, buttermilk, egg, sugar, and oil. Beat well; if time allows, let the batter stand for 5 to 10 minutes for the oatmeal to soften.
3. In a small bowl, combine the flour, baking powder, baking soda, and salt (and nutmeg or cinnamon). Mix well, then combine with the wet ingredients. Stir just until moistened.
4. Gently add the blueberries.
5. Fill the muffin cups. Bake for 15 to 20 minutes or until a toothpick inserted in the middle comes out dry. Cool for 5 minutes, then remove from the pan.

Yield: 12 muffins

Nutrition Information   1,600 total calories; 135 calories per muffin; 18 g carbohydrate; 4 g protein; 5 g fat

Carrot Raisin Muffins

These muffins are a favorite of Evelyn Tribole, RD, sports nutritionist and author of *Healthy Homestyle Desserts*. I can understand why she enjoys these muffins. They're tasty warm from the oven and even tastier on the second day, when the flavors have blended. If you prefer a fat-free muffin, replace the canola oil with 1/3 cup of applesauce, and use 6 egg whites instead of the whole eggs.

1 cup (140 g) whole-wheat flour

1 cup (140 g) white flour

3/4 cup (150 g) sugar

2 teaspoons baking powder

1 teaspoon salt

2 teaspoons cinnamon

1/2 teaspoon baking soda

3 eggs (or substitute) or 6 egg whites

1/2 cup (120 g) buttermilk (or 1/2 cup milk mixed with 1/2 teaspoon vinegar and left to stand for 5 minutes)

1/3 cup (80 ml) oil, preferably canola

2 teaspoons vanilla extract

2 cups (220 g) finely shredded carrot

1 medium apple, peeled and shredded

1/2 cup (80 g) raisins

1/2 cup (60 g) chopped nuts

1. Preheat the oven to 350 °F (180 °C). Prepare 12 muffin tins with papers or cooking spray.
2. In a large bowl, stir together the flours, sugar, baking powder, salt, cinnamon, and baking soda.
3. In a separate bowl, stir together the eggs, buttermilk, oil, and vanilla, then the carrots, apple, raisins, and nuts. Add to the flour mixture, and stir just until blended.
4. Spoon the batter into the muffin cups. Bake about 30 minutes or until a toothpick inserted near the center comes out clean.

Yield: 12 muffins

Nutrition Information 2,750 total calories; 230 calories per muffin; 37 g carbohydrate; 5 g protein; 7 g fat

Adapted with permission. www.EvelynTribole.com

Molasses Muffins With Flax and Dates

Flax is rich in substances that have been shown to protect against heart disease and cancer. It has a very mild taste and is good mixed into muffins and breads as well as sprinkled on cereal. This flax muffin recipe is one way to add a daily tablespoon of flaxseed to your breakfast and snacks. These muffins are remarkably sweet and moist, despite having no added fat. (The 3 grams of fat per muffin are from the health-protective fats in the ground flaxseed meal.)

> 1 egg (or substitute) or 2 egg whites
>
> 1/3 cup (115 g) molasses
>
> 1 cup (240 ml) buttermilk (or 1 cup milk mixed with 1 teaspoon vinegar)
>
> 3/4 cup (120 g) ground flaxseed meal
>
> 1/2 teaspoon salt
>
> 1 cup (175 g) chopped dates
>
> 1 1/2 cups (210 g) flour, preferably half whole wheat and half white
>
> 1 teaspoon baking soda
>
> *Optional:* 1/2 teaspoon cinnamon; 1 teaspoon grated orange rind; 1 teaspoon vanilla extract

1. Preheat the oven to 350 °F (180 °C), and prepare 12 muffin cups with papers or cooking spray.
2. In a large bowl, mix together the egg, molasses, buttermilk, flax, and salt, and add the dates to the batter.
3. In a separate bowl, mix together the flour and baking soda (and cinnamon).
4. Gently stir the flour mixture (and orange rind and vanilla) into the egg mixture.
5. Fill the muffin cups 2/3 full. Bake for 18 to 20 minutes or until a toothpick inserted near the center comes out clean.

Yield: 12 muffins

Nutrition Information   2,000 total calories; 165 calories per muffin; 30 g carbohydrate; 4 g protein; 3 g fat

Cold Cereal With Hot Fruit

This recipe is one of my favorites. I love the combination of hot fruit with cereal and cold milk—reminds me of dessert, similar to a fruit crisp a la mode. Bananas, pears, apples, berries . . . any and all fruits work well as do all types of cereal. Be creative!

In the winter, having warm fruit takes the cold chill away from the quick and easy cereal breakfast. Sometimes I even heat the milk along with the fruit, then add the crunchy cereal. It's easier than making hot oatmeal and has the same warming effect.

This recipe also works well with frozen fruits. For example, I generally stock blueberries in the freezer so that they are ready and waiting to be enjoyed for breakfast. Then I can make "blueberry crisp" for breakfast any day by simply shaking a handful onto the cold cereal and heating the mixture in the microwave.

> 1 cup Life, or other, cereal
>
> 1/2 cup All-Bran
>
> 1/4 cup low-fat granola
>
> 1/2 cup (75 g) blueberries or other fruit
>
> 1 cup (240 ml) low-fat milk

1. In a microwaveable bowl, combine the cereals.
2. Sprinkle with blueberries or other fruit of your choice.
3. Heat in the microwave oven for 20 to 40 seconds, until the blueberries are warm.
4. Pour the cold milk over the top. Dig in!

Yield: 1 serving

Nutrition Information   500 total calories; 85 g carbohydrate; 20 g protein; 7 g fat

Cereal to Go

This is a favorite of Paul Friedman's, a runner and soccer dad who often travels to events. He combines the ingredients in a container that doubles as a bowl, then adds water and shakes: an instant breakfast! Just be sure to pack a spoon.

This recipe can be especially handy for traveling athletes who are on a budget. The cereal, dried milk, and dried fruit won't spoil, and they travel well not only to sports events but also on business trips. You can save yourself great expense (as well as time and hassle) by packing this simple pre-event meal. The trick is to plan ahead and organize your menu so you'll have this breakfast available for a tried-and-true meal.

1/2 cup (70 g) raw rolled oats

1/4 cup Grape-Nuts (or 1/2 cup of your favorite cereal)

1/4 to 1/3 cup (40 to 55 g) raisins or other dried fruit

1/3 to 1/2 cup (40 to 60 g) milk powder

Optional: Brown sugar; diced fresh apple, banana, or other fruit added just before eating

Added later: 1 cup (240 ml) water

Yield: 1 serving

Nutrition Information 520 total calories; 104 g carbohydrate; 15 g protein; 5 g fat

Courtesy of Paul Friedman

Breakfast Fruit Salad With Marmalade Yogurt

This fruit salad can be made with a mixture of fresh, canned, and dried fruits of your choice. Be creative, and buy some fruits that may not be a part of your standard fare—mango, papaya, kiwi.

For the dressing, Greek-style yogurt works well because it is thicker and sweeter than regular yogurt and tastes rich and creamy. If you are not familiar with Greek-style yogurt, it's worth looking for at larger grocery stores or natural-food stores. Vanilla-flavored yogurt also works well.

3 cups cut-up fruit of your choice:
- Apple
- Banana
- Mango
- Pineapple (fresh or canned)
- Berries
- Dried apricots

1/2 cup (115 g) plain low-fat yogurt, preferably Greek style

1 tablespoon orange marmalade

Optional: Dash of nutmeg or cinnamon; slivered almonds or chopped walnuts

1. In a small bowl, combine cut-up fruit.
2. Blend together the yogurt and marmalade.
3. Mix together the yogurt and the fruit (add seasoning and nuts), and serve.

Yield: 2 servings

Nutrition Information   Dressing: 120 total calories; 60 calories per serving; 8 g carbohydrate; 5 g protein; 1 g fat

With fruit: 220 to 280 total calories; 33 to 48 g carbohydrate; 5 g protein; 1 g fat

Honey Nut Granola

The nice thing about making your own granola is you can avoid the unhealthful saturated fat that is found in commercially made granolas. Instead, this recipe offers healthful fat from nuts and canola oil, with a nice blend of carbohydrate-rich whole oats, dried fruits, and other add-ins of your choice to add crunch and goodness.

Mixed with fresh fruit and yogurt, this recipe offers a delicious and healthful way to start the morning or to recover after a tiring workout. The milk powder and nuts add a protein boost.

---

3 cups (420 g) rolled oats (not instant oatmeal)

1 cup (120 g) chopped almonds

2 teaspoons cinnamon

1 cup (120 g) powdered milk

1/3 cup (115 g) honey

1/3 cup (80 ml) canola oil

1 cup (165 g) dried fruit bits (raisins, dried cranberries, chopped dates, and so on)

Optional: 1 teaspoon salt; 1/2 cup (60 g) sesame seeds (untoasted); 1/2 cup (60 g) sunflower seeds (unsalted, untoasted); 1/2 cup (60 g) wheat germ; 1/2 cup (80 g) ground flaxseed meal

---

1. In a large bowl, combine the oats, almonds, cinnamon, and powdered milk (and salt, sesame seeds, and sunflower seeds, as desired).
2. In a saucepan or microwaveable bowl, combine the honey and oil. Heat until almost boiling. Pour the honey mixture over the oat mixture and stir well.
3. Spread the mixture onto two large baking sheets.
4. Bake at 300 °F (150 °C) for 20 to 25 minutes, stirring every 5 minutes.
5. After the granola has cooled, add the dried fruit (and wheat germ and flaxseed meal, as desired). Store in an airtight container.

Yield: 10 1/2-cup servings

Nutrition Information   3,300 total calories; 330 calories per 1/2 cup; 40 g carbohydrate; 10 g protein; 14 g fat

Baked Apple French Toast

This is a beautiful dish with a wonderful aroma, perfect for a postevent brunch with your buddies. The dish can be prepared the night before and baked the next morning.

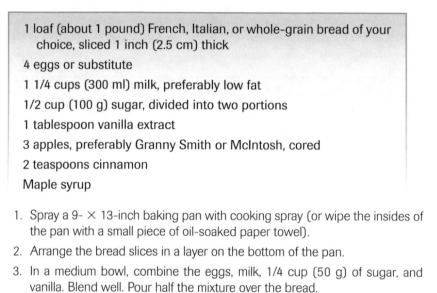

1 loaf (about 1 pound) French, Italian, or whole-grain bread of your choice, sliced 1 inch (2.5 cm) thick

4 eggs or substitute

1 1/4 cups (300 ml) milk, preferably low fat

1/2 cup (100 g) sugar, divided into two portions

1 tablespoon vanilla extract

3 apples, preferably Granny Smith or McIntosh, cored

2 teaspoons cinnamon

Maple syrup

1. Spray a 9- × 13-inch baking pan with cooking spray (or wipe the insides of the pan with a small piece of oil-soaked paper towel).
2. Arrange the bread slices in a layer on the bottom of the pan.
3. In a medium bowl, combine the eggs, milk, 1/4 cup (50 g) of sugar, and vanilla. Blend well. Pour half the mixture over the bread.
4. Slice the apples, and arrange them over the bread.
5. Pour the remaining liquid over the apples.
6. Combine 1/4 cup sugar and the cinnamon and sprinkle over the apples. The dish can be covered and refrigerated overnight at this point, if desired.
7. Bake at 400 °F (200 °C) for 35 to 40 minutes. Let cool for 5 to 10 minutes before serving. Serve with maple syrup.

Yield: 5 servings

Nutrition Information   2,250 total calories; 450 calories per serving (without maple syrup); 77 g carbohydrate; 17 g protein; 8 g fat

Maple syrup: add 60 calories and 15 g carbohydrate per tablespoon.

Courtesy of Jenny Hegmann

Oatmeal Pancakes

These pancakes are light and fluffy prizewinners, perfect for carbohydrate loading or recovering from a hard workout. For best results, let the batter stand for 5 minutes before cooking.

1/2 cup (70 g) uncooked oats, quick or old fashioned

1/2 cup (115) plain yogurt, buttermilk, or milk mixed with 1/2 teaspoon vinegar

1/2 to 3/4 cup (120 to 180 ml) milk

1 egg or 2 egg whites, beaten

1 tablespoon oil, preferably canola

2 tablespoons packed brown sugar

1/2 teaspoon salt, as desired

1 teaspoon baking powder

1 cup (140 g) flour, preferably half whole wheat and half white

Optional: dash cinnamon

1. In a medium bowl, combine the oats, yogurt, and milk. Set aside for 15 to 20 minutes to let the oatmeal soften.
2. When the oatmeal is finished soaking, beat in the egg and oil, and mix well. Add the sugar and salt (and cinnamon), then the baking powder and flour. Stir until just moistened.
3. Heat a lightly oiled or nonstick griddle over medium-high heat (375 °F [190 °C] for electric frying pan).
4. For each pancake, pour about 1/4 cup batter onto the griddle.
5. Turn when the tops are covered with bubbles and the edges look cooked. Turn only once.
6. Serve with syrup, honey, applesauce, yogurt, or other topping of your choice.

Yield: 6 6-inch pancakes

Nutrition Information   1,000 total calories; 330 calories per serving (2 pancakes); 57 g carbohydrate; 10 g protein; 7 g fat

Wheat Germ and Cottage Cheese Pancakes

These pancakes are a tasty way to add protein and satiety to a carbohydrate-rich sports breakfast. Although cottage cheese may sound like an unusual addition to pancakes, you won't even notice it. The wheat germ adds vitamin E, B vitamins, and fiber.

1/2 cup (115 g) cottage cheese, preferably low fat

1/2 cup (60 g) wheat germ

2 to 4 tablespoons firmly packed brown sugar or honey

1 egg or 2 egg whites

1 to 2 tablespoons oil, preferably canola

1 cup (240 ml) milk, preferably low fat

1 teaspoon vanilla extract

1 teaspoon baking powder

1/2 teaspoon baking soda

1 cup (140 ml) flour, preferably half whole wheat and half white

Optional: 1/2 teaspoon cinnamon or 1/4 teaspoon nutmeg

1. In a medium bowl, beat together the cottage cheese, wheat germ, brown sugar, egg, and oil.
2. Beat in the milk and vanilla, then the baking powder and soda (and cinnamon or nutmeg). Gently stir in the flour.
3. For each pancake, pour about 1/4 cup of batter onto a hot griddle. Cook pancakes until the edges are done and bubbles form on the top. Turn and cook until golden.
4. Serve plain or with maple syrup, applesauce with cinnamon, or yogurt.

Yield: 3 servings

Nutrition Information   1,200 total calories; 400 calories per serving; 54 g carbohydrate; 19 g protein; 12 g fat

CHAPTER 18

Pasta, Rice, and Potatoes

Although some weight-conscious people mistakenly try to stay away from dinner starches such as pasta, rice, and potatoes, these carbohydrate-rich foods are important for a high-energy sports diet.

PASTA.   When trying to decide which shape of pasta to use for a meal, the rule of thumb is to use twisted and curved shapes (such as twists and shells) with meaty, beany, and chunky sauces. The shape will trap more sauce than the straight strands of spaghetti or linguini.

Perfectly cooked pasta is tender yet firm when bitten with the teeth—"al dente," as the Italians say. The quickest-cooking pastas include angel hair, alphabets, and little stars (stelline). Here are some tips for cooking pasta perfectly.

- Allow 4 quarts (4 liters) of water per pound (500 grams) of dry pasta. Allow 10 minutes for the water to reach a rolling boil before adding pasta. (If you are rushed for time, you can cook the pasta in half the amount of water, and it will cook OK—in less time.) Plan to cook no more than 2 pounds of pasta at a time; otherwise, you may end up with a gummy mess.

- To keep the water from boiling over, add 1 tablespoon of oil to the cooking water.

- Add the pasta in small amounts to avoid cooling the water too much or causing the pieces to clump. When cooking spaghetti or lasagna, push down the stiff strands as they soften, using a long-handled spoon.

- If the water stops boiling, cover the pan, turn up the heat, and bring the water to a boil again as soon as possible.

- Cooking time will depend on the shape of the pasta. Pasta is done when it starts to look opaque. To tell if it is done, lift a piece of pasta with a fork from the boiling water, let it cool briefly, then carefully pinch or bite it, being sure not to burn yourself. The pasta should feel flexible but still firm inside.

- When the pasta is done, drain it into a colander set in the sink, using potholders to protect your hands from the steam. Shake the pasta briefly to remove excess water, then return it to the cooking pot or to a warmed serving bowl.

- To prevent the pasta from sticking together as it cools, toss the pasta with a little oil or sauce.

The following quick and easy pasta toppings are a change of pace from the standard tomato sauce straight from the jar.

- Steamed chopped broccoli
- Salsa, plain or heated, and then mixed with cottage cheese
- Red pepper flakes
- Low-fat salad dressings of your choice
- (Low-fat) Italian salad dressing with tamari, chopped garlic, and steamed vegetables
- Low-fat sour cream and Italian seasonings
- Italian seasonings and cottage cheese or Parmesan cheese
- Chicken breast sauteed with oil, garlic, onion, and basil
- Chili with kidney beans (and cheese)
- Lentil soup (thick)
- Spaghetti sauce with a spoonful of grape jelly
- Spaghetti sauce with added protein: canned chicken or tuna, tofu cubes, canned beans, cottage cheese, ground beef or turkey
- Spaghetti sauce with added fresh diced tomato and parsley

RICE.   Rice is the world's third-leading grain, after wheat and corn. Brown rice is made into white rice when the fiber-rich bran is removed during the refining process. This also removes some of the nutrients, but you can compensate for this loss (if you prefer white to brown rice) by eating other whole grains such as bran cereals and whole-wheat breads at your other meals. Here are some tips for cooking rice.

- For each 1 cup of rice, put 2 cups of water and 1 teaspoon salt, as desired, into a saucepan. Bring to a boil, then cover and turn the heat down low. Let the rice cook undisturbed until it is tender and all the water has been absorbed. Then, stir gently with a fork. (Stirring too much results in a sticky mess.) This method retains vitamins that otherwise could be lost in the cooking water.
- Because of its tough bran coat and germ, brown rice needs about 45 to 50 minutes to cook; white rice needs only about 20 to 30 minutes.
- Consider cooking rice in the morning while you are getting ready for work so that it will only need to be reheated when you get home.
- When cooking rice, cook double amounts to have leftovers that you can freeze or refrigerate.
- Use the following portion guides when cooking rice:

  1 cup raw white rice = 3 cups cooked = 700 calories

  1 cup raw brown rice = 3 to 4 cups cooked = 700 calories

Here are a few rice suggestions for hungry athletes. For variety, try cooking rice in these liquids:

- Chicken or beef broth
- Mixture of orange or apple juice and water
- Water with seasonings: cinnamon, soy sauce, oregano, curry, chili powder, or whatever might nicely blend with the menu

You can also combine rice with these foods:

- Leftover chili
- Toasted sesame seeds and chopped nuts
- Steamed vegetables
- Chopped mushrooms and green peppers, either raw or sautéed
- Low-fat sour cream, raisins, tuna, and curry powder
- Raisins, cinnamon, and applesauce
- Soy sauce and diced scallions
- Honey, raisins, and toasted sliced almonds

POTATOES. The potato is a carbohydrate-rich vegetable that offers more vitamins and minerals than plain rice or pasta. To help you include more potatoes in your sports diet, here are some tips.

- Potatoes come in different varieties. Some varieties are best suited for baking (russets), others for boiling (red or white rounds). Ask the produce manager at your grocery store for guidance.

- Potatoes are best stored in a cool, humid (but not wet) place that is well ventilated, such as your cellar. Do not refrigerate potatoes because they will become sweet and off-colored.

- Rather than peel the skin (and remove some fiber), scrub the skin well and cook the potato skin and all. Yes, even mashed potatoes can be made with unpeeled potatoes.

- One pound of potatoes equals three medium or two large potatoes. A large "restaurant-size" potato has about 200 calories.

- To bake a potato in the oven, allow about 40 minutes at 400 °F (200 °C) for a medium potato, closer to an hour for a large potato. Because potatoes can be baked at any temperature, you can adjust the cooking time to whatever else is in the oven.

- The potato is done when you can easily pierce it with a fork.

- To cook a potato in the microwave oven, prick its skin in several places with a fork, place it on a paper towel on the bottom of the microwave, and cook it for about 4 minutes if it is medium sized or 6 to 10 minutes if it's large. Cooking time will vary according to the size of the potato, the power of your oven, and the number of potatoes being cooked. Turn the potato over halfway through cooking. Remove the potato from the oven, wrap it in a towel, and allow it to finish cooking outside the oven for about 3 to 5 minutes.

To spice up your potato, try the following toppings:

- Plain yogurt
- Imitation butter granules (such as Molly McButter) and milk
- Mustard (and Worcestershire sauce)
- White and flavored vinegars or low-fat salad dressing
- Soy sauce
- Pesto
- Herbs such as dill, parsley, and chives
- Steamed broccoli or other cooked vegetables

- Chopped jalapeno peppers
- Low-fat sour cream, chopped onion, and grated low-fat cheddar cheese
- Low-fat cottage cheese and garlic powder or salsa
- Chili and grated low-fat cheddar cheese
- Cooked chopped spinach and crumbled feta cheese
- Soup broth or milk mashed into the potato
- Baked beans, refried beans, lentils, or lentil soup
- Applesauce

RECIPE FINDER

See also: Pasta and white bean soup with sun-dried tomatoes, Chicken with pasta and spinach, Country pasta with turkey sausage and white beans, Ground turkey mix for spaghetti sauce or chili, Shrimp pasta, Tofu lo mein, Sweet and spicy orange beef, Minestrone soup, Chicken broccoli fettucini Alfredo, Pasta with spinach and garbanzo beans, Honey-glazed sweet potatoes

Pasta With Spinach and Feta

This goes nicely as a side dish with chicken or fish and a salad. A tasty way to eat your spinach—and be strong to the finish!

8 ounces (250 g) uncooked pasta, such as orzo or small shells

1 to 3 tablespoons olive oil

1 cup (160 g) chopped onion

1 to 2 cloves garlic, minced, or 1/8 to 1/4 teaspoon garlic powder

1 10-ounce (300 g) package frozen chopped spinach, thawed, squeezed to remove excess moisture

1/2 teaspoon dried red chili flakes

1/2 cup (125 g) crumbled feta cheese

Salt and pepper, as desired

Optional: 1/4 cup (34 g) chopped kalamata olives; 1/4 cup (14 g) chopped sun-dried tomatoes

1. Cook pasta in a large pot of boiling water according to package directions. Drain and then rinse with cold water.
2. While the pasta is cooking, heat a skillet over medium heat and then add the oil. Add the onions and garlic, and saute 3 to 5 minutes.
3. Add the spinach and saute another 4 minutes or until tender.
4. Add the red chili flakes and cooked pasta. Saute until entire dish is heated through.
5. Remove from the heat and add the feta (and olives and sun-dried tomatoes, as desired) and stir to combine. Season with salt and pepper, as desired.

Yield: 6 servings as a side dish

Nutrition Information   1,400 total calories; 230 calories per serving; 35 g carbohydrate; 9 g protein; 7 g fat

Adapted from Petusevsky, Steve. "Spinach and Feta a Lively Couple." *South Florida Sun-Sentinel* 12 April 2007: Food News.

Skillet Lasagna

This is a much quicker version of the classic Italian lasagnas, and it offers all the taste. Because it is so simple to make, you'll be able to enjoy lasagna more often. For a vegetarian dish, replace the ground beef with crumbled tofu. To fuel your muscles with more carbohydrate, serve this with crusty whole-grain rolls and fruit for dessert.

1/2 to 1 lb (250 to 500 g) extra-lean ground beef or ground turkey

1 26-ounce (740 ml) jar spaghetti sauce

3 cups (720 ml) water

8 ounces (250 g) egg noodles, uncooked

1 cup (230 g) cottage cheese, preferably low fat

1/4 cup (25 g) grated Parmesan cheese

1/2 to 1 cup (120 to 240 g) shredded part-skim mozzarella cheese

1. In a large skillet, brown the ground beef. Drain.
2. Add the jar of spaghetti sauce and the 3 cups of water. (Rinse out the jar using some of the water.) Bring to a boil.
3. Stir in uncooked noodles. Bring to a boil, stirring occasionally. Reduce heat, cover, and simmer for about 10 minutes or until the noodles are done.
4. Add the cottage, Parmesan, and mozzarella cheeses; stir gently into the noodle mixture. Cover and cook for 5 minutes more.
5. *Optional:* Sprinkle with additional mozzarella. Serve.

Yield: 4 hefty servings

Nutrition Information   2,100 total calories; 525 calories per serving; 60 g carbohydrate; 35 g protein; 16 g fat

Courtesy of Karin Daisy

Gourmet Vegetarian Lasagna

This "company is coming" lasagna has a wonderful flavor and is a nice variation from standard lasagnas. The sun-dried tomatoes and pine nuts make the difference—well worth the effort of buying them if you have none stocked.

15 lasagna noodles

1/2 cup (60 g) pine nuts (pignoli nuts)

8 to 9 sun-dried tomatoes

1 to 3 cloves garlic, peeled and finely chopped

1 teaspoon oil, preferably olive or canola

1 pound (500 g) ricotta cheese, part skim or nonfat

4 to 8 ounces (125 to 250 g) shredded low-fat mozzarella cheese

1 to 2 dashes nutmeg

1/4 teaspoon oregano

1 10-ounce (300 g) package frozen spinach, thawed and drained

1 28-ounce (840 ml) jar spaghetti sauce

Optional: 1/4 cup grated Parmesan cheese

1. Preheat oven to 350 °F (180 °C).
2. Cook the lasagna noodles in a large pot of boiling water according to the package directions. Drain and rinse with cold water and set aside.
3. Spread the pine nuts in a shallow baking pan and toast in the oven for 5 minutes (or toast on the stovetop in a nonstick skillet over medium-high heat for 2 to 3 minutes).
4. Place the sun-dried tomatoes in a small bowl and cover with boiling water. Soak oil packed tomatoes for 5 minutes or dried tomatoes for 10 to 15 minutes. Drain, cool, and chop finely.
5. Saute the garlic in oil for 2 minutes. Do not brown. Remove the pan from heat.
6. In a large mixing bowl, combine the ricotta, mozzarella, nutmeg, oregano, spinach, sun-dried tomatoes, pine nuts, and garlic.
7. Pour enough tomato sauce into a 9- × 13-inch pan to coat the bottom. Layer on five lasagna noodles, cutting or folding to fit. Then add one-third of the ricotta mixture and then one-third of the remaining spaghetti sauce. Repeat twice, making three layers of ricotta. On last layer, end with noodles and tomato sauce. Sprinkle with Parmesan, if desired.
8. Cover with foil. Bake for 30 to 40 minutes or until hot.

Yield: 8 servings

Nutrition Information   3,600 total calories; 450 calories per serving; 53 g carbohydrate; 21 g protein; 17 g fat

Adapted from recipe contributed by Linda Press Wolfe.

Mock Pasta Alfredo

Alfredo sauces tend to be loaded with cream and butter, but this version is low in fat yet rich in flavor. For added color and nutrition, top the pasta with chopped tomatoes, peppers, steamed broccoli, or other vegetable of your choice.

8 ounces (250 g) pasta, such as corkscrew, penne, or shells

1 1/2 cups (345 g) cottage cheese, preferably low fat

1 cup (240 ml) milk, preferably nonfat or low fat

1 to 2 garlic cloves, cut in pieces, or 1/8 to 1/4 teaspoon garlic powder

2 tablespoons flour

1 tablespoon lemon juice

1 teaspoon dried basil or oregano

1/2 teaspoon dry mustard

Salt and pepper, as desired

Optional: 1/4 cup (25 g) Parmesan cheese; dash of chili pepper

1. Cook pasta according to package directions.
2. While the pasta cooks, process cottage cheese, milk, and garlic in a blender or food processor until smooth.
3. Add flour, lemon juice, basil (or oregano), mustard, and salt, pepper, parmesan, and chili pepper as desired; process to mix.
4. Pour the mixture into a saucepan, and cook over medium heat until thickened. Do not boil.
5. Mix into the noodles.

Yield: 3 servings

Nutrition information   1,200 total calories; 400 calories per serving; 70 g carbohydrate; 25 g protein; 2 g fat

Adapted from *Taste of Home* magazine. www.tasteofhome.com

Southwestern Rice and Bean Salad

This makes a nice side dish with barbequed chicken. If you do not have lime juice on hand, you can use lemon juice, rice vinegar, or white vinegar.

2 cups cooked rice, cooled (about 2/3 cup, or 135 g, uncooked)

1 15-ounce (450 g) can black beans, drained and rinsed

1 large tomato, chopped

3 ounces (90 g) low-fat cheddar cheese, diced into small 1/4-inch cubes

Dressing

1 tablespoon oil, preferably olive or canola

2 tablespoons lime juice, lemon juice, or vinegar

1 tablespoon taco seasoning mix (or 1 teaspoon cumin and 1/8 teaspoon cayenne pepper)

Optional: 2 tablespoons chopped cilantro; 1/4 cup diced onion; salt and pepper

1. In a large bowl, combine the cooked rice, beans, tomato, and cheese (and cilantro and onion).
2. In a small bowl, whisk together the oil, lime juice, and taco seasonings. Pour over the rice mixture and mix well. Adjust the seasonings to the desired taste. Refrigerate until ready to serve.

Yield: 4 servings (as a side dish)

Nutrition Information   960 total calories; 240 calories per serving; 27 g carbohydrate; 15 g protein; 8 g fat

Oven French Fries

This healthful French fry recipe is a popular family favorite—and no one will realize it is low in fat. For added flavor, dip the fries in salsa, nonfat yogurt mixed with fresh herbs, or ketchup.

1 large baking potato, cleaned, unpeeled

1 teaspoon oil, preferably canola or olive

Salt and pepper to taste

Optional: red pepper flakes; dried basil; oregano; minced garlic; Parmesan cheese; replace oil with prepared pesto

1. Cut the potato lengthwise into 10 or 12 pieces. Place in a large bowl; cover with cold water, and let stand for 15 to 20 minutes. (This soaking can be eliminated, but it shortens the cooking time and improves the final product.)
2. Drain the potatoes, dry them on a towel, then put them in a bowl or ziplock bag. Drizzle them with the oil, and sprinkle with the salt and pepper, as desired. Toss to coat evenly.
3. Place the potatoes evenly on a nonstick shallow baking pan.
4. Bake at 425 °F (220 °C) for 15 minutes. Turn the potatoes over, sprinkle with the optional seasonings, as desired, and continue baking for another 10 to 15 minutes. Serve immediately. Be careful; the potatoes will be very hot.

Yield: 1 serving

Nutrition Information 260 calories per potato; 52 g carbohydrate; 4 g protein; 4 g fat

Courtesy of Ann LeBaron, RD

Egg-Stuffed Baked Potato

If you let the potato bake while you are exercising, dinner will be ready when you are. Or, cook it in the microwave oven.

One of these potatoes alone may not provide adequate calories for a dinner. Plan to supplement it with soup and salad, or eat two potatoes.

1 large baking potato (1/2 pound or 250 g)

1 egg

1 ounce (30 g) shredded cheese, preferably low fat

Salt and pepper as desired

Optional: 1 to 2 tablespoons milk

1. Prick the potato in several places with a fork. Bake in a 400 °F (200 °C) oven for an hour or until done; the potato should be tender when pierced with a fork. Or cook the potato for about 8 minutes in a microwave oven, letting it rest for an additional 3 minutes.
2. Cut an X on top of the baked potato. Fluff up the insides and make a well.
3. *Optional:* For moistness add 1 to 2 tablespoons of milk.
4. Break the egg into the well. Top with cheese and salt and pepper as desired.
5. Return to the oven until the egg is cooked, about 10 minutes. Or microwave at medium power for 1 to 2 minutes, being sure to pierce the yolk (otherwise it will explode).

Yield: 1 serving

Nutrition Information   375 calories per potato; 53 g carbohydrate; 18 g protein; 10 g fat

CHAPTER 19 ————————

Vegetables and Salads

Vegetables are perfectly delicious when served plain, without added flavorings. That's why you won't find many vegetable recipes in this section. Carefully cook vegetables just until they are tender-crisp and still flavorful. Limp, overcooked veggies lose their appeal as well as some of their nutrients.

Most vegetables contain negligible amounts of protein and fat but offer carbohydrate, fiber, and abundant vitamins and minerals. Eating vegetables is the best way to boost your vitamin intake—preferable to taking vitamin pills.

The first five recipes offer basic advice about cooking methods. Since you will choose your own vegetable combinations in the earlier recipes, nutrition information is provided only for the remaining recipes. Table 1.2 on page 14 and table 4.1 on page 79 provide more nutrition information.

RECIPE FINDER

See also: Minestrone soup, Skillet lasagna, Gourmet vegetarian lasagna, Tofu lo mein, Fish and spinach bake, Carrot cake, Carrot raisin muffins

Steamed Vegetables

Vegetables of your choice. Examples of good choices include the following:

- Broccoli
- Spinach
- Carrots
- Green beans
- Brussels sprouts

Optional: Sprinkle vegetables with herbs before or after cooking. Add basil and oregano to zucchini squash, ginger to carrots, and garlic powder to green beans. With carrots, add a teaspoon of honey afterward. Be creative!

1. Wash the vegetables thoroughly. Cut into the desired size.
2. Put 1/2 inch (just over 1 cm) of water in the bottom of a pan with a tight lid. Bring to a boil, then add the vegetables. Cover tightly. Or put the vegetables in a steamer basket and put the basket into a saucepan with 1 inch (2.5 cm) of water (or enough to prevent the water from boiling away). Cover tightly and bring to a boil.
3. Cook over medium heat until tender-crisp, about 3 to 10 minutes, depending on the type and size of vegetable.
4. Drain the vegetables, reserving the cooking liquid for soup, sauces, or even for drinking as vegetable broth.

Stir-Fried Vegetables

A large nonstick skillet is useful for stir-frying vegetables. The goal is to end up with vegetables that are cooked until tender-crisp and flavorful. By combining only two or three vegetables, you'll get more distinguished flavors. Plus, this makes it easier to time the cooking so they are all done at the right time.

Olive and canola oils are among the heart-healthiest choices for stir-frying. For a wonderful flavor, add a little sesame oil (available in the Chinese food section of larger supermarkets or health food stores). If you are watching your weight, be sure to add only a little oil.

Vegetables of your choice. Popular combinations include the following:

- Carrots, broccoli, and mushrooms
- Onions, zucchini, and tomatoes
- Chinese cabbage and water chestnuts
- Sugar snap peas Chinese pea pods, and green peas

Cooking oil of your choice: canola, olive, sesame

Optional: toasted sesame seeds; nuts; mandarin orange sections; pineapple chunks

1. Wash the vegetables and drain well (to prevent oil from spattering when the vegetables are added to the hot skillet, wok, or pan). Cut into bite-sized pieces or 1/8-inch slices. When possible, slice the vegetables diagonally to increase the surface area; this allows faster cooking. Try to make the pieces uniform so they will cook evenly.

2. Heat a nonstick skillet, wok, or large frying pan over high heat until very hot, then add 1 to 3 teaspoons of canola, olive, or sesame oil—just enough to coat the bottom of the pan. For interesting flavor, try adding a slice of ginger root or minced garlic to the oil. Stir-fry for a minute to flavor the oil.

3. First add vegetables that take the longest to cook (carrots, cauliflower, broccoli); a few minutes later, add the remaining veggies (mushrooms, bean sprouts, cabbage, spinach). Rather than stir constantly (as the name would imply), wait about 30 seconds between each stirring so the pan can regain its heat. Adjust the heat to prevent scorching.

4. Don't overcrowd the pan. Cook small batches at a time. The goal is to cook the vegetables until they are tender but still crunchy, about 2 to 5 minutes.

5. *Optional:* Garnish the vegetables with toasted sesame seeds, toasted nuts (almonds, cashews, peanuts), mandarin orange sections, or pineapple chunks.

Baked Vegetables

If the oven is already hot because you are baking potatoes, chicken, or a casserole, you might as well make good use of the heat and bake the vegetables, too. Roasting vegetables evaporates much of their water, concentrates their natural sugars, and yields a rich, sweet taste and meaty texture.

Vegetables of your choice. Here are some popular combinations:
- Eggplant halves sprinkled with garlic powder
- Zucchini or summer squash halves covered with onion slices
- Carrot chunks
- Sweet potato slices and apples

1. Cut vegetables into equal-sized chunks, rub with a little canola or olive oil, and spread them on a nonstick baking sheet, uncovered.
2. Bake at 350 °F (180 °C) for 30 to 45 minutes, until tender.

Alternatively:

1. Wrap the vegetables in foil, or put them in a covered baking dish with a small amount of water. (This actually steams them rather than roasts them.)
2. Bake at 350 °F (180 °C) for 20 to 30 minutes (depending on the size of the chunks) until tender-crisp.
3. When you open the foil, be careful of escaping steam so that you don't get burned.

Microwaved Vegetables

Microwave cookery is ideal for vegetables because it cooks them quickly and without water, retaining a greater percentage of nutrients than with conventional methods.

Vegetables of your choice. All cook fine in the microwave oven, but these are some nice options:

- Green beans
- Peas
- Broccoli
- Cauliflower
- Carrots

Optional: Sprinkle vegetables with herbs (basil, parsley, oregano, garlic powder), soy sauce, or whatever suits your taste.

1. Wash the vegetables and cut them into bite-sized pieces.
2. Put them in a microwaveable dish, and cover with plastic wrap. If the vegetables vary in thickness (as stalks of broccoli do), arrange them in a ring with the thicker portions toward the outside of the dish.
3. Microwave until tender-crisp. The amount of time will vary according to your particular oven and the amount of vegetables you are cooking. You'll learn by trial and error. Start off with 3 minutes for a single serving; larger quantities take longer. The vegetables will continue cooking after they are removed from the microwave, so plan that into the time allotment.

Grilled Vegetables

When grilling your entree (chicken, fish, meats), plan to save space for grilling vegetables as well. Grilled vegetables have a wonderful flavor; the heat evaporates their water content, and in the process, the flavor of the vegetables becomes more concentrated. Ideally, vegetables should be cooked over a medium-hot fire—you should be able to hold your hand 5 inches (13 cm) above the cooking surface for 4 seconds.

Vegetables of your choice, such as:

- Asparagus
- Eggplant
- Mushrooms
- Onions
- Peppers

1. Slice vegetables such as summer squash, peppers, potato, and eggplant into "steaks." For smaller pieces of vegetables (cherry tomatoes, onion chunks, mushroom tops), use skewers or a grilling basket.

2. To prevent the outside of the vegetables from getting charred, first microwave the cut-up veggies for 1 to 2 minutes, then brush with olive oil. Put smaller pieces in a plastic bag, add a little oil, and shake to coat.

3. Arrange on the grill, skewer, or grilling basket. Cook until tender, turning with tongs or a metal spatula. Allow about 5 to 10 minutes for the vegetables to cook.

Spinach Salad
With Sweet and Spicy Dressing

Spinach is a powerhouse vegetable, rich in potassium, folate, beta-carotene, and many other nutrients. You can easily incorporate more spinach into your diet with tasty spinach salads. Here is one version.

1 10-ounce (300 g) package or large bunch fresh spinach, rinsed well and cut up

Optional: 1 cup (250 g) sliced mushrooms; 2 fresh tomatoes, cut into wedges; 2 hard-boiled eggs, sliced; 1/2 cup (60 g) broken walnuts

Sweet and Spicy Dressing

3 tablespoons olive oil

2 tablespoons red wine vinegar

1 tablespoon sugar

1 teaspoon salt, as desired

1 tablespoon ketchup

1. Place the spinach in a salad bowl (combine with the mushrooms and tomatoes, as desired).
2. In a jar combine the olive oil, vinegar, sugar, salt, and ketchup. Cover and shake until well blended.
3. Pour the dressing over the salad; toss well, then garnish with eggs and walnuts, as desired.

Yield: 4 large salads

Nutrition Information 480 total calories; 120 calories per serving; 7 g carbohydrate; 2 g protein; 9 g fat

Spinach Salad With Oriental Dressing

This recipe goes nicely with a simple baked fish or chicken meal and some fresh whole-grain bread.

1 10-ounce (300 g) package or large bunch fresh spinach, rinsed well and cut up

Optional: 4 ounces (125 g) water chestnuts, sliced; 1/2 pound (250 g) mushrooms, sliced; 1/2 pound (250 g) bean sprouts; 1 11-ounce (325 ml) can mandarin oranges; 1/2 teaspoon toasted sesame seeds

Oriental Dressing

1 tablespoon soy sauce, light or regular

1/4 cup (60 ml) vinegar, preferably rice vinegar

2 teaspoons fresh lemon juice (or 2 teaspoons more vinegar)

1 teaspoon sugar

1/2 teaspoon grated ginger

1/4 teaspoon garlic powder

2 tablespoons sesame oil

1. Place the spinach in a salad bowl (combine with the water chestnuts, mushrooms, bean sprouts, and mandarin oranges, as desired).
2. In a jar combine the soy sauce, vinegar, lemon juice, sugar, ginger, garlic powder, and sesame oil. Cover and shake until well blended.
3. Pour the dressing over the salad and toss well.
4. Garnish with sesame seeds, as desired.

Yield: 4 large salads

Nutrition Information 320 total calories; 80 calories per serving; 4 g carbohydrate; 2 g protein; 6 g fat

Brenda's Greek Salad

This recipe is a favorite of Brenda Ponichtera's, RD, cookbook author of *Quick and Healthy Recipes and Ideas*. Brenda says the combination of red and yellow peppers gives the salad an especially good flavor.

If time allows, let it marinate for several hours—and make enough for leftovers because it'll be great the next day. (I like to make it into a wrap for lunch.) The salad can be made with only green peppers; it'll taste just fine. For a richer flavor, you can add a drizzle of olive oil.

1 green pepper, sliced or in rings

1 red pepper, sliced or in rings

1 yellow pepper, sliced or in rings

1 unpeeled cucumber, sliced

2 tablespoons lemon juice

3 tablespoons red wine vinegar

1/4 teaspoon dried oregano

4 ounces (125 g) fat-free feta cheese, crumbled

1. Mix peppers and cucumber in a bowl.
2. Add lemon juice, vinegar, and oregano. Mix well.
3. Top with crumbled feta cheese.

Yield: 4 servings

Nutrition Information   250 total calories; 60 calories per serving; 10 g carbohydrate; 5 g protein; 0 g fat

Honey-Glazed Sweet Potatoes

Carbohydrate-rich and colorful, sweet potatoes offer lots of health-protective beta-carotene. Enjoy sweet potatoes with chicken, fish, and beef meals, and plan to make extra so you'll have leftovers to enjoy cold as a preexercise snack. Sweet potatoes are healthier than a cookie—but just as sweet!

2 pounds sweet potatoes (about 4 medium)

1/4 (60 ml) cup water

2 tablespoons brown sugar

2 tablespoons honey

1 tablespoon olive oil

1. Preheat the oven to 375 °F (190 °C).
2. Lightly coat bottom and sides of a 9- × 13-inch (23 × 33 cm) baking pan with cooking spray; set aside.
3. Peel (if desired) and cut the sweet potatoes into 3/4-inch-thick (2 cm) chunks.
4. In a small bowl, stir together the water, brown sugar, honey, and olive oil.
5. Transfer the sweet potatoes to the baking pan and spread into a single layer. Pour the sauce over the potatoes and turn the potatoes to coat thoroughly.
6. Cover with foil and bake about 30 to 45 minutes or until tender, stirring gently twice to ensure sweet potatoes are coated.
7. When sweet potatoes are tender, remove the foil and bake an additional 15 minutes or until the glaze is set.

Yield: 4 servings

Nutrition Information   1,050 total calories; 260 calories per serving; 55 g carbohydrate; 3 g protein; 3 g fat

Adapted from recipe at www.mayoclinic.com

CHAPTER 20

Chicken and Turkey

The white and dark meat of chicken and turkey are excellent examples of muscle physiology. They represent two types of muscle fibers. The white breast meat is primarily fast-twitch muscle fibers used for bursts of energy. Athletes such as elite gymnasts, basketball players, and others who do sprint types of exercise tend to have a high percentage of fast-twitch fibers.

The dark meat in the legs and wings is primarily slow-twitch muscle fibers that function best for endurance exercise. Elite marathoners, long-distance cyclists, and other successful endurance athletes tend to have a high percentage of slow-twitch fibers. The dark meat of poultry contains more fat than the white meat because the fat provides energy for greater endurance; the dark meat also has slightly more fat calories than light meat:

3 oz (90 g) chicken breast (white meat) = 120 calories

3 oz (90 g) chicken thigh (dark meat) = 150 calories

The dark meat also has more iron, zinc, B vitamins, and other nutrients. I recommend that athletes who don't eat beef select skinless dark-meat poultry to boost their intake of these important nutrients. Because the highest source of fat in chicken is in the skin, be sure to remove the skin before cooking. This eliminates the temptation to eat it.

For a basic chicken meal, put 1/2 inch (just over 1 cm) of water in a saucepan, add the chicken, cover tightly, and bring just to a boil. Turn down heat; gently simmer over medium-low heat for 20 to 25 minutes or until the juices run clear when the chicken is poked with a fork. You may prefer to place the skinless chicken on a rack in a baking pan. Bake uncovered at 350 °F (180 °C) for 20 to 30 minutes or until the juices run clear when the meat is poked with a fork. For easy cleanup when baking chicken, use a nonstick pan or a regular baking pan treated with cooking spray, or line the pan with aluminum foil.

Some of my clients eat so much chicken that they claim they'll turn into one! If that sounds familiar, here are some ways to add variety to your chicken meals:

- Replace cooking water with orange juice, white wine, or a can of stewed tomatoes.
- Add seasonings to the cooking water: a low-sodium chicken bouillon cube, lite soy sauce, curry, basil, or thyme.
- Cook rice along with the chicken (add extra water).
- Make stuffing with the chicken broth and stuffing mix.
- Add vegetables in the last 5 minutes.
- Dice the cooked chicken and wrap it in a tortilla with salsa, shredded lettuce, and grated low-fat cheese.
- Spread a teaspoon of Dijon mustard on raw chicken, add a generous sprinkling of Parmesan cheese, and bake until done.
- Spread a teaspoon of honey on raw chicken, then sprinkle on curry powder, and bake until done.
- Wrap a raw chicken breast around a piece of string cheese sliced in half lengthwise; secure with toothpicks, then bake until done.
- Marinate the chicken for 10 to 60 minutes in a ziplock bag with soy sauce, a shake of ground ginger, mustard, and garlic powder, then bake or saute in a little oil in a frying pan.
- Dip in olive or canola oil, then in sesame seeds, cracker crumbs, or Corn Flake crumbs, and bake or saute in a little oil in a frying pan.
- Place a chicken breast on a piece of foil, cover with vegetables (your choice of onion, mushrooms, carrots, potato, tomato) and seasonings (your choice of garlic, rosemary, thyme, basil). Wrap well by folding the edges of the foil together, and then bake at 375 °F (190 °C) for about 20 minutes. Be careful to not get burned by the steam that escapes when you open the foil packet.

RECIPE FINDER ────────────────────────────

See also: Stir-fried vegetables; Skillet lasagna; Pasta and white bean soup with sun-dried tomatoes; Tofu lo mein; Fish in foil, Mexican style; Quick and easy chili; Meatballs by the gallon; Pasta with spinach and garbanzo beans; Enchilada casserole

Oven-Fried Chicken

Deep-fried chicken is popular with many athletes but is certainly not the healthiest of sports foods. This recipe offers a lower-fat alternative that will get "thumbs up" from even fussy eaters; it rates a thumbs up for the cook, too. The wire rack allows air to circulate on all sides; you'll get crisper chicken, and you won't have to turn it during cooking. Meanwhile, the foil pan lining speeds your clean-up time.

1 box (5 ounces) Melba toast

2 to 4 tablespoons olive or canola oil

2 egg whites or 1 egg

4 boneless, skinless chicken breasts

Optional: 1 tablespoon Dijon mustard; salt and pepper as desired

1. Heat oven to 400 °F (200 °C).
2. Place a wire rack in a shallow baking pan lined with foil.
3. Add the Melba toast to a heavy-duty plastic bag, seal, and crush with a rolling pin (or other hard object) into crumbs, leaving some crumbs as large as small corn kernels.
4. Pour the crumbs into a shallow dish and drizzle the oil over them. Toss well to distribute the oil evenly.
5. Beat the egg in a medium bowl. Add mustard, salt, and pepper if desired.
6. Dip each piece of chicken into the egg mixture, allow excess to drip off, and then place each coated breast in the crumbs. Sprinkle the crumbs over the chicken and press them in. Shake off excess crumbs and place the chicken on the rack.
7. Bake for 40 minutes. The coating should be deep brown and the juices should run clear when the meat is cut.

Yield: 4 servings

Nutrition Information   1,200 total calories; 300 calories per serving; 12 g carbohydrate; 40 g protein; 10 g fat

Adapted from *Cook's Illustrated* magazine, May/June 1999.

Sauteed Chicken With Mushrooms and Onions

This simple recipe is tasty enough for an impromptu gourmet dinner. It includes common ingredients that are easy to keep stocked: (frozen) chicken breasts, (canned) mushrooms, onions, low-fat cheese, and wine. Enjoy it with (brown) rice, crusty whole-grain rolls, and a green vegetable.

1 to 2 tablespoons oil, preferably olive or canola

4 boneless, skinless chicken breasts

1 medium onion, diced

1 cup (240 ml) dry white wine

2 6-ounce (175 ml) cans sliced mushrooms, drained

2 ounces (60 g) low-fat Swiss cheese

Optional: 1 to 2 cloves garlic, minced, or 1 teaspoon ground thyme

1. In a large nonstick skillet, heat the oil and add the chicken breasts and onion (and garlic). Cook for about 5 minutes per side.
2. Add the wine and drained mushrooms (and thyme).
3. Cover and simmer for about 10 minutes or until the chicken is done and the juices run clear when the meat is slit with a knife.
4. Place 1/2 ounce of cheese on top of each cooked chicken breast. Cover the pan and simmer for another 3 minutes or until the cheese is melted.
5. Serve by placing the chicken on top of a bed of mushrooms.

Yield: 4 servings

Nutrition Information   1,200 total calories; 300 calories per serving; 10 g carbohydrate; 42 g protein; 10 g fat

Courtesy of Molly Curran

Chicken With Pasta and Spinach

This recipe is not only quick and easy but also includes three different food groups (grain, protein, and vegetable), creating a well-balanced meal. Food variety can help you be strong to the finish—as can the spinach itself.

---

1 pound (500 g) pasta, such as fettuccine

2 tablespoons oil, preferably olive or canola

1 pound (500 g) boneless, skinless chicken breasts, thinly sliced

1 to 4 cloves garlic, finely chopped, or 1/4 to 1 teaspoon garlic powder

1 10-ounce (300 ml) can chicken broth

1 pound (500 g) fresh spinach, washed, drained, and roughly chopped

Salt and pepper to taste

Optional: 10 ounces (300 g) mushrooms, sliced; 1/4 cup Parmesan cheese

---

1. Cook the pasta according to the package directions.
2. While the pasta is cooking, in a large skillet heat the oil and saute the sliced chicken breasts for 30 seconds.
3. Toss in the garlic (and mushrooms) and stir well. Cook for about 5 minutes.
4. Pour in the chicken broth and bring it to a simmer. Add the spinach, stirring until it wilts.
5. Drain the pasta and return it to the cooking pot. Pour in the chicken and spinach mixture and toss well. Heat for 2 minutes.
6. Season to taste with salt and pepper (and Parmesan cheese, as desired).

Yield: 5 servings

Nutrition Information   2,800 total calories; 560 calories per serving; 75 g carbohydrate; 40 g protein; 11 g fat

Chicken Broccoli Fettuccini Alfredo

This quick and easy recipe is a favorite of Suzie Dorner, a soccer goalie and daughter of dietitian Becky Dorner, RD. She likes this to be ready and waiting after a hard game so she can refuel her muscles.

> 8 ounces (250 g) uncooked fettuccine or other pasta
>
> 1 10-ounce (300 g) box frozen chopped broccoli or 2 cups fresh
>
> 8 ounces (250 g) boneless, skinless chicken breast
>
> 1 to 3 teaspoons olive oil
>
> 1 10-ounce (300 ml) can condensed cream of chicken soup, regular, low fat, or low sodium
>
> 1/2 cup (120 ml) milk, preferably low fat or nonfat
>
> 1/2 cup (50 g) grated Parmesan cheese

1. Cook pasta according to package directions. Add the broccoli for the last 4 minutes of cooking. Drain.
2. Meanwhile, cut the chicken breast meat into bite-sized pieces, trimming off any skin or fat in the process.
3. In a large skillet, heat a little bit of olive oil over medium heat. Add the chicken and saute until well browned.
4. Add the soup, milk, and cheese, and stir all together. Add the pasta and broccoli mixture and heat through. Serve hot.

Yield: 3 hearty servings

Nutrition Information   1,600 total calories; 530 calories per serving; 70 g carbohydrate; 36 g protein; 12 g fat

Courtesy of Suzie Dorner

Chicken Salad With Almonds and Mandarin Oranges

This is nice served on a bed of salad greens with whole-grain bread.

---

1 pound (500 g) boneless, skinless chicken breasts

1/4 to 1/2 (60 to 120 g) cup slivered almonds

1 11-ounce (325 ml) can mandarin oranges, drained

Optional: 1 8-ounce (250 ml) can pineapple chunks; 1 6-ounce (175 ml) can sliced water chestnuts; 1/2 cup raisins or chopped dates

Lemon Dressing

1/2 to 1 (115 to 230 g) cup low-fat lemon yogurt, or a mixture of half yogurt, half low-fat mayonnaise

Oriental Dressing

2 tablespoons hoisin sauce

2 tablespoons juice from the mandarin oranges

4 tablespoons low-fat mayonnaise

Optional: 1/2 teaspoon dry mustard; 1/4 teaspoon garlic powder

Alternate Dressing

1/2 cup (115 g) low-fat mayonnaise

---

1. Simmer the chicken in 1 cup water in a covered pan for about 20 minutes or until the juices run clear when chicken is pricked with a fork. Cool, then dice and place in a large bowl along with the almonds and oranges (and pineapple, water chestnuts, and raisins or dates).
2. For the lemon dressing: Add the lemon yogurt and mix well. For the Oriental dressing: In a small bowl, mix the hoisin sauce, mandarin orange juice, and low-fat mayonnaise (and mustard and garlic).
3. If time allows, chill. Serve on a bed of salad greens.

Yield: 4 servings

Nutrition Information   1,100 total calories with lemon dressing; 275 calories per serving; 12 g carbohydrate; 40 g protein; 7 g fat

1,200 total calories with Oriental dressing; 300 calories per serving; 17 g carbohydrate; 40 g protein, 8 g fat

Courtesy of Barbara Day, RD

Chicken Black Bean Soup

Fitness enthusiast and chef Peter Herman gave me this simple yet delicious and nutritious recipe. It's a tasty way to add more fiber-rich beans to your diet. You can make it a heartier meal by adding cooked pasta.

---

4 boneless, skinless chicken breasts

5 cups chicken broth or water

2 carrots, peeled and sliced

2 tomatoes, chopped

1/2 onion, chopped

3 to 5 cloves garlic, crushed

2 16-ounce (480 ml) cans black beans, rinsed and drained

1 tablespoon fresh oregano leaves or 1 teaspoon dried oregano

Optional: 1/2 cup (120 ml) marsala wine; 2 to 4 cups cooked pasta, shells or bow ties; 2 ounces (60 g) grated cheddar cheese; hot red pepper flakes

---

1. In a large stock pot, place the chicken breasts, broth or water, carrots, tomatoes, onion, garlic, beans, and seasonings (and wine). Cover and bring to a boil, reduce the heat, and simmer for about 20 minutes or until done.
2. Remove the chicken pieces from the broth and set them aside to cool. Keep the broth warm over low heat. (*Optional:* Add the cooked pasta.)
3. Dice the chicken into small pieces. Return it to the soup and heat it through.
4. Garnish with grated cheese and red pepper flakes, if desired.

Yield: 4 servings

Nutrition Information   1,200 total calories; 300 calories per serving; 33 g carbohydrate; 35 g protein; 3 g fat

Courtesy of Peter Herman

Turkey Cran-Apple Wrap

Simple to make, yet different and tasty, this wrap is a favorite lunch or supper for Boston-area registered dietitian Heidi McIndoo. You can make it with a wrap, pita, crusty whole-grain baguette, or sliced bread. It's a perfect recovery food—a nice combination of protein, carbohydrate, and good taste. On a winter day, zap it briefly in the microwave oven. Yum!

Per sandwich:

1 to 2 tablespoons cranberry sauce

1 wrap or whole-grain roll or 2 slices whole-grain bread

1 ounce (30 g) sliced cheddar cheese, preferably low fat

2 ounces (60 g) turkey breast, sliced

1/4 apple, such as Granny Smith, sliced very thinly

1. Spread the cranberry sauce on the wrap, bottom of roll, or slice of bread.
2. Add the sliced cheese, turkey breast, and very thinly sliced apple.
3. Roll up the wrap, or add top of roll or second slice of bread
4. If desired, heat briefly in the microwave oven.

Yield: 1 sandwich

Nutrition Information   400 total calories; 400 calories per serving; 60 g carbohydrate; 25 g protein; 6 g fat

Courtesy of Heidi McIndoo

Country Pasta With Turkey Sausage and White Beans

This recipe is versatile and allows for being creative: You can make it without the turkey sausage, without the beans, or with different protein sources, such as ground beef, diced chicken, tofu, or seafood. When I make this, I like to remove the casing from the sausage by cutting it with a sharp knife and then scrambling the sausage meat. The alternative is to cook the sausage whole, then cut it into coins.

1 pound (500 g) turkey sausage, casing removed

12 ounces (345 g) uncooked pasta, such as shells, ziti, or rotini

1 14-ounce (420 ml) can diced tomatoes, drained

1 15-ounce (450 ml) can white cannellini beans, drained

1 1/2 tablespoons cornstarch mixed into

1 1/2 cups (360 ml) low-fat milk or evaporated milk

1/4 cup grated Parmesan or Romano cheese

Optional: 1 small onion, diced; 1 to 2 cloves garlic, minced; 1/8 teaspoon crushed red pepper flakes; salt and pepper

1. Heat a large nonstick skillet, and add the turkey sausage (and onion, garlic, and red pepper flakes). Cook over medium heat for about 10 minutes or until done.
2. While the sausage is cooking, cook the pasta according to package directions; drain.
3. To the scrambled sausage, add the drained diced tomatoes and cannellini beans. Heat through, then add the cornstarch and milk mixture. Stir until thickened, then add the Parmesan cheese.
4. Add the cooked pasta; toss well and let sit for a few minutes for the flavors to blend. Season as desired with salt and pepper.

Yield: 5 large servings

Nutrition Information   2,500 total calories; 500 calories per serving; 75 g carbohydrate; 25 g protein; 11 g fat

Turkey Meatballs or Turkey Burgers

This recipe works well for either meatballs or burgers. Adding oatmeal makes the burgers juicier than when they're made with plain ground turkey. The recipe also works well with extra-lean ground beef, but when feeding people who don't eat red meat, these turkey burgers or meatballs will appeal to everyone.

1/3 cup (45 g) oatmeal, uncooked

1/2 cup (120 ml) chicken broth, canned, homemade, or from bouillon cubes

1 pound (500 g) ground turkey

1 egg or 2 egg whites

2 tablespoons grated onion

Salt and pepper as desired

Optional: 1/8 teaspoon nutmeg or 1/4 teaspoon allspice

1. In a medium bowl, combine the oatmeal, broth, turkey, egg, onion, and seasonings.
2. For meatballs: Shape into 1 1/2 inch (4 cm) meatballs, place on a nonstick cooking sheet, and bake at 350 °F (180 °C) for 20 to 25 minutes. (Or cook them in a nonstick skillet on the stovetop.) For burgers: Shape into four patties. Cook over medium-high heat in a nonstick skillet for about 5 minutes per side.

Yield: 4 servings

Nutrition Information   760 total calories; 190 calories per serving; 5 g carbohydrate; 26 g protein; 7 g fat

Ground Turkey Mix
for Spaghetti Sauce or Chili

This recipe is popular with Sue Luke, RD, sports nutritionist in Charlotte, North Carolina. She makes double or triple this recipe and stores the extra in the freezer to use as needed. It's a simple way to add protein to spaghetti sauce or soups. It also works well for sloppy joes and tacos.

1 1/2 pounds (750 g) ground turkey

1 tablespoon oil, preferably olive or canola

1 small onion, chopped

1 small green pepper, chopped

8 ounces (250 g) fresh mushrooms, chopped

1. In a large nonstick skillet, saute the ground turkey until cooked. Transfer the turkey to a colander, and let any excess fat drip away. Wipe the skillet.
2. In the same skillet, heat the oil and saute the onion and green pepper until tender-crisp.
3. Add the mushrooms and continue cooking until the mushrooms are softened.
4. Return the turkey to the pan and mix well.
5. Either use immediately for spaghetti sauce or chili, or divide the mixture into the desired portion size, place in resealable plastic bags, and freeze for future use.

Yield: 4 servings

Nutrition Information   900 total calories; 225 calories per serving; 5 g carbohydrate; 35 g protein; 7 g fat

Courtesy of Sue Luke

Mexican Baked Chicken with Pinto Beans

A spicy favorite! When cooking for myself, I wrap one piece of chicken, a quarter of a can of beans, and 1/2 cup of salsa in a piece of foil, bake it in the oven, and have no dishes to wash.

2 16-ounce (480 ml) cans pinto beans

4 pieces chicken, skinned

1 cup salsa

1. Drain the beans and put in the bottom of a baking dish.
2. Put the skinless chicken on top; pour salsa over beans and chicken.
3. Cover and bake in a 350 °F (180 °C) oven for 25 to 30 minutes. If desired, bake uncovered the last 10 minutes to thicken the pan juices.

Yield: 4 servings

Nutrition Information   1,350 total calories; 340 calories per serving; 31 g carbohydrate; 45 g protein; 4 g fat

CHAPTER 21 ————

Fish and Seafood

Fish meals tend to be more popular in restaurants than at home because many people don't know how to buy or prepare fish. The following tips will take the mystique out of fish cookery; fish is actually one of the easiest foods to prepare.

Fresh fish, when properly handled, has no fishy odor whether it is raw or cooked. The odor comes with aging and bacterial contamination. Whenever possible, ask to smell the fish you want to buy. Signs of freshness to look for are bulging eyes, reddish gills, and shiny scales that adhere firmly to the skin. After buying fresh fish, use it quickly, preferably within a day. Keep it in the coldest part of the refrigerator.

When buying commercially frozen fish, be sure the box is firm and square, showing no sign of thawing and refreezing. To thaw, defrost the fish in the refrigerator or microwave oven. Do not refreeze.

For each serving, allow 1 pound (500 grams) of uncooked whole fish (such as trout or mackerel) or 1/3 to 1/2 pound (175 to 250 grams) uncooked fish fillets or steaks (such as salmon, swordfish, halibut, or sole). To rid your hands of any fishy smell, rub them with lemon juice or vinegar. Wash cooking utensils with 1 teaspoon of baking soda per quart of water.

Here are a few tips to help you prepare your "catch":

- If possible, cook fish in its serving dish; fish is fragile, and the less it is handled, the more attractive it is.

- Seasonings that go well with fish include lemon, dill, basil, rosemary, and parsley. Add paprika for color.

- To test for doneness, gently pull the flesh apart with a fork. It should flake easily and not be translucent.

- Use leftover fish, warm or cold, in sandwiches as a change from chicken or turkey.

Here are four different ways to cook fish.

Broiling. Place fish on a broiling pan that has been lightly oiled or treated with cooking spray to prevent sticking. Sprinkle with a little olive oil and seasonings (if desired), and place 4 to 6 inches (10 to 15 centimeters) from the heat source. Thin fillets (such as sole or bluefish) can be cooked in 5 minutes without turning; thicker fillets (such as salmon or swordfish) may require about 5 or 6 minutes per side. Before broiling, spread with a mixture of equal parts low-fat mayonnaise and Dijon mustard.

Baking. Set the fish in a baking dish that has been lightly oiled or treated with cooking spray, season as desired, cover, and bake at 400 °F (200 °C) for 15 to 20 minutes, depending on thickness.

Poaching. Set the fish in a nonstick skillet, and cover the fillets with water, white wine, or milk. Season as desired with herbs and garlic, cover, and gently simmer on the stovetop for about 10 minutes. For an Asian twist, add scallions and a little soy sauce.

Microwaving. If possible, place the thickest part of the fillet toward the outside of the dish, overlapping thin portions to prevent overcooking. Season as desired, cover with waxed paper, and microwave for the minimum amount of time to prevent the fish from becoming tough and dry. Remove from the oven before the fish is totally cooked, and allow it to stand for 5 minutes to finish cooking before serving. Whitefish fillets may need 4 minutes, salmon steaks 6 to 7 minutes.

RECIPE FINDER

See also: Country pasta with turkey sausage and white beans, Tofu lo mein

Mustard Dill Salmon

Enjoying oily fish such as salmon once or twice a week is a smart choice because it is rich in health-protective omega-3 fat. This simple recipe, a favorite of marathon champ Joan Benoit Samuelson, can help you reach that dietary goal. Salmon goes nicely with green peas and potatoes.

1 pound (500 g) fresh salmon fillets or steaks

1/4 cup (60 ml) of your favorite mustard

2 tablespoons lemon juice (or juice from half a lemon)

Dill, preferably fresh

Optional: Slivered almonds

1. Cut the salmon into three serving pieces. Place the salmon in a baking dish. Spread each piece with mustard.
2. Squeeze lemon juice over the salmon, and top with (fresh) dill.
3. Bake at 325 °F (170 °C) for 20 to 25 minutes, or grill for 3 to 7 minutes on each side, depending on thickness. Top with slivered almonds, if desired.

Yield: 3 servings

Nutrition Information   660 total calories; 220 calories per serving; 2 g carbohydrate; 30 g protein; 10 g fat

Courtesy of Joan Benoit Samuelson

Simple Salmon Patties

These salmon patties are made with canned salmon, an inexpensive source of health-protective omega-3 fat. Enjoy them with Pasta With Spinach and Feta (page 334) or brown rice and a green vegetable for a complete meal.

1 14-ounce (420 g) can pink salmon, drained and flaked (remove the skin, but keep the bones for added calcium)

1 cup (70 g) crushed whole-wheat saltine crackers or bread crumbs

1 egg or substitute, slightly beaten

1 cup (150 g) diced pepper, green or red

1/2 diced onion, preferably a sweet onion such as a Vidalia

1/4 cup (60 ml) milk, preferably low fat

Lemon pepper or black pepper, as desired

1 to 2 tablespoons olive or canola oil, for cooking

Optional: 1 teaspoon Worcestershire sauce or soy sauce; dash of hot pepper sauce; 1/2 teaspoon dried dill or 2 teaspoons fresh dill

1. In a large bowl, stir together salmon, cracker or bread crumbs, egg, bell pepper, and onion. Mix in milk (and Worcestershire sauce and hot pepper sauce, as desired). Add pepper (and dill), and mix well with your hands. Lightly press the mixture into eight patties.

2. Heat oil in large saute pan on medium heat. Once oil is hot, place the patties in the pan and cook on both sides until lightly browned, about 3 to 5 minutes.

Yield: 4 servings (8 patties)

Nutrition Information   1,200 total calories; 300 calories per serving (2 patties); 24 g carbohydrate; 27 g protein; 11 g fat (2 g omega-3)

Courtesy of Kelly Leonard, MS, RD

Fish and Spinach Bake

This recipe goes nicely with rice and a loaf of crusty whole-grain bread. If you want a fancier recipe, saute 1/2 teaspoon of minced garlic, 1/2 pound (250 g) of sliced mushrooms, and 1/4 teaspoon of oregano in a little olive oil, then add that to the spinach before placing it in the baking dish.

1 10-ounce (300 g) box frozen chopped spinach

2 ounces (60 g) shredded mozzarella cheese

1 pound (500 g) fish fillets

Salt, pepper, and lemon juice as desired

1. Preheat the oven to 400 °F (200 °C).
2. Thaw the spinach, and squeeze out excess moisture. Spread on the bottom of a small baking dish.
3. Sprinkle with the cheese and top with the fish. Season as desired.
4. Cover with foil. Bake for 20 minutes or until the fish flakes easily.

Yield: 2 servings

Nutrition Information   560 total calories (made with cod); 280 calories per serving; 6 g carbohydrate; 50 g protein; 6 g fat

Shrimp Pasta

Yum! This is quick and easy, yet tasty enough to be a special company meal. Serve it with green vegetables (such as peas, green beans, or broccoli) that you steam while the pasta is cooking.

6 ounces (175 g) pasta, preferably fettuccine

1 tablespoon margarine or olive oil

1 8-ounce (250 g) package frozen, peeled, and deveined shrimp

1/2 teaspoon instant chicken bouillon granules or 1 bouillon cube

1 tablespoon cornstarch mixed into

1 cup (240 ml) milk, preferably low fat

2 tablespoons grated Parmesan cheese

Optional: 1 clove garlic, minced, or 1/8 teaspoon garlic powder; 2 tablespoons white wine; tomatoes and parsley for garnish

1. Cook the pasta according to package directions.
2. As the pasta cooks, melt the margarine in a large nonstick skillet.
3. Add the shrimp and chicken bouillon. Add the garlic, if using. Stir-fry until the shrimp turn pink, about 3 to 4 minutes.
4. Add the cornstarch to the milk and stir. Pour the mixture into the skillet. Stir constantly while the mix cooks. When it's thick and bubbly, sprinkle in the cheese and add the wine, if desired.
5. Drain the pasta and toss with the sauce.
6. Top with parmesan, chopped tomatoes, and parsley and serve.

Yield: 2 large servings

Nutrition Information   1,100 total calories; 550 calories per serving; 70 g carbohydrate; 40 g protein; 12 g fat

Adapted from recipe contributed by Helen Baker.

Greek Shrimp With Feta and Tomatoes

Quick and easy, this goes nicely served over rice. Start the rice before you start making the shrimp.

> 1 tablespoon oil, preferably olive
>
> 2 to 4 cloves garlic, chopped, or 1/4 teaspoon garlic powder
>
> 1 pound (500 g) cleaned, deveined shrimp
>
> 1 28-ounce (840 ml) can crushed or diced tomatoes
>
> 4 ounces (125 g) feta cheese, crumbled
>
> *Optional:* 1/2 teaspoon dried oregano; 1/2 cup chopped fresh parsley

1. In a nonstick skillet, heat the oil; saute the garlic and shrimp until the shrimp turns pink, about 1 minute.
2. Add the tomatoes (and oregano), and simmer for 2 to 5 minutes.
3. Add the crumbled feta. Add the parsley just before serving.

Yield: 4 servings

Nutrition Information   1,000 total calories; 250 calories per serving; 9 g carbohydrate; 28 g protein; 11 g fat

With one cup of rice: 450 calories; 53 g carbohydrate; 30 g protein; 13 g fat

Shrimp Marinara

I adapted this recipe from sports nutritionist Eileen Stellefson Myers, MPH, RD, of Nashville. It makes a quick and easy—yet somewhat special—dinner. It's light and easy to digest—good for carbohydrate loading!

Eileen recommends letting the tomato sauce simmer for about 25 minutes, to thicken it. I get impatient and settle for 5 minutes.

Serve with salad and whole-grain rolls.

1 28-ounce (840 ml) can diced tomatoes that come seasoned with basil, garlic, and oregano

1/4 teaspoon red pepper

3 tablespoons olive oil

1 pound (500 g) raw shrimp, shelled and deveined

12 ounces (350 g) pasta, preferably whole wheat

Optional: 1 to 2 cloves minced garlic; 2 tablespoons parsley, cut fine

1. Cook pasta according to package directions.
2. While the pasta water is coming to a boil, in a large skillet combine the olive oil, red pepper, and diced tomatoes. Heat on a low boil, then let simmer for 5 to 25 minutes while the pasta cooks.
3. Add shrimp and cook until just pink. Garnish with parsley, as desired.
4. Serve over pasta.

Yield: 4 hearty servings

Nutrition Information   2,400 total calories; 600 calories per serving; 82 g carbohydrate; 35 g protein; 12 g fat

Sauce only: 1100 total calories; 275 calories per serving; 20 g carbohydrate; 25 g protein; 11 g fat

Adapted from recipe contributed by Eileen Stellefson Myers, MPH, RD.

Fish in Foil, Mexican Style

Fish always comes out moist and flavorful when cooked in foil. For variety, you can bake the fish Oriental style (with soy sauce, sesame oil, and scallions) or Italian style (with tomatoes, onions, and oregano). The recipe also works well with boneless, skinless chicken breasts.

The amount below is for two servings. Be sure to double it if you're feeding the family.

2 18-inch (46 cm) pieces of heavy-duty foil

1 pound (500 g) white fish fillets

1/2 cup (120 ml) salsa

Optional: 1 diced green pepper and 1 diced small onion, sauteed in 1 teaspoon olive oil; 1/8 teaspoon garlic powder; salt and pepper; low-fat grated cheddar cheese

1. If desired, saute the onion and pepper in olive oil.
2. In the middle of each piece of foil, place 1/2 pound (250 g) of fish. Cover with 1/4 cup salsa (add peppers, onions, and other ingredients or seasonings, as desired).
3. Wrap by bringing together two edges of the foil, folding them over, then folding up the ends and crimping the edges.
4. Bake or grill the packets for 15 to 20 minutes. Lift with a spatula and open carefully, being sure to not burn yourself on escaping steam.

Yield: 2 servings

Nutrition Information   400 total calories; 200 calories per serving; 4 g carbohydrate; 42 g protein; 2 g fat

CHAPTER 22

Beef and Pork

Despite popular belief, lean beef and pork can be a part of a heart-healthy diet. They are excellent sources of protein, iron, and zinc—nutrients important for everyone, particularly athletes. The main health concern about red meat is its fat content. The solution is to choose lean cuts, trim the fat, and eat smaller portions. To protect against cancer, limit red meat intake to 18 ounces (560 g) per week (4 small servings).

These are the leanest cuts of beef:

- Top round roast and steak
- Bottom round roast
- Eye of round
- Boneless rump roast
- Tip roast and steak
- Round, strip, and flank steak
- Lean stew beef

And here are the leanest cuts of pork:

- Sirloin roast and chops
- Loin chops
- Top loin roast

- Tenderloin
- Cutlets

Finally, the leanest cuts of ham:

- Lean and extra-lean cured ham (labeled 93 to 97 percent fat free)
- Center-cut ham
- Canadian bacon

RECIPE FINDER ⎯⎯⎯⎯⎯⎯⎯⎯⎯⎯⎯⎯⎯⎯⎯⎯

See also: Quick and easy chili, Ground turkey mix for spaghetti sauce or chili, Skillet lasagna

Meatballs by the Gallon

Sports dietitian Sue Luke of Charlotte, North Carolina, always likes to have these meatballs in her freezer. When all else fails for dinner, spaghetti and meatballs or a meatball sub are readily available, accompanied by cut-up peppers and baby carrots or a salad.

2 lb (1 kg) extra-lean ground beef or ground turkey

4 eggs, slightly beaten, or egg substitute

1 1/2 cups (180 g) seasoned bread crumbs

2 medium onions, finely chopped

2 teaspoons Italian seasoning

1 teaspoon pepper

Optional: 2 to 6 cloves garlic, minced

1. Put all the ingredients in a large bowl.
2. Wash your hands, then mix the ingredients with your hands.
3. Shape into meatballs of whatever size you desire.
4. Place on a large cookie sheet sprayed with cooking spray (or lined with foil that you have oiled), and bake at 350 °F (180 °C) for 25 to 30 minutes.
5. Cool. Place in a 1-gallon freezer bag and freeze.
6. When you are ready to eat the meatballs, take out the number needed. Thaw in the microwave or in a pot of simmering spaghetti sauce.

Yield: 28 2-inch (5 cm) meatballs

Nutrition Information   2,800 total calories; 200 calories per serving (2 meatballs); 10 g carbohydrate; 22 g protein; 8 g fat

Courtesy of Sue Luke

Enchilada Casserole

This particular recipe is made with beef, but you could just as easily make it with ground turkey, diced tofu, or kidney beans. For color, top the casserole with diced peppers.

1 pound (500 g) extra-lean ground beef

1 28-ounce (840 ml) can diced tomatoes, drained, or fresh tomatoes, chopped

1 10-ounce (300 ml) can enchilada sauce

1 16-ounce (480 ml) can refried beans, preferably low fat

6 ounces (175 g) baked corn chips

4 ounces (125 g) cheddar cheese, preferably reduced fat

Optional: 1 medium onion, chopped; 1 teaspoon chili powder; 1/2 teaspoon dried basil; 1 green pepper, diced

1. Brown the ground beef (and onion) in a large nonstick skillet.
2. Drain any fat, then add the diced tomatoes, enchilada sauce, and refried beans (and chili powder and basil, as desired). Heat until bubbly.
3. Preheat the oven to 350 °F (180 °C). Crumble the corn chips, and spread all but 1 cup in the bottom of a 9- × 13-inch baking pan.
4. Pour the beef and enchilada mixture over the chips.
5. Grate the cheese and sprinkle it over the top. Sprinkle with 1 cup corn chips (and diced green pepper, if desired).
6. Bake for 15 minutes or until the cheese is melted.

Yield: 6 servings

Nutrition Information   2,800 total calories; 470 calories per serving; 52 g carbohydrate; 30 g protein; 16 g fat

Mexican Meal in a Skillet

This Mexican-style carbohydrate–protein combination is simple to prepare and tastes even better as "planned-overs" the next day. You'll enjoy having it ready and waiting when you arrive home hungry and eager to refuel after a hard workout.

For a vegetarian meal, delete the beef.

> 1 cup (195 g) uncooked rice, preferably brown
>
> 1 pound (500 g) extra-lean ground beef or ground turkey
>
> 1 package (about 1.2 oz or 33 g) taco seasoning mix
>
> 1 16-ounce (480 ml) jar salsa, mild or medium
>
> 1 16-ounce (480 ml) can black or red beans, rinsed and drained
>
> 1/2 to 1 cup (120 to 240 ml) water
>
> *Optional:* 1 cup (150 g) diced green or red pepper; 1 11-ounce (312 g) can corn or 1 cup (164 g) frozen corn; grated low-fat cheddar cheese for a garnish

1. Cook rice according to package directions.
2. While the rice is cooking, brown the extra-lean ground beef in a nonstick skillet (along with peppers, if desired). Drain any grease, then sprinkle the taco seasoning mix over the beef.
3. Add the salsa, beans (and corn), and water in the same skillet; cook for 3 to 5 minutes or until heated. Add the cooked rice. If desired, garnish with grated low-fat cheddar cheese.

Yield: 4 hearty servings

Nutrition Information   2,000 total calories; 500 calories per serving; 60 g carbohydrate; 30 g protein; 15 g fat

Sweet and Spicy Orange Beef

Here's a welcome treat after a hard workout when you're hankering for something sweet but healthful. This goes nicely with cooked carrots and peas.

1 cup (195 g) uncooked rice

1 pound (500 g) extra-lean ground beef

1/4 cup (55 g) orange marmalade

1/4 teaspoon red pepper flakes or dash cayenne pepper

Optional: cooked peas; diced celery; green peppers; pineapple chunks

1. Cook the rice according to package directions.
2. In a skillet, cook the beef until browned; drain fat.
3. To the beef, add the marmalade, red pepper flakes, and cooked rice. Mix well. Add optional ingredients as desired.

Yield: 3 servings

Nutrition Information   1,500 total calories; 500 calories per serving; 70 g carbohydrate; 42 g protein; 6 g fat

Honey-Glazed Pork Chops

The combination of honey, cinnamon, and applesauce makes a nice glaze for pork chops. Enjoy these with rice, using the pan juices as a gravy.

---

4 extra-lean pork chops or pork cutlets, well trimmed (about 5 ounces, or 150 g, each, raw)

Honey Glaze

2 tablespoons honey

1/4 cup (55 g) applesauce

1/4 teaspoon cinnamon

Salt and pepper, as desired

---

1. In a small bowl, combine the honey, applesauce, and cinnamon (and salt and pepper, as desired).
2. Heat a nonstick skillet, then brown the pork for 3 minutes on one side.
3. Turn the pork, then spoon the glaze on top. Cover and cook for 3 minutes.
4. Uncover and cook over medium-low heat for 10 minutes or until done, turning once.
5. Serve the pork with rice, spooning the glaze over both the rice and the pork.

Yield: 4 servings

Nutrition Information   1,000 total calories; 250 calories per serving; 10 g carbohydrate; 30 g protein; 10 g fat

Stir-Fried Pork With Fruit

This is a popular family food that appeals to children and adults alike. Pineapple is a nice alternative or addition to the mandarin oranges.

---

1 teaspoon oil

1 pound (500 g) boneless pork cutlets, trimmed and sliced into
  thin strips

1/2 cup (120 ml) water

1/4 cup (60 ml) vinegar

2 tablespoons molasses or honey

2 tablespoons soy sauce

1 11-ounce (325 ml) can mandarin oranges

1 tablespoon cornstarch mixed in

1 tablespoon water

Optional: 1/2 cup (125 g) pineapple chunks; 1 green pepper cut into chunks; 1 medium apple, diced; 1/4 cup (40 g) raisins; 1/4 cup (30 g) chopped toasted nuts

---

1. In a large nonstick skillet, heat the oil and add the sliced pork. Stir until browned.
2. Add the water, vinegar, molasses, soy sauce, and mandarin oranges (and pineapple, green pepper, apple, and raisins, as desired).
3. Bring to a boil; cover and simmer for 5 minutes.
4. Thicken the broth by slowly adding the cornstarch and water mixture and cooking until thickened to the desired consistency.
5. Sprinkle with chopped nuts, as desired.

Yield: 4 servings

Nutrition Information   1,200 total calories; 300 calories per serving; 30 g carbohydrate; 25 g protein; 8 g fat

CHAPTER 23

Beans and Tofu

Beans are some of nature's greatest foods; they are rich in protein and contain little fat and no cholesterol. They help lower blood cholesterol, control blood sugar, fight cancer, reduce problems with constipation, build muscles (with their protein), fuel muscles (with their carbohydrate), and nourish muscles (with lots of B vitamins, iron, zinc, magnesium, copper, folic acid, and potassium).

Because beans are a healthful source of both protein and carbohydrate, vegetarian meals such as chili, hummus, bean and rice casseroles, and other bean meals are perfect for a sports diet. When beans are the only protein source, be sure to eat them in large quantities to consume adequate protein (see chapter 7). If you are a meat eater who wants to become more of a vegetarian, replace part or all of the meat in recipes with more beans, such as replacing ground beef in chili or lasagna with kidney beans.

Here are some suggestions for preparing and serving beans:

- In a blender, mix black or pinto beans, salsa, and cheese. Heat in the microwave and use as a dip or on top of tortillas or potatoes.
- Saute garlic and onions in a little oil; add canned beans (whole or mashed), and heat together. Eat with rice or rolled in a tortilla.
- Add beans to salads, spaghetti sauce, soups, and stews for a protein booster.

- Top a tortilla with 1/2 can (225 g) heated vegetarian refried beans, 1/2 cup (115 g) cottage cheese, salsa, chopped lettuce, and tomato, as desired. Roll into a burrito.
- Combine black beans, refried beans, and salsa to taste. Spoon onto a tortilla, and top with more salsa and cheese, as desired.

For more information about preparing homemade beans and creating bean dishes, read cookbooks that specialize in vegetarian cookery. Appendix A has some suggestions.

Tofu, also known as bean curd, is made from an extract of soybeans. It is a complete protein that contains all the essential amino acids and healthful fat. Tofu has no cholesterol and is relatively low in calories and sodium. It is a popular alternative to meat and can be a source of calcium for people who limit their intake of dairy foods.

Tofu is found in most supermarkets in the refrigerated vegetable section. You can buy soft or firm tofu cakes that are packaged in water; be sure to check the "sell by" date, and buy the freshest brand. Soft or silken tofu is preferable for blending into a smooth cream; firm tofu is good to crumble or slice.

Tofu itself has very little flavor; it takes on the flavors of the foods it's prepared with. For example, tofu mixed with soy sauce takes on a Chinese flavor; with chili, a Mexican flavor. Because of this versatility, tofu lends itself to many recipes: spaghetti, salads, chili, Chinese stir-fry, and even salad dressings. To achieve an interesting, spongy texture, freeze the tofu for at least two days. After it has thawed, squeeze out the water (as if it were a kitchen sponge), tear the tofu into chunks, and add them to spaghetti sauce, chili, soups, or other dishes.

RECIPE FINDER

See also: Chicken and black bean soup, Country pasta with turkey sausage and white beans, Mexican baked chicken with pinto beans, Diana's supersoy and phytochemical shake, Protein shake, Quick and easy chili, Mexican meal in a skillet, Skillet lasagna, Enchilada casserole

Minestrone Soup

This soup offers an enjoyable way to boost your intake of not only beans but also vegetables. Feel free to vary the ingredients, depending on what's available. Serve with crusty whole-grain rolls.

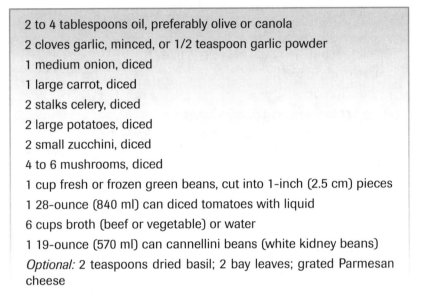

2 to 4 tablespoons oil, preferably olive or canola

2 cloves garlic, minced, or 1/2 teaspoon garlic powder

1 medium onion, diced

1 large carrot, diced

2 stalks celery, diced

2 large potatoes, diced

2 small zucchini, diced

4 to 6 mushrooms, diced

1 cup fresh or frozen green beans, cut into 1-inch (2.5 cm) pieces

1 28-ounce (840 ml) can diced tomatoes with liquid

6 cups broth (beef or vegetable) or water

1 19-ounce (570 ml) can cannellini beans (white kidney beans)

Optional: 2 teaspoons dried basil; 2 bay leaves; grated Parmesan cheese

1. In a large pot, heat the oil and add the garlic and onion; saute until the onions are softened.
2. Add the carrot, celery, potato, zucchini, mushrooms, green beans, tomatoes, broth (and basil and bay leaves). Bring to a boil, reduce the heat, and simmer for about 30 minutes.
3. Add the cannellini beans and heat through. Add seasonings as desired.
4. Serve and sprinkle with Parmesan cheese, as desired.

Yield: 6 large servings

Nutrition Information   1,300 total calories; 220 calories per serving; 36 g carbohydrate; 10 g protein; 4 g fat

Pasta and White Bean Soup With Sun-Dried Tomatoes

This soup is delicious—worth the trip to the store to get the sun-dried tomatoes. If desired, add more beans and pasta—and even diced chicken—to the soup, and you'll have a heartier meal.

1 tablespoon oil, preferably olive or canola

1 large onion, diced

1 medium carrot, diced

1/4 to 1/2 teaspoon red pepper flakes

1 12-ounce (360 ml) can cannellini beans, drained

5 cups (1.2 L) chicken or vegetable broth, homemade, canned, or from bouillon

3 ounces (about 2/3 cup or 85 g) dry bowtie or shell pasta

1/3 cup (35 g) sun-dried tomatoes, diced

Salt and pepper, as desired

3 tablespoons fresh parsley

Optional: 1 clove garlic, minced, or 1/4 teaspoon garlic powder; 1 bay leaf; grated Parmesan cheese

1. In a large nonstick pot, heat the oil over medium heat. Saute the onion, carrot, and red pepper flakes (and garlic).
2. Cover and cook for 10 minutes, stirring occasionally.
3. Pour in the broth and add the beans (and bay leaf). Bring the mixture to a boil.
4. Add the pasta and sun-dried tomatoes. Reduce the heat and simmer for about 10 minutes (or until the pasta is tender).
5. Season with salt and pepper, and add the parsley.
6. Serve with grated Parmesan cheese, if desired.

Yield: 4 servings

Nutrition Information   900 total calories; 225 calories per serving; 38 g carbohydrate; 9 g protein; 4 g fat

Adapted from recipe contributed by Terri Smith, RD.

Quick and Easy Chili

This is a simple family favorite. Although using packaged chili seasonings may seem like cheating, it actually simplifies the cooking process and perhaps enhances the likelihood you'll even make the recipe. Adding a second can of beans and halving the meat makes this a higher-carbohydrate meal. You can also eliminate the beef and turkey and add tofu, if desired.

> 1 pound (500 g) extra-lean ground beef or ground turkey
>
> 1 16-ounce (480 ml) can stewed tomatoes, preferably Cajun style
>
> 1 16-ounce (480 ml) can beans, kidney or pinto
>
> 1 package chili seasonings, hot or mild
>
> 1 2/3 cups (330 g) rice, uncooked
>
> *Optional:* 1 11-ounce (325 ml) can corn, drained; 1 green pepper, diced

1. In a skillet with high sides, brown the beef or turkey. Drain the fat, if any.
2. Add the stewed tomatoes, beans, and chili seasonings (and corn and green pepper). Bring the mixture to a boil, then reduce the heat.
3. Simmer for 5 to 50 minutes, depending on how much time you have.
4. While the chili is simmering, cook the rice according to package directions.
5. Serve the chili over rice.

Yield: 6 servings

Nutrition Information   1,650 total calories without rice; 275 calories per serving; 20 g carbohydrate; 24 g protein; 11 g fat

With 1 cup rice: 480 calories per serving; 64 g carbohydrate; 27 g protein; 13 g fat

Courtesy of John McGrath

Pasta With Spinach and Garbanzo Beans

Made with ingredients you can easily keep stocked, this sports meal is simple to prepare and delicious to eat. It's a balanced vegetarian meal in a bowl, representing four food groups. Nonvegetarians can enjoy this meal as is or with cooked chicken, if desired.

3 to 6 teaspoons olive oil

1 large onion, chopped

1 to 4 garlic cloves, minced, or 1/8 to 1/2 teaspoon garlic powder

1 14-ounce (420 ml) can chicken broth, regular or low sodium

1 15-ounce (450 g) can garbanzo beans (chickpeas), rinsed and drained

1 10-ounce (300 g) package frozen leaf spinach, thawed and squeezed dry, or 1 bag fresh baby spinach

12 ounces (350 g) pasta, such as shells

Salt and pepper to taste

1/4 cup (25 g) grated Parmesan cheese

Optional: Diced cooked chicken

1. Cook pasta according to package directions.
2. While the pasta is cooking, heat 1 to 2 teaspoons oil in large, heavy nonstick skillet over medium heat. Add onion and garlic; saute until tender, about 10 minutes.
3. Pour in chicken broth and simmer until liquid is reduced by half, about 4 minutes.
4. Add garbanzo beans and spinach; boil 1 minute. Transfer spinach mixture to large bowl.
5. Add pasta. Drizzle pasta with remaining 2 to 4 teaspoons olive oil and toss.
6. Season pasta generously with pepper; sprinkle with salt, as desired, and grated Parmesan, and toss well.

Yield: 4 hearty servings

Nutrition Information   2,000 total calories; 500 calories per serving; 87 g carbohydrate; 20 g protein; 8 g fat

Hummus Roll-Ups

Traditional hummus, made with olive oil and tahini, can be a surprisingly high-fat meal. This recipe reduces the fat. The secret ingredient in hummus is tahini, or sesame paste. You can buy tahini in the ethnic food section of larger supermarkets or health-food stores. Store leftover tahini in the refrigerator, and use it for other dishes.

---

1 16-ounce (480 ml) can chickpeas

1 to 2 tablespoons lemon juice, bottled or fresh

1 clove garlic or 1/4 teaspoon garlic powder to taste

2 to 4 tablespoons tahini or peanut butter

Salt and pepper, as desired

8-inch (20 cm) tortillas or wraps, preferably whole wheat

Optional: dash of cayenne; 1 tablespoon parsley; 1/4 teaspoon cumin; diced or shredded vegetables for topping

---

1. Drain the chickpeas, saving 1/4 cup of the liquid.
2. In a blender or food processor, mix the chickpeas, 1/4 cup reserved liquid, lemon juice, garlic, tahini, and seasonings.
3. Blend until smooth. If you don't have a blender, mash the chickpeas with the back of a fork.
4. Spread 1/3 cup hummus on a tortilla. Add 1/2 cup diced or shredded vegetables of your choice: tomato, pepper, scallion, beans, nuts, carrot, lettuce.

Yield: About 1 1/2 cups hummus; about 5 servings

Nutrition Information   625 total calories; 125 calories per serving (1/3 cup); 18 g carbohydrate; 5 g protein; 4 g fat
In tortilla roll-up (with 1/2 cup hummus): 300 calories per serving; 49 g carbohydrate; 8 g protein; 8 g fat

Tofu Lo Mein

This versatile recipe can be made according to your tastes—with extra veggies, hot pepper, or garlic. You can also replace the tofu with chicken, shrimp, beef, or just vegetables. If the noodles seem dry, add a little water or broth.

9 ounces (275 g) Chinese noodles or 4 ounces (125 g) dry spaghetti

4 teaspoons oil, preferably half sesame, half canola

1/2 to 3/4 teaspoon ground ginger or 2 teaspoons fresh chopped ginger

1/4 to 1/2 teaspoon garlic powder or 1 to 2 cloves garlic, minced

2 to 4 cups shredded napa cabbage or bok choy

1 large carrot, grated

2 tablespoons soy sauce or tamari sauce

8 ounces (250 g) extra-firm tofu, drained and cut into 1/2 inch (1 cm) cubes

Optional: 1/8 teaspoon sugar (adds a nice hint of sweetness); dash hot pepper flakes; 4 scallions, chopped; 1 to 2 cups (250 to 500) diced mushrooms, onions, pea pods, peppers, or other vegetables of your choice; sunflower seeds or sliced almonds for garnish

1. Cook the noodles according to the package directions. Drain, return to the pot, and using two knives as scissors, cut them into smaller, more manageable pieces.

2. While the noodles are cooking, in a large nonstick skillet heat the oil, then add the ginger, garlic powder, cabbage, and carrot (and sugar, hot pepper, and vegetables). Stir-fry over medium-high heat for 1 to 2 minutes.

3. Add the soy sauce and cubed tofu. Stir-fry for another 1 to 2 minutes or until the vegetables are tender-crisp.

4. Add the noodles, toss well, adjust the seasonings, then serve.

Yield: 5 servings as a side dish; 3 large servings as a main dish

Nutrition Information   1,500 total calories; 300 calories per serving (side dish); 35 g carbohydrate; 10 g protein; 13 g fat

Tofu Burritos

This is a simple lunch, dinner, or even breakfast. I like it with a dollop of hummus.

> 2 teaspoons margarine or olive oil
>
> 1 small onion, diced
>
> 1 green pepper, diced
>
> 1 14-ounce (400 g) cake firm tofu, crumbled
>
> 4 tortillas, white, whole wheat, or corn, warmed
>
> Salt and pepper, as desired
>
> *Optional:* raisins, chopped walnuts, and curry powder; sesame seeds, sesame oil (instead of margarine), and soy sauce; garlic powder; hummus

1. In a nonstick skillet, melt the margarine, then add the onion and green pepper. Saute until tender.
2. Add the crumbled tofu and desired seasonings; heat thoroughly.
3. Place 1/4 of the mixture in the middle of a tortilla, fold over one end, fold in the sides, and roll up.

Yield: 4 small servings (or 2 large)

Nutrition Information   1,200 total calories; 300 calories per serving (small); 40 g carbohydrate; 15 g protein; 9 g fat

CHAPTER 24

Beverages and Smoothies

Beverages are not only a way to quench your thirst and replace fluids lost through sweat but also a way to refuel your muscles with carbohydrate and boost recovery with protein. Some smoothies can be a quick meal that you pour into a portable coffee mug and sip on the way to work. Others are an easy way to boost your fruit intake with minimal effort.

To spur your creativity, here are a few smoothie suggestions. If you don't have frozen fruit handy, you can add ice cubes to the smoothie for that cool and frosty feeling.

- Frozen strawberries, banana, milk powder, and orange juice
- Vanilla yogurt, instant coffee powder (decaf or regular), and ice cubes
- Frozen raspberries, silken tofu, cranberry juice, and honey
- Frozen banana chunks, orange juice, pineapple juice, and protein powder
- Soy milk, peaches, and vanilla low-fat frozen yogurt
- Orange juice, cantaloupe chunks, and vanilla yogurt

RECIPE FINDER

Homemade Sports Drink

The nutrition profile of commercial sports drinks is 50 to 70 calories per 8 ounces (250 ml), with about 110 milligrams of sodium. Below is a simple recipe that offers this profile, but at a much lower cost than the expensive store-bought brands. You can make it without the lemon juice, but the flavor will be weaker.

You can be creative when making your own sports drink. You can dilute many combinations of juices (such as cranberry and lemonade) to 50 calories per 8 ounces (250 ml) and then add a pinch of salt. More precisely, add 1/4 teaspoon salt per quart (liter) of liquid. Some people use flavorings such as sugar-free lemonade to enhance the flavor yet leave the calories in the 50 to 70 per 8-ounce range. The trick is to always test the recipe during training, not during an important event. You want to be sure it tastes good when you are hot and sweaty and settles well when you're working hard.

> 1/4 cup (50 g) sugar
>
> 1/4 teaspoon salt
>
> 1/4 cup (60 ml) hot water
>
> 1/4 cup (60 ml) orange juice (not concentrate) plus 2 tablespoons lemon juice
>
> 3 1/2 cups (840 ml) cold water

1. In the bottom of a pitcher, dissolve the sugar and salt in the hot water.
2. Add the juice and the remaining water; chill.
3. Quench that thirst!

Yield: 1 quart (1 L)

Nutrition Information   200 total calories; 50 calories per 8 ounces (250 ml); 12 g carbohydrate; 110 mg sodium

Fruit Smoothie

Fruit smoothies are popular for breakfasts and snacks. The ingredients can vary according to individual tastes. Some tried-and-true combinations include banana and strawberries in orange juice and melon and pineapple in pineapple juice. Almost any combination works.

For a thick, frosty shake, use fruit that has been frozen. To have fruit ready for blending into a smoothie, simply slice a surplus of ripe fresh fruit (that might otherwise spoil) into chunks, then freeze the chunks on a flat sheet. When frozen, pack them into ziplock bags. (If you freeze them in the bag, you'll end up with one big chunk of frozen fruit that is hard to break apart.)

1/2 cup (115 g) low-fat yogurt (plain or flavored) or milk

1 cup (240 ml) fruit juice

1/2 to 1 cup (80 to 160 g) fruit, fresh, frozen, or canned

Optional: 1/4 cup (30 g) milk powder; dash cinnamon or nutmeg; sweetener as desired

---

1. Place all ingredients in a blender, cover, and whip until smooth.

Yield: 1 serving

Nutrition Information   220-290 calories per serving; 50-60 g carbohydrate; 5 g protein; 0-3 g fat

Diana's SuperSoy and Phytochemical Shake

Diana Dyer, RD, a nutritionist and three-time cancer survivor, swears by this smoothie. It's full of vitamins, minerals, fiber, calcium, and health-protective phytochemicals. Diana enjoys it for breakfast every day. She drinks about half the shake right away, often with a whole-grain bagel. Then she puts the rest of the shake in an insulated coffee mug to carry with her "on the go." Many people have told her how tasty the shake is and additionally how "energizing" it is. She invites you to drink to your health and enjoy it!

3/4 cup (180 ml) soy milk, preferably calcium fortified

3/4 cup (180 ml) orange juice, preferably calcium fortified

1 to 2 tablespoons* wheat or oat bran

1 to 2 tablespoons* wheat germ

1 to 2 tablespoons* whole flaxseed or ground flaxseed meal

2 to 3 ounces (60-90 g) soft tofu

6 to 8 baby carrots or one large raw carrot, chopped

3/4 cup (120 g) fresh or frozen fruit

*Increase the fiber content gradually, starting with a scant tablespoon each of the wheat bran, wheat germ, and flaxseed. Take a few weeks to work up to 2 tablespoons of each.

---

1. Pour the milk and juice into a blender. Turn on the blender, and carefully add the bran, wheat germ, and flax. (This keeps the dry ingredients from sticking to the side of the blender.)
2. Stop the blender, then add the tofu, carrots, and fruit. Cover and blend on high until smooth.
3. If the shake is too thick, thin it with a little juice, soy milk, milk, water, or even iced green tea.

Yield: about 3 cups

Nutrition Information 450 approximate calories; 65 g carbohydrate; 25 g protein; 10 g fat

Courtesy of Diana Dyer

Protein Shake

This shake is a simple way to boost not only protein and calcium but also your intake of health-protective tofu. This recipe uses silken tofu, which has about 5 grams of protein per quarter-cake. Extra-firm tofu has more protein (10 grams per quarter-cake), but it blends poorly. Dry milk powder, with 8 grams of protein per quarter-cup, boosts protein as well.

4 ounces (125 g) silken tofu

1/3 cup (45 g) dried milk powder

1 cup (240 ml) low-fat milk

2 tablespoons chocolate milk powder or chocolate syrup

1. Combine ingredients in a blender.
2. Cover and blend for 1 minute or until smooth.

Yield: 1 serving

Nutrition Information   350 total calories; 52 g carbohydrate; 26 g protein; 4 g fat

Thick and Frosty Milk Shake

This thick and tasty milk shake is a healthful alternative to ones made with ice cream. The instant pudding adds a thick texture, and the ice cubes make it frosty and refreshing. I like to make these for my kids—an enjoyable way to boost their protein and calcium intake.

By varying the flavor of the pudding (vanilla, lemon, chocolate), you can create numerous variations. You can also add fruit (preferably frozen chunks) for extra nutritional value. Note: The shake thickens upon standing; you can add more (or less) pudding mix, depending on how thick you like your shakes. If there are pieces of ice cubes remaining in the shake, worry not—they'll just keep the beverage cool.

1 cup (240 ml) low-fat milk

1/4 cup (35 g) instant pudding

1/4 cup (30 g) powdered milk

3 ice cubes

Optional: 1/2 to 1 cup (80 to 160 g) (frozen) fruit chunks

1. Place all ingredients in a blender, and blend until smooth.

Yield: 1 serving

Nutrition Information 280 total calories; 55 g carbohydrate; 15 g protein; 0 g fat

Courtesy of Annie and David Bastille

Reese's Shake

If you like peanut butter cups, you'll love this shake! For a light-tasting and refreshing recovery shake, use 1/4 cup each of peanut butter and chocolate syrup. For a heavy-duty weight gainer, use 1/2 cup of each.

> 2 cups (480 ml) milk, preferably low fat or nonfat
>
> 1/2 cup (60 g) powdered milk
>
> 1/4 to 1/2 cup (65 to 130 g) peanut butter
>
> 1/4 to 1/2 cup (60 to 125 ml) chocolate syrup

1. Combine all the ingredients in a blender.
2. Cover and blend for 1 minute or until smooth.

Yield: 1 serving

Nutrition Information   890 to 1,500 total calories; 105-170 g carbohydrate; 45-60 g protein; 32-64 g fat

CHAPTER 25 —————

Snacks and Desserts

Many athletes enjoy snacks and desserts as part of their daily food plans. Fresh fruits are ideal choices for either, yet there is a time and a place for other sweets. The trick is to choose snacks and desserts that are low in fat and high in carbohydrate. These recipes provide healthy alternatives to empty-calorie temptations.

Remember that peanut butter is a staple for hungry athletes who want a satisfying, wholesome snack. Although peanut butter is fat laden, it can healthfully fit into the fat budget for most sports diets. If you are a peanut butter lover, you can spread peanut butter on bread or tortillas and add any of the following ingredients to put some variety in your sports snacks:

- Jelly (of course!)
- Honey
- Cinnamon or cinnamon sugar
- Applesauce, raisins, and cinnamon
- Raisins
- Banana slices
- Apple slices
- Sprouts
- Granola or sunflower seeds

- Cottage cheese
- Dill pickle slices (no kidding!)

You can also make yourself a homemade milk shake by combining 1 cup milk, 1 banana, 1 tablespoon peanut butter, and sweetener as desired.

RECIPE FINDER

Oatmeal cookies	405
Peanutty energy bars	406
Sugar and spice trail mix	407
Peanut butter banana roll-up	408
Apple crisp	409
Rainbow fruit salad	410
Peach and gingersnap sundaes	411
Carrot cake	412
Chocolate lush	413

See also: Fruit smoothies, Thick and frosty milk shake, Reese's shake

Oatmeal Cookies

These cakey, low-fat cookies digest easily and are good for a preexercise snack or recovery food. The recipe makes about 5 dozen cookies—enough to feed the whole team. If you are cooking for yourself, you might want to cut the recipe in half.

3 cups flour (420 g), preferably half whole wheat and half white

2 teaspoons baking soda

2 teaspoons salt

2 teaspoons cinnamon

1 1/4 cups (300 ml) milk

1 cup (240 ml) oil, preferably canola

3/4 cup (150 g) white sugar

1 cup (200 g) packed brown sugar

4 cups (320 g) uncooked oatmeal

2 eggs or 4 egg whites

2 teaspoons vanilla

1 cup (165 g) raisins

1. Preheat the oven to 350 °F (180 °C).
2. In a medium bowl, combine the soda, salt, cinnamon, and flour. Set aside.
3. In a large bowl, mix together the milk, oil, sugar, oatmeal, eggs, and vanilla. Beat well.
4. Gradually add flour mixture to large bowl and combine thoroughly. Then gently stir in raisins.
5. Drop by rounded tablespoons onto ungreased baking sheet.
6. Bake for 15 to 18 minutes. Cookies should be firm when tapped with a finger.

Yield: 5 dozen cookies

Nutrition Information   6,500 total calories; 110 calories per cookie; 16 g carbohydrate; 2 g protein; 4 g fat

Adapted from recipe contributed by Natalie Updegrove Partridge.

Peanutty Energy Bars

This prizewinning recipe offers a yummy alternative to commercial energy bars. These homemade bars are perfect for when you are hiking or biking, as well as for a satisfying afternoon snack. They are relatively high in fat, but it's healthful fat from peanuts and sunflower seeds. For variety, you can make this recipe with cashews and cashew butter and add a variety of dried fruits (cranberries, cherries, and dates).

1/2 cup (60 g) salted dry-roasted peanuts

1/2 cup (60 g) roasted sunflower seed kernels, or use more peanuts or other nuts

1/2 cup (80 g) raisins or other dried fruit

2 cups (160 g) uncooked oatmeal, old-fashioned or instant

2 cups (50 g) toasted rice cereal, such as Rice Krispies

1/2 cup (130 g) peanut butter, crunchy or creamy

1/2 cup (100 g) packed brown sugar

1/2 cup (120 ml) light corn syrup

1 teaspoon vanilla

Optional: 1/4 cup toasted wheat germ

1. In a large bowl, mix together the peanuts, sunflower seeds, raisins, oatmeal, and toasted rice cereal (and wheat germ). Set aside.

2. In a medium microwaveable bowl, combine the peanut butter, brown sugar, and corn syrup. Microwave on high for 2 minutes. Add vanilla and stir until blended.

3. Pour the peanut butter mixture over the dry ingredients; stir until coated.

4. For squares, spoon the mixture into an 8- × 8-inch pan coated with cooking spray; for bars spoon it into a 9- × 13-inch pan. Press down firmly. (It helps to coat your fingers with margarine, oil, or cooking spray.)

5. Let stand for about an hour, then cut into squares or bars.

Yield: 16 squares or bars

Nutrition Information   3,600 total calories; 225 calories per serving; 30 g carbohydrate; 6 g protein; 9 g fat

Recipe courtesy of The Peanut Institute

Sugar and Spice Trail Mix

Shannon Weiderholt, RD, likes this recipe as a snack for calming the afternoon munchies on the trail, at home, or at work. Keep this in a resealable plastic bag in your desk drawer or gym bag, and you'll have energy to enjoy your day. It's sweet, but not too sweet.

3 cups (165 g) oat squares cereal

3 cups mini pretzels, salted or unsalted, as desired

2 tablespoons tub margarine, melted

1 tablespoon packed brown sugar

1/2 teaspoon cinnamon

1 cup (165 g) dried fruit bits or raisins

1. Preheat oven to 325 °F (170 °C).
2. Combine the oat squares and pretzels in a large resealable plastic bag or a plastic container with a lid. Set aside.
3. Melt the margarine in a small microwaveable bowl.
4. Add the brown sugar and cinnamon to the margarine and mix well.
5. Pour the cinnamon and sugar mixture over the cereal and pretzels, and seal the bag or container. Shake gently until the mixture is coated. Pour onto a baking sheet and spread evenly.
6. Bake for 15 to 20 minutes, stirring once or twice.
7. Remove from the oven, allow to cool, and then mix in the dried fruit.
8. Store in an airtight container or single-serving resealable bags.

Yield: 10 servings

Nutrition Information   2,000 total calories; 200 calories per serving; 40 g carbohydrate; 5 g protein; 2 g fat

Adapted from American Heart Association. www.deliciousdecisions.org

Peanut Butter Banana Roll-Up

This snack is popular with the family of Anne Fletcher, RD, author of *Sober for Good*. Kids of all ages enjoy it, not only for an afternoon energy booster but also for a simple breakfast or dinner.

1 10-inch (25 cm) flour tortilla, white or whole wheat

2 tablespoons peanut butter

1/2 medium banana, sliced into coins

1 tablespoon raisins

1. Warm tortilla in the microwave oven for 20 to 30 seconds or until soft.
2. Spread with peanut butter to within 1/2 inch of the edges.
3. Place the banana coins in the middle of the tortilla, sprinkle with raisins, and roll it up like a burrito.

Yield: 2 servings for a snack; 1 serving for a quick breakfast or supper

Nutrition Information   500 total calories (whole recipe); 70 g carbohydrate; 12 g protein; 19 g fat

Courtesy of Anne Fletcher

Apple Crisp

When making apple crisp, I prefer to leave the peels on the apples for added fiber and nutrients. The small amount of spices allows for a nice apple flavor to shine through the "crisp." For a crisp topping, the margarine or butter should be thoroughly worked into the flour, coating each granule.

> 6 cups sliced apples, preferably half Granny Smith, half McIntosh
>
> 1/4 cup (50 g) sugar
>
> 1/2 cup (70 g) flour
>
> 1/3 to 1/2 cup (65 to 100 g) sugar, preferably half white, half packed brown sugar
>
> 1/4 teaspoon cinnamon
>
> 3 to 4 tablespoons margarine or butter, cold from the refrigerator
>
> *Optional:* 3/4 cup chopped almonds or pecans; 1/4 teaspoon nutmeg; 1/4 teaspoon salt

1. Core, slice, and place the apples in an 8- × 8-inch baking pan. Coat with 1/4 cup sugar.
2. Heat oven to 375 °F (190 °C).
3. In a medium bowl, mix together the flour, sugar, and cinnamon (and nutmeg and salt). Add the margarine or butter, pinching it into the flour with your fingers until it looks like crumbly wet sand. Add nuts, as desired.
4. Distribute the topping evenly over the apples.
5. Bake for 40 minutes. If you want a crisper topping, turn the oven up to 400 °F (200 °C) for the last 5 minutes.

Yield: 6 servings

Nutrition Information 1,560 total calories; 260 calories per serving; 50 g carbohydrate; 1 g protein; 6 g fat

Courtesy of Janice Clark

Rainbow Fruit Salad

A pretty fruit salad is always a welcome dessert. This fruit salad is particularly healthful because it offers a variety of nutrients from the variety of colorful fruits. This recipe is one of many healthy recipes found at www.nhlbi.nih.gov/health. Click on the Stay Young at Heart Recipe Collection.

1 large mango, peeled and diced

1 cup (145 g) fresh blueberries

1 banana, sliced

1 cup (150 g) strawberries, halved

1 cup (160 g) seedless grapes

1 nectarine or peach, sliced

1 kiwi fruit, peeled and sliced

Honey-Orange Sauce

1/3 cup (75 ml) orange juice

2 tablespoons lemon juice

1 1/2 teaspoons honey

1/4 teaspoon ground ginger

Dash nutmeg

1. Prepare and combine the fruits in a large bowl.
2. Combine all the ingredients for the sauce and mix.
3. Just before serving, pour the sauce over the fruit.

Yield: 6 servings

Nutrition Information   600 total calories; 100 calories per serving; 25 g carbohydrate; 0 g protein; 0 g fat

Peach and Gingersnap Sundaes

Delightfully different and yummy good, this is a welcome snack for kids as well as an easy dessert for company dinner. You can prepare the yogurt and gingersnaps ahead of time, and then add the warm peaches at the last minute. You can easily cut the recipe to make a single serving just for yourself. This is just one of many recipes found at www.eatsmart.org and can be easily adapted using various fruits and flavors of yogurt.

---

1 tablespoon margarine or butter

1 15-ounce (450 ml) can diced peaches or 2 cups (340 g) fresh or frozen peaches, diced

2 tablespoons brown sugar

1/4 teaspoon cinnamon

12 gingersnap cookies

4 6-ounce (175 g) containers vanilla or peach yogurt, low fat or nonfat

---

1. Add the margarine or butter to a skillet and melt over medium heat.
2. Add the peaches, brown sugar, and cinnamon to the skillet. Cook until the peaches are hot (2 to 5 minutes), stirring occasionally.
3. As the fruit cooks, place the gingersnaps in a heavy-duty plastic bag, seal, and pound with rolling pin (or other hard object) until cookies are broken into coarse crumbs.
4. Spoon the yogurt into four bowls. Top with a layer of gingersnap crumbs and then add warm peaches over the top.

Yield: 4 servings

Nutrition Information   1,100 total calories; 275 calories per serving; 47 g carbohydrate; 8 g protein; 6 g fat

Adapted from Washington State Dairy Council.

Carrot Cake

Sports nutritionist Jenny Hegmann, RD, suggests that if you are destined to eat cake, at least have one filled with fruit, vegetables, and nuts. This carrot cake recipe fills that bill. Unlike most carrot cakes that are extremely high in fat, Jenny's recipe offers a lower-fat option—with a heart-healthful fat at that, canola oil.

1 1/2 cups (300 g) sugar
3/4 cup (180 ml) oil, preferably canola
3 eggs or 6 egg whites
2 cups (220 g) grated carrot, lightly packed
1 cup (250 g) crushed canned pineapple with juice
2 teaspoons vanilla extract
1 teaspoon salt
1 teaspoon cinnamon
1 teaspoon baking powder
1/2 teaspoon baking soda
2 1/2 cups (350 g) flour
Optional: 1 cup (120 g) chopped walnuts; 1 cup (165 g) raisins

Frosting
4 ounces (125 g) low-fat cream cheese, at room temperature
2 1/2 cups (250 g) confectioners' sugar, sifted
1 teaspoon vanilla extract or 2 teaspoons grated orange peel
1 to 2 tablespoons milk or orange juice

1. Treat a 9- × 13-inch baking pan with cooking spray, or line with waxed paper.
2. Preheat the oven to 350 °F (180 °C).
3. In a medium mixing bowl, beat together the sugar and oil, then the eggs.
4. Add the grated carrot, pineapple and its juice, and vanilla. Mix well.
5. Add the salt, cinnamon, baking powder, and baking soda (and nuts and raisins, if desired). Gently blend in the flour, being careful not to overbeat.
6. Pour the batter into the prepared pan. Bake for 35 to 40 minutes. Cool completely before frosting.
7. In a small mixing bowl, beat the cream cheese and confectioners' sugar. Add vanilla and milk (or orange juice and grated orange peel), and beat until smooth, creamy, and the desired consistency. Spread the frosting on the cake.

Yield: 24 pieces

Nutrition Information   4,200 total calories (plain cake); 175 calories per serving; 26 g carbohydrate; 2 g protein; 7 g fat

With frosting: 5,500 total calories; 230 calories per serving; 37 g carbohydrate; 3 g protein, 8 g fat

Courtesy of Jenny Hegmann, RD

Chocolate Lush

What I like best about this brownie pudding is that it's a low-fat yet tasty treat for those who want a chocolate fix. It forms its own sauce during baking. If you need to rationalize eating chocolate, remember it does contain some health-protective phytochemicals.

1 cup (140 g) flour

3/4 cup (150 g) sugar

2 tablespoons unsweetened dry cocoa

2 teaspoons baking powder

1 teaspoon salt

1/2 cup (120 ml) milk

2 tablespoons oil, preferably canola

2 teaspoons vanilla

3/4 cup (150 g) brown sugar

1/4 cup (35 g) unsweetened dry cocoa

1 3/4 cups (420 ml) hot water

Optional: 1/2 cup (60 g) chopped nuts.

1. Preheat the oven to 350 °F (180 °C).
2. In a medium bowl, stir together the flour, white sugar, 2 tablespoons cocoa, baking powder, and salt; add the milk, oil, and vanilla (and nuts). Mix until smooth.
3. Pour into an 8- × 8-inch square pan that is nonstick, lightly oiled, or treated with cooking spray.
4. Combine the brown sugar, 1/4 cup cocoa, and hot water. Gently pour this mixture on top of the batter in the pan.
5. Bake for 40 minutes or until lightly browned and bubbly.

Yield: 9 servings

Nutrition Information   2,100 total calories; 230 calories per serving; 46 g carbohydrate; 3 g protein; 4 g fat

Courtesy of Sue Westin

APPENDIX A

For More Information

Publications and Web Sites

This list provides a variety of sources, including books, Web sites, and newsletters, where you can find additional information about many of the topics discussed in this book. Some of the books listed are classics; some are new releases. A few titles are primarily for professionals, but most are appropriate for the public. You can look for the books in your local library or bookstore. Alternatively, many are available through the following sources of reliable nutrition materials:

Nutrition Counseling and Education Services (NCES)
www.ncescatalog.com
877-623-7266

Gurze Eating Disorders Resource Catalogue
www.bulimia.com
800-756-7533

The Web sites and newsletters listed provide quality nutrition, sports nutrition, and health information. The list reflects information gathered in July 2007. It is by no means complete; many other excellent resources and Web sites are available.

Because I am frequently asked how to become a sports nutritionist, I have included at the end of this appendix some information on starting down that road. Health professionals who want sports nutrition teaching materials can find handouts and slides on my Web site, www.nancyclarkrd.com, and online courses at www.sportsnutritionworkshop.com.

Aging

Nelson, M. 1999. *Strong Women Stay Slim.* New York: Random House.

www.healthandage.com An exceptional resource to help you or your aging parents find answers to the nutrition, fitness, and health questions and concerns of older people.

Alcohol

Garner, A., and J. Woititz. 1990. *Lifeskills for adult children.* Deerfield Beach, FL: Health Communications.

Woititz, J. 2002. *The complete adult children of alcoholics sourcebook: Adult children at home, at work and in love.* Deerfield Beach, FL: Health Communications.

www.smartrecovery.org, www.AddictionAlternatives.com, www.alcoholics-anony-mous.org, www.secularsobriety.org, www.unhooked.com, www.moderation.org All these Web sites offer helpful resources for people who want to stop their problem drinking and for their loved ones.

Body Image (See Also Eating Disorders)

Clairborn, J., and C. Pedrick. 2002. *The BDD workbook: Overcome body dysmorphic disorder and end body image obsessions.* Oakland, CA: New Harbinger.

Freedman, R. 2002. *Bodylove: Learning to like our looks and ourselves.* Carlsbad, CA: Gurze Books.

Johnson, C. 2001. *Self-esteem comes in all sizes: How to be happy and healthy at your natural weight.* Carlsbad, CA: Gurze Books.

Pope, H., K. Phillips, and R. Olivardia. 2000. *The Adonis complex: The secret crisis of male body obsession.* New York: Free Press.

www.bodypositive.com Dedicated to boosting body image at any weight.

www.about-face.org This Web site promotes positive self-esteem in women of all ages.

Calories (See Also Dietary Analysis and Nutrition Assessment)

Netzer, C. 2005. *The complete book of food counts.* 7th ed. New York: Dell.

Pennington, J., and R. Douglass. 2004. *Bowes & Church's food values of portions commonly used.* 18th ed. Philadelphia: Lippincott.

www.calorieking.com www.ars.usda.gov/services/docs.htm?docid=8964

Cancer (See Also Healthy Eating; Herbs, Medicinal; Supplements)

Dyer, D. 2002. *The dietitian's cancer story: Information and inspiration for recovery and healing.* Ann Arbor, MI: Swan Press.

Weihofen, D., and C. Marino. 2002. *The cancer survival cookbook: 200 quick and easy recipes with helpful eating tips.* New York: Wiley.

www.cancer.org The American Cancer Society's site has answers to all your questions about prevention and treatment.

www.aicr.org The American Institute for Cancer Research offers dietary information about eating for a healthier life.

www.CancerRD.com Diana Dyer, MS, RD offers nutrition information and inspiration for people with cancer.

www.cancernutritioninfo.com Suzanne Dixon, MPH, MS, RD, helps people understand the link between nutrition and cancer.

www.dietandcancerreport.org The Food, Nutrition, Physical Activity and the Prevention of Cancer; a Global Perspective provides the latest information from The World Cancer Research Fund and the American Institute for Cancer Research.

Celiac Disease

Case, S. 2006. *Gluten-free diet: A comprehensive resource guide.* Regina, Saskatchewan: Case Nutrition Consulting.

www.glutenfreediet.ca Shelley Case, RD, has a helpful Web site for people with celiac disease.

www.glutenfreemeals.com This site is for people with celiac disease who don't like to cook.

www.iansnaturalfoods.com This site identifies kids' foods that are free of the top eight allergens.

www.celiac.org, www.gluten.net, www.niddk.nih.gov Visit the Web sites for the Celiac Disease Foundation, The Gluten Intolerance Group of North America, and the National Institute of Diabetes and Digestive and Kidney Diseases for more information, resources, and links about celiac disease.

Childhood Obesity

www.nhlbi.nih.gov/health/public/heart/obesity/wecan We Can! is a national education program that offers parents and families tips and fun activities to encourage healthy eating, increase physical activity, and reduce sedentary or screen time.

www.cdc.gov/growthcharts Growth charts for assessing children's weight are available at the Center for Disease Control's Web site.

Children and Nutrition

Friedman, S. 2001. *When girls feel fat: Helping girls through adolescence.* Toronto: HarperCollins.

Litt, A. 2005. *The college student's guide to eating well on campus.* Bethesda, MD: Tulip Hill Press.

Satter, E. 2000. *Child of mine: Feeding with love and good sense.* Palo Alto, CA: Bull.

Satter, E. 2005. *Secrets of feeding a healthy family.* Madison, WI: Kelcy Press.

Ward, E. 2002. *Healthy foods, healthy kids: A complete guide to nutrition for children from birth to six years old.* Avon, MA: Adams Media.

www.kidnetic.com This site was designed to promote healthful eating and physical activity among kids and parents.

Clothing

www.raceready.com This site has running shorts and other exercise apparel with pockets for holding sports foods.

Complementary and Alternative Medicine (See also Herbs, Medicinal)

www.nccam.nih.gov, http://dietary-supplements.info.nih.gov The Web sites for the National Center for Complementary and Alternative Medicine and The Office of Dietary Supplements provide more information about alternative medicine, herbs, and dietary supplements.

Cookbooks and Cooking Magazines (See also Vegetarian Nutrition, Recipes)

American Heart Association. 2000. *AHA meals in minutes cookbook: Over 200 all new quick and easy low-fat recipes.* New York: Crown.

Bissex, J., and L. Weiss. 2003. *The mom's guide to meal makeovers: Improving the way your family eats, one meal at a time.* New York: Broadway.

Foco, Z. 2007. *Lickety-split meals for health conscious people on the go!* Walled Lake, MI: ZHI.

Molt, M. 2005. *Food for fifty.* 12th ed. Upper Saddle River, NJ: Prentice Hall.

Pivanka, E., and B. Berry. 2002. *5 a day: The better health cookbook.* Emmaus, PA: Rodale.

Ponichtera, B. 2008. *Quick and healthy recipes and ideas.* Small Steps Press

Tribole, E. 1994. *Healthy homestyle cooking.* Emmaus, PA: Rodale.

www.cookinglight.com, www.cooksillustrated.com, www.eatingwell.com, www.lightandtasty.com Visit these sites for recipes and additional cooking information.

Diabetes

American Diabetes Association. 2006. *The American Diabetes Association's complete guide to diabetes.* Alexandria, VA: Author.

Colberg, S. 2000. *The diabetic athlete.* Champaign, IL: Human Kinetics.

www.ndep.nih.gov The National Diabetes Education Program, part of the NIDDK, offers abundant information on how to improve diabetes care.

www.diabetes.org The American Diabetes Association offers abundant information and resources for diabetes care.

Dietary Analysis and Nutrition Assessment (See also Calories)

www.fitday.com, www.mypyramidtracker.gov, www.nutrimaps.com, www.nutritiondata.com, www.sparkpeople.com Enjoy these sites for tracking your food intake.

www.usda.gov/cnpp Created by the USDA's Center for Nutrition Policy and Promotion, this Web site offers an interactive healthy eating index. You can assess 25 nutrients in your diet and see how your food choices stack up against the food guide pyramid.

www.ars.usda.gov/services/docs.htm?docid=7783 This USDA site provides a search tool you can use to view the nutrient profiles of thousands of foods.

http://hin.nhlbi.nih.gov/menuplanner/menu.cgi This menu planner lets you select a calorie level and plan meals with portions of the correct size.

Dietitian (How to find one locally)

www.eatright.org The American Dietetic Association's referral network can help you find a registered dietitian (RD). You can also call 1-800-366-1655.

www.SCANdpg.org The referral network of the ADA's Sports, Cardiovascular, and Wellness Nutritionists, a dietetic practice group, is a good resource for finding an RD.

You can also find an RD by calling the nutrition department at your local hospital or sports medicine clinic or by looking in a general telephone directory under dietitian or nutritionist. Select a name followed by RD.

Eating Disorders

Beals, K. 2004. *Disordered eating among athletes.* Champaign, IL: Human Kinetics.

Heffner, M., and G. Eifert. 2004. *The anorexia workbook: How to accept yourself, heal your suffering and reclaim your life.* Carlsbad, CA: Gurze Books.

Hirschmann, J., and C. Munter. 2000. *Overcoming overeating: Living free in a world of food.* London: Vermillion.

Koenig, K. 2007. *Food and feelings workbook: A full course meal on emotional health.* Carlsbad, CA: Gurze Books.

LoBue, A., and M. Marcus. 1999. *The don't diet, live-it! workbook: Healing food, weight and body issues.* Carlsbad, CA: Gurze Books.

McCabe, R., T. McFarlane, and M. Olmsted. 2003. *Overcoming bulimia workbook: Your comprehensive step-by-step guide to recovery.* Carlsbad, CA: Gurze Books.

Pope, H. 2000. *The Adonis complex: The secret crisis of male body obsession.* New York: Free Press.

Prussin, R. 1992. *Hooked on exercise.* New York: Fireside

Roth, G. 2003. *Breaking free from emotional eating.* New York: Plume.

Siegel, M., J. Brisman, and M. Weinshel. 1997. *Surviving an eating disorder: Perspectives and strategies for family and friends.* New York: Harper Perennial.

www.eatright.org, www.SCANdpg.org The American Dietetic Association and the sports nutrition dietary practice group of the ADA offer a referral service for sports nutritionists skilled in handling eating disorders. You can also call 800-877-1600.

www.anad.org, www.nationaleatingdisorders.org The National Eating Disorders Association offers information about eating disorders and body image and provides a referral network and educational materials for schools. You can also call 800-931-2237.

www.bulimia.com This Web site offers information about eating disorders and a bookstore with more than 200 titles on eating disorders.

www.findingbalance.com This site offers excellent information, including videos with helpful information from leading health professionals.

www.somethingfishy.org Inspired by a woman who recovered from anorexia, this site offers a wellspring of hope and inspiration as well as a referral network.

Eating Disorders (Primarily for Professionals)

Katrina, K., N. King, and D. Hayes. 2003. *Moving away from diets: New ways to heal eating problems and exercise resistance.* 2nd ed. Lake Dallas, TX: Helm.

Thompson, R., and R. Trattner Sherman. 1993. *Helping athletes with eating disorders.* Champaign, IL: Human Kinetics.

Woolsey, M. 2002. *Eating disorders: A clinical guide to counseling and treatment.* Chicago: American Dietetic Association.

Ergogenic Aids

Bahrke, M., and C. Yesalis. 2002. *Performance-enhancing substances in sport and exercise.* Champaign, IL: Human Kinetics.

Exercise and Exercise Physiology (See Also Weight Management)

McArdle, W., F. Katch, and V. Katch. 2006. *Exercise physiology: Energy, nutrition and human performance.* 3rd ed. Philadelphia: Lippincott, Williams & Wilkins.

Wilmore, J., and D. Costill. 2008. *Physiology of sport and exercise.* Champaign, IL: Human Kinetics.

www.acsm.org The American College of Sports Medicine is the largest group of sports medicine and sports science professionals.

www.fitlinxx.com This site offers a plethora of exercise advice for beginner and experienced exercisers alike.

www.choosetomove.org Sponsored by the American Heart Association, this site offers a 12-week program to improve the fitness and health of people who want to start an exercise program.

Food Information

www.ific.org The International Food Information Council offers information about all aspects of food.

Food Labels

www.cfsan.fda.gov/~dms/foodlab.html Sponsored by the USDA Center for Food Safety and Applied Nutrition, this site offers a comprehensive guide to understanding food labels.

Healthy Eating (See Also Recipes)

Carpenter, R.A., and C. Finley. 2005. *Healthy eating every day.* Champaign, IL: Human Kinetics.

Duyff, R. 2006. *The American Dietetic Association's complete food and nutrition guide.* 3rd ed. New York: Wiley.

Lichten, J. 2007. *Dining lean: How to eat healthy when you're not at home.* Houston, TX: Nutrifit.

Nelson, M., A. Lichtenstein, and L. Linder. 2005. *Strong women, strong hearts.* London: Aurum Press.

Nestle, M. 2006. *What to eat: An aisle-by-aisle guide to savvy food choices and good eating.* New York: North Point Press.

Tribole, E. 2004. *Eating on the run*. 3rd ed. Champaign, IL: Human Kinetics.

www.americanheart.org (click on Healthy Lifestyle, then Diet & Nutrition) The American Heart Association Web site allows you to determine how a specific food can fit into a heart-healthy food plan. Search for "eating out" to find recommendations for healthy eating away from home.

www.nal.usda.gov/fnic (click on Consumer Corner, then Lifecycle Nutrition) The National Agricultural Library's Food and Nutrition Information Center features dietary guidelines for infants, children, teens, adults, and seniors.

www.fruitsandveggiesmatter.gov The Center for Disease Control's Web site offers practical advice for eating better.

www.mayoclinic.com (click on Healthy Living) The Mayo Clinic offers information on nutrition, fitness, sports nutrition, and sports medicine—and even recipes.

www.health.gov/dietaryguidelines This site provides information on how to eat for health.

Herbs, Medicinal (See Also Complementary and Alternative Medicine)

www.herbmed.org The nonprofit Alternative Medicine Foundation provides a consumer-friendly scientific database regarding the use of herbs for health.

www.mskcc.org/aboutherbs The Memorial Sloan-Kettering Cancer Center offers reliable information about herbs, botanicals, supplements, and more.

www.herbs.org The Herb Research Foundation offers accurate science-based information on the health benefits and safety of herbs.

Hoaxes

www.quackwatch.com This site offers an excellent guide to health fraud and quackery and enhances your ability to make intelligent decisions regarding sports supplements and herbs.

www.healthfactsandfears.com Sponsored by the American Council on Science and Health, this site provides answers to a multitude of nutrition and health concerns.

Hypertension and the DASH Diet

www.nhlbi.nih.gov (click on Health Information and Publications, then High Blood Pressure) Sponsored by the National Heart, Lung, and Blood Institute of the National Institutes of Health, this site offers abundant information on how to control high blood pressure.

Locally Grown Food

www.localharvest.com This site can help you find farm stands and farmers' markets in your area.

Medical Information

www.WebMD.com This site offers the latest medical information and helpful nutrition information.

www.medem.com Sponsored by the nation's medical societies, this site provides a full range of patient information.

Menopause

Boston Women's Health Book Collective and Vivian Pinn. 2006. *Our bodies, ourselves: Menopause.* New York: Touchstone.

Nelson, M., and S. Wernick. 2006. *Strong women, strong bones: Everything you need to know to prevent, treat, and beat osteoporosis.* New York: Perigree.

www.menopause.org Sponsored by the North American Menopause Society, this site is devoted to promoting women's health through menopause and beyond.

www.power-surge.com This site has been praised as a powerfully effective support group for perimenopausal women.

Newsletters

Environmental Nutrition
P.O. Box 420235, Palm Coast, FL 32142-0235
800-829-5384; on the Web: www.environmentalnutrition.com

Tufts University Health & Nutrition Letter
P.O. Box 420235, Palm Coast, FL 32142-0235
800-274-7581; on the Web: www.healthletter.tufts.edu

University of California, Berkeley Wellness Letter
P.O. Box 420235, Palm Coast, FL 32142
800-829-9170; on the Web: www.WellnessLetter.com

Osteoporosis

www.nof.org The National Osteoporosis Foundation offers a variety of information and resources.

Pesticides

www.ams.usda.gov/science/pdp, www.EPA.gov/pesticides, www.ewg.org, www.beyondpesticides.org The Web sites for the USDA Pesticide Data Program, the Environmental Protection Agency (EPA), the Environmental Working Group, and Beyond Pesticides (formerly the National Commission Against the Misuse of Pesticides) provide extensive information about pesticides.

www.foodnews.org Sponsored by the Environmental Working Group, this site provides a complete list of the pesticide loads of 43 fruits and vegetables.

Pregnancy

Erick, M. 2004. *Managing morning sickness: A survival guide for pregnant women.* Palo Alto, CA: Bull.

Luke, B., and T. Eberlein. 2004. *When you are expecting twins, triplets or quads.* New York: Harper Collins.

Swinney, B. 2006. *Eating expectantly: A practical and tasty approach to prenatal nutrition.* Minnetonka, MN: Meadowbrook Press.

Waterhouse, D. 2003. *Outsmarting the female fat cell—after pregnancy: Every woman's guide to shaping up, slimming down, and staying sane after the baby.* New York: Hyperion.

www.morningsickness.net This site is by Miriam Erick, RD, an expert in prenatal nutrition and morning sickness.

Recipes (See Also Cookbooks, Vegetarian Nutrition)

www.eatchicken.com, www.eatturkey.com, www.beef.org, www.otherwhitemeat. com, www.aboutseafood.com Visit these sites for chicken, turkey, beef, pork, and seafood recipes.

www.foodfit.com This site offers an array of healthful recipes; cooking classes; and information on family fitness, calorie expenditure, and nutrition.

www.fruitsandveggiesmorematters.org, www.fruitsandveggiesmatter.gov These sites provide abundant recipes with vegetables and fruits.

www.ilovepasta.org, www.usarice.com, www.potatohelp.com Visit these sites for pasta, rice, and potato recipes.

www.mealsforyou.com You can search for recipes according to calories, nutrition concerns (allergies, diabetes), preparation time, and more.

www.mealmakeovermoms.com Visit this site for family-friendly recipes as well as cooking demonstrations.

www.mealtime.org This site provides numerous healthy and easy-to-prepare recipes using canned foods to make healthful eating easy and accessible for everyone.

www.nal.usda.gov/fnic (click on Consumer Corner) The National Agricultural Library's Food and Nutrition Information Center offers an extensive list of links to sites for healthful recipes and information about meal planning, shopping, food, and cooking.

Self-Improvement

Prochaska, J., J. Norcross, and C. DiClemente. 1995. *Changing for good: A revolutionary six-stage program for overcoming bad habits and moving your life positively forward.* New York: Harper Collins.

Rollnick, S. 1999. *Health behavior change: A guide for practitioners.* Edinburgh: Churchill Livingstone.

Sports Nutrition

Benardot, D. 2006. *Advanced sports nutrition.* Champaign, IL: Human Kinetics.

Burke, L. 2007. *Practical sports nutrition.* Champaign, IL: Human Kinetics.

Clark, N. 2005. *The cyclist's food guide: Fueling for the distance.* Newton, MA: Sports Nutrition.

Clark, N. 2007. *Nancy Clark's food guide for marathoners: Tips for everyday champions.* Aachen, Germany: Meyer & Meyer Sport.

Coleman, E. 2003. *Eating for endurance.* Palo Alto, CA: Bull.

Dunford, M., ed. 2006. *Sports nutrition: A practice manual for professionals.* 4th ed. Chicago: American Dietetic Association.

Gerard Eberle, S. 2007. *Endurance sports nutrition.* Champaign, IL: Human Kinetics.

Ivy, J., and R. Poortman. 2004. *Nutrient timing: The future of sports nutrition.* North Bergen, NJ: Basic Health.

Kleiner, S.M., and M. Greenwood-Robinson. 2007. *Power eating.* 3rd ed. Champaign, IL: Human Kinetics.

Larson-Meyer D.E. 2007. *Vegetarian sports nutrition.* Champaign, IL: Human Kinetics.

Litt, A. 2004. *Fuel for young athletes.* Champaign, IL: Human Kinetics.

Volpe S., S. Sabelawski, and C. Mohr. 2007. *Fitness nutrition for special dietary needs.* Champaign, IL: Human Kinetics

www.ais.org.au (click on Sports Science/Sports Medicine, then on Nutrition) The Australian Institute of Sport Web site offers excellent sports nutrition information, including advice about sports supplements.

www.SCANdpg.org This is the professional Web site of the American Dietetic Association's practice group of Sports, Cardiovascular, and Wellness Nutritionists (SCAN).

www.gssiweb.com The Web site for the Gatorade Sports Science Institute offers an excellent and extensive resource for both professionals and the public.

www.nlm.nih.gov (click on PubMed, then search on your topic of interest) The National Library of Medicine offers access to the latest research in medical and scientific journals.

Stress Management and Relaxation

www.meditationcenter.com The World Wide Online Meditation Center, designed for both novices and experienced meditators, includes different types of meditation rooms complete with audio for stress reduction, healing, and centering.

www.learningmeditation.com This site includes a meditation room with audio and meditations to help you heal food issues.

Supplements (See Also Herbs, Medicinal; Sports Nutrition)

www.nlm.nih.gov/medlineplus (click on Drugs & Supplements) Here's an A to Z list of herbs and other supplements, including background information as well as information about dose, safety, interactions, and references.

www.nal.usda.gov/fnic (click on Dietary Supplements) The National Agricultural Library's Food and Nutrition Information Center offers abundant information on the safe use of supplements as well as links to sites and sources with credible information.

www.cfsan.fda.gov The FDA's Center for Food Safety and Applied Nutrition provides helpful information about supplements.

http://ods.od.nih.gov/databases/ibids.html Sponsored by the International Bibliographic Information on Dietary Supplements (IBIDS) Database, this site contains published, peer-reviewed scientific literature on dietary supplements, including vitamins, minerals, and herbs. The site is a joint effort between the NIH's Office of Dietary Supplements and the National Agricultural Library's Food and Nutrition Information Center.

www.ncaa.org (click on Academics and Athletes) The Web site for the National Collegiate Athletic Association provides information about supplements that have been banned for use by college athletes. It also provides information on sports nutrition for student athletes.

www.drugabuse.gov The National Institute on Drug Abuse offers a program on the dangers of steroids.

www.supplementwatch.com This site contains up-to-date scientific information about dietary supplements. Some of the information is free; some requires an access fee.

www.ConsumerLab.com ConsumerLab provides the results of dietary supplement testing for quality and purity.

Vegetarian Nutrition

Krizmanic, J. 2000. *The teen's vegetarian cookbook*. New York: Viking Press.

Lappe, F.M. 2002. *Hope's edge: The next diet for a small planet*. New York: Tarcher.

Melina, V., and B. Davis. 2003. *The new becoming vegetarian: The essential guide to a healthy vegetarian diet*. Summertime, TN: Healthy Living.

www.vrg.org The Vegetarian Resource Group is a nonprofit organization dedicated to educating the public on the interrelated issues of nutrition, ecology, ethics, and world hunger.

www.vegweb.com Sponsored by Veggies Unite!, this Web site offers 4,300 recipes, discussion boards, articles, book reviews, health information, and even veggie poetry.

www.vegancooking.com This Web site provides simple recipes that taste great and contain ingredients you can find in your local grocery or health-food store.

Weight Management

Fletcher, A. 2003. *Thin for life: 10 keys to success from people who have lost weight and kept it off*. Boston: Houghton Mifflin.

Fletcher, A., and H. Wyatt. 2007. *Weight loss confidential: How teens lose weight and keep it off—and what they wish parents knew*. Boston: Houghton Mifflin.

Kostas, G. 2007. *The Cooper Clinic solution to the diet revolution*. Dallas: Good Health Press.

Tribole, E., and E. Resch. 2003. *Intuitive eating: A revolutionary program that works*. New York: St. Martin's Griffin.

www.chasefreedom.com This Web site provides an extensive list of reviews of fad diets from A to Z.

www.shapeup.org The purpose of Shape Up America! is to educate the public on how to eat right and exercise appropriately to achieve a healthy body weight.

www.caloriescount.com, www.cyberdiet.com, www.dietwatch.com, www.weight-lossbuddy.com, www.sparkpeople.com, www.ediets.com, www.miavita.com, www.nutrio.com These sites offer diet and exercise programs, chat rooms, and support.

How to Become a Sports Nutritionist

Every week I receive e-mails from people who have read my books or articles and want to know where they can go to school to learn more about nutrition and exercise. Some even want to become sports nutritionists. Here's what I tell them.

• More and more institutions are creating a sports nutrition major, particularly if they have departments in both nutrition and exercise science. You can often combine the two programs to create a major that suits your needs.

• For a list of sports nutrition degree programs, visit www.SCANdpg. org, the Web site of Sports, Cardiovascular and Wellness Nutritionists (SCAN), a dietetic practice group of the American Dietetic Association. For a list of academic programs in nutrition accredited and approved by the American Dietetic Association, visit www.eatright.org. For a list of academic programs in exercise science, visit www.acsm.org, the Web site of the American College of Sports Medicine.

• If you just want to further your personal knowledge, you can take one or two classes in nutrition or exercise science without committing to four years of advanced education. I recommend the full program, however, to people who want to develop a career in sports nutrition.

• If you want to be a nutrition counselor, you should become a registered dietitian (RD). This means you will be recognized by the American Dietetic Association, the largest organization of nutrition professionals in the United States. Career doors will open up to you. Some people take short certificate courses, but these cannot match the education you receive in four years of undergraduate schooling, plus an internship and perhaps a master's degree in nutrition. Getting proper education and credentials is an important professional responsibility.

• By becoming a registered dietitian, you will also be eligible to join SCAN, the sports nutrition interest group of the American Dietetic Association. SCAN members are the leading sports nutritionists. Once you have experience, you can sit for an exam and become a board certified specialist in sports dietetics (CSSD). See www.SCANdpg.org for more information.

• Although your career goals may be to work with athletes and other active, healthy people, I strongly recommend that students and new graduates work first in a clinical setting, such as a hospital, to learn more about how to handle heart disease, diabetes, cancer, and many of the ailments of aging. This knowledge will help you keep people well and enhance your work experience. One or two years of clinical work is a good investment in your career.

•   Get involved as a volunteer for Little League, youth soccer, the YMCA, or any sport that interests you. Work on nutrition and fitness programs sponsored by the dietetic association or council on physical fitness in your area. Practice what you preach. Write articles for the local newspaper or the newsletter of your local bicycle or running club. By developing networks that will help you meet other local sports nutritionists and sports medicine professionals, you might open doors that eventually lead to paid work.

•   Sports nutrition is now an integral part of most training programs, so job opportunities are becoming more available. Some places to look for (or create) a job include health clubs, training centers, spas, the YMCA, corporate wellness programs, sports medicine practices, high schools, college and university athletic departments, and professional or semiprofessional sports teams. Be creative!

•   Most people knock on several doors before finding a welcoming venue. Or they make their own jobs using their personal contacts. For example, some registered dietitians who are mothers of teenage athletes have started sports nutrition classes targeted to parents, coaches, and students. Some RDs who love tennis, ballet, or gymnastics have become known as the sports nutritionist for their sports. Many who work out at a health club have started to work with the members of their clubs. You can create your dream job, and with lots of hard work and time, you'll achieve your goals.

APPENDIX B

Selected References

Ackermark, C., I. Jacobs, M. Rasmussan, and J. Karlsson. 1996. Diet and muscle glycogen concentration in relation to physical performance in Swedish elite ice hockey players. *Int J Sports Nutr and Exerc Metab* 6(3):272-284.

Affenito, S. 2007. Breakfast: A missed opportunity. *J Amer Diet Assoc* 107(4):565-569.

Ainslie, P., I. Campbell, K. Frayn, et al. 2002. Energy balance, metabolism, hydration, and performance during strenuous hill walking: The effect of age. *J Appl Physiol* 93(2):714-723.

Akerstrom, T.C., and B.K. Pedersen. 2007. Strategies to enhance immune function for marathoners: What can be done? *Sports Med* 37(4-5):416-419.

Alford, B.A., A. Blankenship, and D.R. Hagen. 1990. The effects of variations in carbohydrate, protein, and fat content of the diet upon weight loss, blood values, and nutrient intakes of adult obese women. *J Amer Diet Assoc* 90:534-540.

American College of Sports Medicine (ACSM). 1998. The recommended quantity and quality of exercise for developing and maintaining cardiorespiratory and muscular fitness, and flexibility in healthy adults. *Med Sci Sports Exerc* 30(6):975-991.

American College of Sports Medicine (ACSM). 2007. ACSM position stand on exercise and fluid replacement. *Med Sci Sports Exerc* 39(2):377-390.

American College of Sports Medicine (ACSM). 2007. ACSM position stand on the female athlete triad. *Med Sci Sports Exerc* 39(10):1867-1882.

American College of Sports Medicine (ACSM), American Dietetic Association (ADA), and Dietitians of Canada. 2000. Joint position statement: Nutrition and athletic performance. *Med Sci Sports Exerc* 32(12):2130-2145.

American Psychiatric Association. 2000. *Diagnostic and statistical manual of mental disorders.* 4th ed. Washington, DC: Author.

Armstrong, L. 2002. Caffeine, body fluid-electrolyte balance, and exercise performance. *Int J Sports Nutr and Exerc Metab* 12:189-206.

Armstrong, L., A. Pumerantz, M. Roti, et al. 2005. Fluid, electrolyte, and renal indices of hydration during 11 days of controlled caffeine consumption. *Int J Sport Nutr Exerc Metab* 15:252-265.

Bailey, W., D. Jacobsen, and J. Donnelly. 2002. Changes in total daily energy expenditure as a result of 16 months of aerobic training: The Midwest Exercise Trial. *Am J Clin Nutr* 75 (Suppl. no. 2): 363.

Barr, S. 1999. Vegetarianism and menstrual cycle disturbances: Is there an association? *Am J Clin Nutr* 70 (Suppl. no. 3): 549-554.

Barr, S., K.C. Janelle, and J.C. Prior. 1995. Energy intakes are higher during the luteal phase of ovulatory menstrual cycles. *Am J Clin Nutr* 61:39-43.

Bazzano, L.A., Y. Song, V. Bubes, C. Good, J. Manson, and S. Liu. 2005. Dietary intake of whole and refined grain breakfast cereals and weight gain in men. *Obes Res* 13(11):1952-1960.

Beals, K., and M. Manore. 2000. Behavioral, psychological, and physical characteristics of female athletes with subclinical eating disorders. *Int J Sports Nutr and Exerc Metab* 10(2):128-143.

Beals, K., and M. Manore. 2002. Disorders of the female athlete triad among collegiate athletes. *Int J Sports Nutr and Exerc Metab* 12:281-293.

Bell, D.G. and T.M. McLellan. 2002. Endurance exercise 1, 3 and 6 h after caffeine ingestion on caffeine users and nonusers. *J Appl Physiol* 93(4):1227-1234.

Benardot, D., ed. 1992. *Sports nutrition: A guide for the professional working with active people*. 2nd ed. Chicago: American Dietetic Association.

Bergstrom, J., L. Hermansen, E. Hultman, and B. Saltin. 1967. Diet, muscle glycogen, and physical performance. *Acta Physiol Scand* 71:140-150.

Bjelakovic, G., D. Nikolova, L.L. Gluud, R.G. Simonetti, and C. Gluud. 2007. Mortality in randomized trials of antioxidant supplements for primary and secondary prevention: Systematic review and meta-analysis. *JAMA* 297(8):842-857.

Blackburn, G. 2001. The public health implications of the Dietary Approaches to Stop Hypertension Trial. *Am J Clin Nutr* 74:1-2.

Bolster, D.R., M.A. Pikosky, P.C. Gaine, et al. 2005. Dietary protein intake impacts human skeletal muscle protein fractional synthetic rates after endurance exercise. *Am J Physiol* 289:E678-E683.

Bouchard, C. 1990. Heredity and the path to overweight and obesity. *Med Sci Sports Exerc* 23(3):285-291.

Bray, G., S.J. Nielsen, and B. Popkin. 2004. Consumption of high-fructose corn syrup in beverages may play a role in the epidemic of obesity. *Am J Clin Nutr* 79:537-543.

Brouns, F., W. Saris, and N. Rehrer. 1987. Abdominal complaints and gastro-intestinal function during long lasting exercise. *Int J Sports Med* 8:175-189.

Burke, L. 2007. Training and competition nutrition. In *Practical sports nutrition*. Champaign IL: Human Kinetics.

Burke, L., G. Collier, and M. Hargreaves. 1998. Glycemic index: A new tool in sports nutrition? *Int J Sport Nutr* 8:401-415.

Burke, L.M., A. Classen, J.A. Hawley, and T.D. Noakes. 1998. Carbohydrate intake during prolonged cycling minimizes effect of glycemic index of preexercise meal. *J Appl Physiol* 85(6):2220-2226.

Caan, B., M. Neuhouser, A. Aragaki, et al. 2007. Calcium plus vitamin D supplementation and the risk of postmenopausal weight gain. *Arch Intern Med* 167(9):893-902.

Campbell, C., D. Prince, E. Applegate, and G. Casazza G. 2007. Effect of carbohydrate supplementation type on endurance cycling performance in competitive athletes. *Med Sci Sports Exerc* 39 (Suppl. no. 5): Abstract 1760.

Casa D., L. Armstrong, S. Montain, et al. 2000. National Athletic Trainers' Association position statement: Fluid replacement for athletes. *J Athletic Training* 35(2):212-224.

Center for Science in the Public Interest (CSPI). 2006. Are you deficient? *Nutrition Action Healthletter* 33(9): 3-7.

Center for Science in the Public Interest (CSPI). 2006. Pour better or pour worse: How beverages stack up. *Nutrition Action Healthletter* 33(5):3-7.

Clancy, R.L., M. Gleeson, A. Cox, et al. 2006. Reversal in fatigued athletes of a defect in interferon gamma secretion after administration of Lactobacillus acidophilus. *Br J Sports Med* 40(4):351-354.

Clark, N., M. Nelson, and W. Evans. 1988. Nutrition education for elite women runners. *Phys Sportsmed* 16:124-135.

Clegg, D., D. Reda, C. Harris, et al. 2006. Glucosamine, chondroitin sulfate, and the two in combination for painful knee osteoarthritis. *N Engl J Med* 354(8):795-808.

ConsumerLab.com. 2007. Product review: Joint supplements. [Online.] Available: www.Consumerlab.com/results/gluco.asp.

Cook, N.R., J. Cutler, E. Obarzanek, et al. 2007. Long term effects of dietary sodium reduction on cardiovascular disease outcomes: Observational follow-up of the trials of hypertension prevention (TOHP). *Br Med J* 334(7599):885.

Costill, D., R. Bowers, G. Branam, and K. Sparks. 1971. Muscle glycogen utilization during prolonged exercise on successive days. *J Appl Physiol* 31(6):834-838.

Costill, D.L., D.S. King, R. Thomas, and M. Hargreaves. 1985. Effects of reduced training on muscular power in swimmers. *Phys Sportsmed* 13(2):94-101.

Costill, D.L., W. Sherman, W. Fink, C. Maresh, M. Witten, and J. Miller. 1981. The role of dietary carbohydrate in muscle glycogen resynthesis after strenuous exercise. *Am J Clin Nutr* 34:1831-1836.

Costill, D.L., R. Thomas, R.A. Roberts, et al. 1991. Adaptations to swimming training: Influence of training volume. *Med Sci Sports Exerc* 23(3):371-377.

Couzin, J. 2002. Nutrition research: IOM panel weighs in on diet and health. *Science* 297(5588):1399-1409.

Coyle, E.F., and S.J. Montain. 1992. Benefits of fluid replacement with carbohydrates during exercise. *Med Sci Sports Exerc* 24 (Suppl. no. 9): 324-330.

Cribb, P., and A. Hayes. 2006. Effects of supplement timing and resistance exercise on skeletal muscle hypertrophy. *Med Sci Sports Exerc* 38(1):1918-1925.

Cribb, P., A. Williams, and A. Hayes. 2007. A creatine-protein-carbohydrate supplement enhances responses to resistance training. *Med Sci Sports Exerc* 39(11):1960-1968.

Das, S.K., C. Gilhooly, J. Golden, et al. 2007. Long-term effects of 2 energy-restricted diets differing in glycemic load on dietary adherence, body composition, and metabolism in CALERIE: a 1-y randomized controlled trial. *Am J Clin Nutr* 85:1023-1030.

Davison, G., and M. Gleeson. 2005. Vitamin C and carbohydrate ingestion in prolonged exercise. *Int J Sports Nutr Exerc Metab* 15:465-479.

Davison, G., M. Gleeson, and S. Phillips. 2007. Antioxidant supplementation and immunoendocrine responses to prolonged exercise. *Med Sci Sports Exerc* 39(4):645-652.

Dawson, D., C. Henry, C. Goodman, et al. 2002. Effect of C and E supplementation on biochemical and ultrastructural indices of muscle damage after a 21 km run. *Int J Sports Med* 23(1):10-15.

Demura, S., S. Yamaji, F. Goshi, and Y. Nagasawa. 2002. The influence of transient change of total body water on relative body fats based on three bioelectrical impedance analyses methods. Comparison between before and after exercise with sweat loss, and after drinking. *J Sports Med Phys Fitness* 42(1):38-44.

Deutz, R., D. Benardot, D. Martin, and M. Cody. 2000. Relationship between energy deficits and body composition in elite female gymnasts and runners. *Med Sci Sports Exerc* 32(3):659-668.

Di Carlo, C., G. Tommaselli, A. Sammartino, et al. 2004. Serum leptin levels and body composition in postmenopausal women: Effects of hormone therapy. *Menopause* 11(4):466-473.

Doherty, M., and P. Smith. 2005. Effects of caffeine ingestion on the rating of perceived exertion during and after exercise: A meta-analysis. *Scand J Med Sci Sports* 15(2):69-78.

Dominguez, J., L. Goodman, S. Sen Gupta, et al. 2007. Treatment of anorexia nervosa is associated with increases in bone mineral density, and recovery is a biphasic process involving both nutrition and return of menses. *Am J Clin Nutr* 86(1):92-99.

Drewnowski, A., and F. Bellisle. 2007. Liquid calories, sugar, and body weight. *Am J Clin Nutr* 85:651-661.

Dueck, C., K. Matt, M. Manore, and J. Skinner. 1996. Treatment of athletic amenorrhea with a diet and training intervention program. *Int J Sport Nutr and Exerc Metab* 6(1):24-40.

Ebbeling, C.B., M.M. Leidig, H.A. Feldman, M.M. Lovesky, and D.S. Ludwig. 2007. Effects of a low-glycemic load vs low-fat diet in obese young adults: A randomized trial. *JAMA* 297(19):2092-2102.

Edwards. J., A. Lindeman, A. Mikesky, and J. Stager. 1993. Energy balance in highly trained female endurance runners. *Med Sci Sports Exerc* 25(12):1398-1404.

Environmental Working Group. 2006. When should you buy organic? [Online.] Available: www.foodnews.org/release.php.

Esmarck, B., J. Andersen, S. Olsen, E. Richter, M. Mizuno, and M. Kjaer. 2001. Timing of postexercise protein intake is important for muscle hypertrophy with resistance training in elderly humans. *J Physiol* 535 (Pt. 1): 301-311.

Etnier, J., R. Caselli, E. Reiman, et al. 2007. Cognitive performance in older women relative to Apo-E4 genotype and aerobic fitness. *Med Sci Sports Exerc* 39(1):199-207.

Expert Panel on Detection, Evaluation, and Treatment of High Blood Cholesterol in Adults. 2001. Executive summary of the third report of the National Cholesterol Education Program Expert Panel on detection, evaluation, and treatment of high cholesterol in adults. *JAMA* 285:2486-2497.

Fairchild, T., S. Fletcher, P. Steele, C. Goodman, B. Dawson, and P. Fournier. 2002. Rapid carbohydrate loading after a short bout of near maximal-intensity exercise. *Med Sci Sports Exerc* 34(6):980-986.

Fairfield, K., and R. Fletcher. 2002. Vitamins for chronic disease prevention in adults. *JAMA* 287(23):3116-3126.

Ferreira, S.E., M.T. de Mello, S. Pompeia, and M.L. de Souza-Formigoni. 2006. Effects of energy drink ingestion on alcohol intoxication. *Alcohol Clin Exp Res* 30(4):598-605.

Fields, D., M. Goran, and M. McCrory. 2002. Body-composition assessment via air-displacement plethysmography in adults and children: A review. *Am J Clin Nutr* 75:453-467.

Finnegan, D. 2003. The health effects of stimulant drinks. *Nutrition Bulletin* 28:147-155.

Fitó, M., M. Cladellas, R. de la Torre, et al. 2007. Anti-inflammatory effect of virgin olive oil in stable coronary disease patients: A randomized, crossover, controlled trial. *Eur J Clin Nutr* [Online]. March 21.

Flakoll, P., T. Judy, K. Flinn, C. Carr, and S. Flinn. 2004. Postexercise protein supplementation improves health and muscle soreness during basic military training in marine recruits. *J Appl Physiol* 96(3):951-956.

Flight, I., and P. Clifton. 2006. Cereal grains and legumes in the prevention of coronary heart disease and stroke: A review of the literature. *Eur J Clin Nutr* 60(10):1145-1159.

Food and Nutrition Board, Institute of Medicine. 1998/2000. *Dietary reference intakes.* Lanover, MD: National Academy Press.

Franz, M.J. 2003. Glycemic index: Not the most effective nutrition therapy intervention. *Diabetes Care* 26:2466-2468.

Fredericson, M., and K. Kent. 2005. Normalization of bone density in a previously amenorrheic runner with osteoporosis. *Med Sci Sports Exerc* 37(9):1481-1486.

Gallus, S., L. Scotti, E. Negri, et al. 2007. Artificial sweeteners and cancer risk in a network of case-control studies. *Ann Oncol* 18(1):40-44.

Gardner, C.D., A. Kiazand, S. Alhassan, et al. 2007. Comparison of the Atkins, Zone, Ornish, and LEARN diets for change in weight and related risk factors among overweight premenopausal women: The A to Z Weight Loss Study: A randomized trial. *JAMA* 297(9):969-977.

Garner, D. 1998. The effects of starvation on behavior: Implications for dieting and eating disorders. *Healthy Weight Journal* 12(5):68-72.

Geleijnse, J., L. Launer, D. van der Kuip, A. Hofman, and J. Witteman. 2002. Inverse association of tea and flavonoid intakes with incident myocardial infarction: The Rotterdam Study. *Am J Clin Nutr* 75:880-886.

Getchell, B., and W. Anderson. 1982. *Being fit: A personal guide.* New York: Wiley.

Gibson, A., V. Heyward, and C. Mermier. 2000. Predictive accuracy of Omron Body Logic Analyzer in estimating relative body fat of adults. *Int J Sports Nutr and Exerc Metab* 10:216-227.

Gilhooly, C., S.K. Das, J.K. Golden, et al. 2007. Food cravings and energy regulation: The characteristics of craved foods and their relationship with eating behaviors and weight change during 6 months of dietary energy restriction. *Int J Obes* 31(12):1849-1858.

Godard, M., D. Williamson, and S. Trappe. 2002. Oral amino-acid provision does not affect muscle strength or size gains in older men. *Med Sci Sports Exerc* 34(7):1126-1131.

Goran, M., and E. Poehlman. 1992. Endurance training does not enhance total energy expenditure in healthy elderly persons. *Am J Physiol* 263:E950-E957.

Green, H., M. Ball-Burnett, S. Jones, and B. Farrance. 2007. Mechanical and metabolic responses with exercise and dietary carbohydrate manipulation. *Med Sci Sports Exerc* 39(1):139-148.

Greene, R., S. Godek, A. Burkholder, and C. Peduzzi. 2007. Sweat sodium and total sodium losses in NFL players with exercise associated muscle cramps during training camp vs matched non-crampers. *Med Sci Sports Exerc* 39 (Suppl. no. 5): Abstract 574.

Haller, C., N. Benowitz, and J. Peyton. 2005. Hemodynamic effects of ephedra-free weight-loss supplements in humans. *Am J Med* 118:998-1003.

Hansen, A., C. Fischer, P. Plomgaard, J. Andersen, B. Saltin, and B. Pedersen. 2005. Skeletal muscle adaptation: Training twice every second day vs training once daily. *J Appl Physiol* 98:93-99.

Heymsfield, S., J. Harp, M. Reitman, et al. 2007. Why do obese patients not lose more weight when treated with low-calorie diets? A mechanistic perspective. *Am J Clin Nutr* 85:346-354.

Hickner, R., C. Horswill, J. Welker, J. Scott, J. Roemmich, and D. Costill. 1991. Test development for the study of physical performance in wrestlers following weight loss. *Int J Sports Med* 12(6):557-562.

Hill, J.O., W. McArdle, J. Snook, and J. Wilmore. 1992. *Commonly asked questions regarding nutrition and exercise: What does the scientific literature suggest?* Vol. 9 of *Sports science exchange.* Chicago: Gatorade Sports Science Institute.

Holm, L., B. Esmarck, M. Mizuno, et al. 2006. The effect of protein and carbohydrate supplementation on strength training outcome of rehabilitation in ACL patients. *J Orthop Res* 24(11):2114-2123.

Hooper, S.L., L.T. Mackinnon, A. Howard, R. Gordon, and A. Bachmann. 1995. Markers for monitoring overtraining and recovery. *Med Sci Sports Exerc* 27(1):106-112.

Horowitz, J.F., and E.F. Coyle. 1993. Metabolic responses to preexercise meals containing various carbohydrates and fat. *Am J Clin Nutr* 58:235-241.

Houmard, J.A., D.L. Costill, J.B. Mitchell, S.H. Park, R.C. Hickner, and J.N. Roemmich. 1990. Reduced training maintains performance in distance runners. *Int J Sports Med* 11(1):46-52.

Hu, F., L. Bronner, W. Willett, et al. 2002. Fish and omega-three fatty acid intake and risk of coronary heart disease in women. *JAMA* 287:1807-1814.

Huang, H.Y., B. Caballero, S. Chang, et al. 2006. The efficacy and safety of multivitamin and mineral supplement use to prevent cancer and chronic disease in adults: A systematic review for a National Institutes of Health state-of-the-science conference. *Ann Intern Med* 145(5):372-385.

Institute of Medicine. 1994. *Fluid replacement and heat stress.* Washington, DC: National Academy Press.

Institute of Medicine. 2002. *Dietary reference intakes for energy, carbohydrate, fiber, fat, fatty acids, cholesterol, protein and amino acids.* Washington, DC: National Academy Press.

International Olympic Committee. 2004. Consensus on sports nutrition 2003. *J Sports Sci* 22(1):X.

Ivy, J. 2001. Dietary strategies to promote glycogen synthesis after exercise. *Can J Appl Physiol* 26 (Suppl.): 236-245.

Ivy, J., H. Goforth, B. Damon, T. McCauley, E. Parsons, and T. Price. 2002. Early postexercise muscle glycogen recovery is enhanced with a carbohydrate-protein supplement. *J Appl Physiol* 93(4):1337-1344.

Janssen, G., C. Graef, and W. Saris. 1989. Food intake and body composition in novice athletes during a training period to run a marathon. *Int J Sports Med* 10:S17-21.

Jentjens, R.L., K. Underwood, J. Achten, K. Currell, C.H. Mann, and A.E. Jeukendrup. 2006. Exogenous carbohydrate oxidation rates are elevated after combined ingestion of glucose and fructose during exercise in the heat. *J Appl Physiol* 100(3):807-816.

Jiang, R., J.E. Manson, M.J. Stampfer, S. Liu, W.C. Willett, and F.B. Hu. 2002. Nut and peanut butter consumption and risk of type 2 diabetes in women. *JAMA* 288(20):2554-2560.

Jówko, E., P. Ostaszewski, M. Jank, et al. 2001. Creatine and beta-hydroxy beta-methylbutyrate (HMB) additively increase lean body mass and muscle strength during a weight-training program. *Nutrition* 17(7-8):558-566.

Jung, A., P. Bishop, A. Al-Nawwas, and R. Dale. 2005. Influence of hydration and electrolyte supplementation on incidence and time of onset of exercise associated muscle cramps. *J Athl Train* 40:71-75.

Kant, A., R. Ballard-Barbash, and A. Schatzkin. 1995. Evening eating and its relation to self-reported weight and nutrient intake in women, CSFII 1985-1986. *J Am College Nutr* 14(8):358-363.

Karp, J., J. Johnston, S. Tecklenburg, T. Mickleborough, A. Fly, and J. Stager. Chocolate milk as a post-exercise recovery aid. 2006. *Int J Sports Nutr Exerc Metab* 16:78-91.

Karppanen, H., and E. Mervaala. 2006. Sodium intake and hypertension. *Prog Cardiovasc Dis* 49(2):59-75.

Katz, D., M. Evans, H. Nawaz, et al. 2005. Egg consumption and endothelial function: A randomized controlled crossover trial. *Int J Cardiol* 9(1):65-70.

Keys, A., J. Brozek, A. Henschel, et al. 1950. *The biology of human starvation.* Vols. I and II. Minneapolis: University of Minnesota Press.

Kilduff, L., P. Vidakovic, G. Cooney, et al. 2002. Effects of creatine on isometric bench-press performance in resistance-trained humans. *Med Sci Sports Exerc* 34(7):1176-1183.

Kirk, E.P., J. Donnelly, and D. Jacobsen. 2002. Time course and gender effects in aerobic capacity and body composition for overweight individuals: Midwest Exercise Trial (MET). *Med Sci Sports Exerc* 34 (Suppl. no. 5): 120.

Klibanski, A., B.M.K. Biller, D.A. Schoenfeld, D. Herzog, and V. Saxe. 1995. The effects of estrogen administration on trabecular bone loss in young women with anorexia nervosa. *J Clin Endocrinol Metab* 80:898-904.

Knowler, W.C., E. Barrett-Conner, S.E. Fowler, et al. 2002. Reduction in the incidence of type II diabetes with lifestyle intervention or metformin. *N Eng J Med* 346:393-403.

Kris-Etherton, P., W. Harris, and L. Appel. 2002. American Heart Association scientific statement: Fish consumption, fish oil, omega-3 fatty acids, and cardiovascular disease. *Circulation* 106:2747-2757.

Kris-Etherton, P., G. Zhao, A.E. Binkoski, S.M. Coval, and T.D. Etherton. 2001. The effects of nuts on coronary heart disease. *Nutr Rev* 59(4):103-111.

Kritchevsky, S., and D. Kritchevsky. 2000. Egg consumption and coronary heart disease: An epidemiologic overview. *J Am Coll Nutr* 19 (Suppl. no. 5): 549-555.

Laidlaw, S.A., M. Grosvenor, and J.D. Kopple. 1990. The taurine content of common foodstuffs. *J Par Ent Nutr* 14:183-188.

Lappe, J., D. Travers-Gustafson, K. Davies, R. Recker, and R. Heaney. 2007. Vitamin D and calcium supplementation reduces cancer risk: Results of a randomized trial. *Am J Clin Nutr* 85(6):1586-1591.

Leibel, R.L., M. Rosenbaum, and J. Hirsch. 1995. Changes in energy expenditure resulting from altered body weight. *N Engl J Med* 332:621-628.

Lemon, P. 1995. Do athletes need more protein and amino acids? *Int J Sport Nutr* 5 (Suppl.): 39-61.

Levine J., N. Eberhardt, and M. Jensen. 1999. Role of non-exercise activity thermogenesis in resistance to fat gain in humans. *Science* 282(5399):212-214.

Lichtenstein, A., L. Appel, M. Brands, et al. 2006. American Heart Association scientific statement: Diet and lifestyle recommendations revision 2006: A scientific statement from the American Heart Association Nutrition Committee. *Circulation* 114(1):82-96.

Lim, U., A.F. Subar, T. Mouw, et al. 2006. Consumption of aspartame-containing beverages and incidence of hematopoietic and brain malignancies. *Cancer Epidemiol Biomarkers Prev* 15(9):1654-1659.

Liu, H., D. Bravata, I. Olkin, et al. 2007. Systematic review: The safety and efficacy of growth hormone in the healthy elderly. *Ann Intern Med* 146(2):104-115.

Loucks, A. 2004. Energy balance and body composition in sports and exercise. *J Sport Sci* 22(1):1-14.

Loucks, A., and B. Thuma. 2003. Luteinizing hormone pulsatility is disrupted at a threshold of energy availability in regularly menstruating women. *J Clin Endocrinol Metab* 88(1):297-311.

Luscombe, N., P. Clifton, M. Noakes, B. Parker, and G. Wittert. 2002. The effects of energy-restricted diets containing increased protein on weight loss, resting energy expenditure and the thermic effect of feeding in type 2 diabetes. *Diabetes Care* 25:652-657.

Lutter, J., and S. Cushman. 1982. Running while pregnant. *J Melpomene Institute* 1(1):2-4.

Marchioli, R., C. Schweiger, G. Levantesi, L. Tavassi, and F. Valagussa. 2001. Antioxidant vitamins and prevention of cardiovascular disease: Epidemiological and clinical trial data. *Lipids* 36 (Suppl.): 53-63.

Marczinski, C.A., and M.T. Fillmore. 2006. Clubgoers and their trendy cocktails: Implications of mixing caffeine into alcohol on information processing and subjective reports of intoxication. *Exp Clin Psychopharmacol* 14(4):450-458.

Martin, W., L. Armstrong, and N. Rodriquez. 2005. Dietary protein intake and renal function. *Nutr Metab* (Lond) 20(2):25.

Mason, W.L., G. McConell, and M. Hargreaves. 1993. Carbohydrate ingestion during exercise: Liquid vs. solid feedings. *Med Sci Sports Exerc* 25(8):966-969.

McManus, K., L. Antinoro, and F. Sacks.2001. A randomized controlled trial of a moderate fat, low-energy diet compared with a low-fat, low energy diet for weight loss in overweight adults. *Int J Obes Relat Metab Disord* 25:1503-1511.

Miller, K., E. Lee, E. Lawson, et al. 2006. Determinants of skeletal loss and recovery in anorexia nervosa. *J Endocrinol Metab* 91(8):2931-2937.

Morales, A., R. Haubrich, J. Hwang, H. Asakura, and S. Yen. 1998. The effect of six months treatment with a 100 mg daily dose of dehydroepiandrosterone (DHEA) on circulating sex steroids, body composition and muscle strength in age-advanced men and women. *Clin Endocrinol* 49(4):421-432.

Mosca, L., C. Banka, E. Benjamin, et al. 2007. Evidence-based guidelines for cardiovascular disease prevention in women: 2007 update. *Circulation* 115(7):1481-1501.

Nair, K., R. Rizza, P. O'Brien, et al. 2006. DHEA in elderly women and DHEA or testosterone in elderly men. *New Engl J Med* 355(16):1647-1659.

Napoli, N., J. Thompson, R. Civitelli, and R. Armamento-Villareal. 2007. Effects of dietary calcium compared with calcium supplements on estrogen metabolism and bone mineral density. *Am J Clin Nutr* 85:1428-1433.

National Eating Disorders Association. 2005. No weigh! A declaration of independence from a weight-obsessed world. [Online.] Available: www.NationalEatingDisorders. org.

National Institutes of Health State-of-the-Science Panel. 2007. National Institutes of Health state-of-the-science conference statement: Multi-vitamin and mineral supplements and chronic disease prevention. *Am J Clin Nutr* 85(1):257S-264S.

Nattiv, A. 2000. Stress fractures and bone health in track and field athletes. *J Sci Med Sport* 3(3):268-279.

Nattiv, A., A. Loucks, M. Manore, C. Sanborn et al. 2007. Position Stand of the American College of Sports Medicine: The Female Athlete Triad. *Med Sci Sports Exerc* 39 (10):1867-1882

Nelson, M., E. Fisher, P. Catsos, C. Meredith, R. Turksoy, and W. Evans. 1986. Diet and bone status in amenorrheic runners. *Am J Clin Nutr* 43:910-916.

Neumark-Sztainer, D., M. Wall, J. Guo, M. Story, J. Haines, and M. Eisenhberg. 2006. Obesity, disordered eating, and eating disorders in a longitudinal study of adolescents: How do dieters fare five years later? *J Amer Diet Assoc* 106:559-568.

Nieman, D., D. Henson, S. McAnulty, et al. 2002. Influence of vitamin C supplementation on oxidative and immune changes after an ultramarathon. *J Appl Physiol* 92(5):1070-1077.

Nieman, D., D. Henson, S. McAnulty, et al. 2004. Vitamin E and immunity after the Kona Triathlon World Championship. *Med Sci Sports Exerc* 36(8):1328-1335.

Noakes, T. 2003. *Lore of running*. 4th ed. Champaign, IL: Human Kinetics.

O'Dea, J., and P. Rawstorne. 2001. Male adolescents identify their weight gain practices, reasons for desired weight gain, and sources of weight gain information. *J Amer Diet Assoc* 101(1):105-107.

Ode, J., J. Pivarnik, M. Reeves, and J. Knous. 2007. Body mass index as a predictor of percent fat in college athletes and nonathletes. *Med Sci Sports Exerc* 39(3):403-409.

Olivardia, R. 2002. Body image obsession in men. *Healthy Weight Journal* 16(4):59-63.

Pasman, W., M. van Baak, A. Jeukendrup, and A. de Haan. 1995. The effects of different dosages of caffeine on endurance performance time. *Int J Sports Med* 16:225-230.

Pedersen, S., J. Kang, and G. Kline. 2007. Portion control plate for weight loss in obese patients with type 2 diabetes mellitus: A controlled clinical trial. *Arch Intern Med* 167:1277-1283.

Pennington, J. 2004. *Bowes & Church's food values of portions commonly used*. 18th ed. Philadelphia: Lippincott Williams & Wilkins.

Pereira, M., D. Jacobs, J. Pins, et al. 2002. Effect of whole grains on insulin sensitivity in overweight hyperinsulinemic adults. *Am J Clin Nutr* 75:848-855.

Peterson, J., W. Repovich, M. Eash, D. Notrica, and C. Hill. 2007. Accuracy of consumer grade bioelectrical impedance analysis devices compared to air displacement plethysmography. *Med Sci Sports Exerc* 39 (Suppl. no. 5): Abstract 2105.

Phillips, P., B. Rolls, J. Ledingham, et al. 1984. Reduced thirst after water deprivation in healthy elderly men. *N Engl J Med* 311:753-759.

Pomerleau, M., P. Imbeault, T. Parker, and E. Doucet. 2004. Effects of exercise intensity on food intake and appetite in women. *Am J Clin Nutr* 80:1230-1236.

Rasmussen, B., K. Tipton, S. Miller, et al. 2000. An oral essential amino acid-carbohydrate supplement enhances muscle protein anabolism after resistance exercise. *J Appl Physiol* 88:386-392.

Rauch, L.H.G., I. Rodger, G. Wilson, et al. 1995. The effects of carbohydrate loading on muscle glycogen content and cycling performance. *Int J Sports Nutr* 5(1):25-35.

Reichenbach, S., R. Sterchi, M. Schere, et al. 2007. Meta-analysis: Chondroitin for osteoarthritis of the knee or hip. *Ann Int Med* 146(8):580-590.

Reyner, L., and J. Horne. 2002. Efficacy of a "functional energy drink" in counteracting driver sleepiness. *Physiol Behav* 75(3):331-335.

Ribisl, P. 2002. A slim chance in a fat world: Beating the odds on weight control. *ACSM's Health Fit J* 6(4):33.

Rock, C. 2007. Primary dietary prevention: Is the fiber story over? *Recent Results Cancer Research*. 174:171-177

Roffe, C., S. Sills, P. Crome, and P. Jones. 2002. Randomised, cross-over, placebo controlled trial of magnesium citrate in the treatment of chronic persistent leg cramps. *Med Sci Monit* 8(5):CR326-330.

Roti, M.W., D.J. Casa, A.C. Pumerantz, et al. 2006. Thermoregulatory responses to exercise in the heat: Chronic caffeine intake has no effect. *Aviat Space Environ Med* 77(2):124-129.

Saarni, S., A. Rissanen, S. Sarna, M. Koskenvuo, and J. Kaprio. 2006. Weight cycling of athletes and subsequent gain in middle age. *Int J Obes* 30(11):1639-1644.

Sacks, F.M., A. Lichtenstein, L. Van Horn, W. Harris, P. Kris-Etherton, and M. Winston; American Heart Association Nutrition Committee. 2006. Soy protein, isoflavones, and cardiovascular health: An American Heart Association Science Advisory for professionals from the Nutrition Committee. *Circulation* 113(7):1034-1044.

Sallis, R., M. Longacre, and L. Morris. 2007. Gastrointestinal symptoms in Hawaiian Ironman Triathletes. *Med Sci Sports Exerc* 39 (Suppl. no. 5): Abstract 2080.

Sanborn, C., M. Horea, B. Siemers, and K. Dieringer. 2000. Disordered eating and the female athlete triad. *Clin Sports Med* 19(2):199-213.

Saunders, M., M. Kane, and K. Todd. 2004. Effects of a carbohydrate-protein beverage on cycling endurance and muscle damage. *Med Sci Sports Exerc* 36:1233-1238.

Schabort, E., A. Bosch, S. Welton, and T. Noakes. 1999. The effect of a preexercise meal on time to fatigue during prolonged cycling exercise. *Med Sci Sports Exerc* 31(3):464-471.

Schlundt, D.G., J.O. Hill, T. Sbrocco, J. Pope-Cordle, and T. Sharp. 1992. The role of breakfast in the treatment of obesity: A randomized clinical trial. *Am J Clin Nutr* 55(3):645-651.

Schwellnus, M.P., J. Nicol, R. Laubscher, and T.D. Noakes. 2004. Serum electrolyte concentrations and hydration status are not associated with exercise associated muscle cramping (EAMC) in distance runners. *Br J Sports Med* 38(4):488-492.

Sellmeyer, D., M. Schloetter, and A. Sebastian. 2002. Potassium citrate prevents increased urine calcium secretion and bone resorption induced by a high sodium chloride diet. *J Clin Endocrinol Metab* 87(5):2008-2012.

Sesso H., R. Pfaffenbarger, and I. Lee. 2000. Physical activity and coronary heart disease in men: The Harvard Alumni Health Study. *Circulation* 102(9):975-980.

Sherman, W., G. Brodowicz, D. Wright, W. Allen, J. Simonsen, and A. Dernbach. 1989. Effects of 4 h preexercise carbohydrate feedings on cycling performance. *Med Sci Sports Exerc* 21(5):598-604.

Sherman, W., D. Costill, W. Fink, and J. Miller. 1981. Effect of exercise-diet manipulation on muscle glycogen and its subsequent utilization during performance. *Int J Sports Med* 2:114-118.

Sherman, W., M. Pedan, and D. Wright. 1991. Carbohydrate feedings 1 hour before exercise improves cycling performance. *Am J Clin Nutr* 54:866-870.

Sherman, W.M., and E.W. Maglischo. 1991. Minimizing athletic fatigue among swimmers: Special emphasis on nutrition. *Sports Sci Exchange* 4(35): 1-4.

Sherriffs, S., and R. Maughan. 1997. Restoration of fluid balance after exercise-induced dehydration: Effects of alcohol consumption. *J Appl Physiol* 83(40):1152-1158.

Shields, D., K. Corrales, and K. Metallinos-Katsaras. 2004. Gourmet coffee beverage consumption among college women. *J Amer Diet Assoc* 104:650-653.

Shing, C.M., J. Peake, K. Suzuki, et al. 2007. Effects of bovine colostrum supplementation on immune variables in highly trained cyclists. *J Appl Physiol* 102:1113-1122.

Sims, E. 1976. Experimental obesity, dietary induced thermogenesis, and their clinical implications. *J Clin Endocrinol Metab* 5:377-395.

Sims, E., and E. Danforth. 1987. Expenditure and storage of energy in man. *J Clin Invest* 79:1-7.

Sims, S.T., L. van Vliet, J. Cotter, and N. Rehrer. 2007. Sodium loading aids fluid balance and reduces physiological strain of trained men exercising in the heat. *Med Sci Sports Exerc* 39(1):123-130.

Siris, E.S., P.D. Miller, E. Barrett-Connor, et al. 2001. Identification and fracture outcomes of undiagnosed low bone mineral density in postmenopausal women: Results of the National Osteoporosis Risk Assessment. *JAMA* 286(22):2815-2822.

Slater, G., A. Rice, K. Sharpe, D. Jenkins, and A. Hahn. 2007. The influence of nutrient intake after weigh-in on lightweight rowing performance. *Med Sci Sports Exerc* 39(1):184-191.

Song, W., O. Chun, S. Obayashi, S. Cho, and C. Chung. 2005. Is consumption of breakfast associated with body mass index in US adults? *J Amer Diet Assoc* 105:1373-1382.

Staten, M. 1991. The effect of exercise on food intake in men and women. *Am J Clin Nutr* 53:27-31.

Sternfeld, B., H. Wang, C. Quesenberry, et al. 2004. Physical activity and changes in weight and waist circumference in midlife women: Findings from the study of women's health across the nation. *Am J Epidemiol* 160(9):912-922.

Stevenson E., C. Williams, and H. Biscoe. 2005. The metabolic responses to high carbohydrate meals with different glycemic indices consumed during recovery from prolonged strenuous exercise. *Int J Sports Nutr Exerc Metab* 15(3):291-307.

Stevenson, E., C. Williams, G. McComb, and C. Oram. 2005. Improved recovery from prolonged exercise following the consumption of low glycemic index carbohydrate meals. *Int J Sport Nutr Exerc Metab* 15(4):333-349.

Stout, R., J. Eckerson, T. Housch, G. Johnson, and N. Betts. 1994. Validity of body fat estimations in males. *Med Sci Sports Exerc* 26(5): 262.

Taheri, S., L. Lin, D. Austin, T. Young, and E. Mignot. 2004. Short sleep duration is associated with reduced leptin, elevated ghrelin, and increased body mass index. *PLoS Med* 1(3):E62.

Taubert, D., R. Roesen, C. Lehmann, N. Jung, and E. Schömig. 2007. Effects of low habitual cocoa intake on blood pressure and bioactive nitric oxide: A randomized controlled trial. *JAMA* 298:49-60.

Terjung R.L., P. Clarkson, R. Eichner, et al. 2000. American College of Sports Medicine roundtable. The physiological and health effects of oral creatine supplements. *Med Sci Sports Exerc* 32(3):706-717.

Thompson, J., M. Manore, J. Skinner, E. Ravussin, and M. Spraul. 1995. Daily energy expenditure in male athletes with differing energy intakes. *Med Sci Sports Exerc* 27(3):347-354.

Tipton, K., T. Elliot, M. Cree, S. Wolf, A. Sanford, and R. Wolfe. 2004. Ingestion of casein and whey proteins result in muscle anabolism after resistance exercise. *Med Sci Sports Exerc* 36(12):2073-2081.

Torres, I.C., L. Mira, C.P. Ornelas, and A. Melim. 2000. Study of the effects of dietary fish intake on serum lipids and lipoproteins in two populations with different dietary habits. *Br J Nutr* 83(4):371-379.

Tremblay, A., J. Despres, C. Leblanc, et al. 1990. Effect of intensity of physical activity on body fatness and fat distribution. *Am J Clin Nutr* 51:153-157.

Tucker, K.L., K. Morita, N. Qiao, M.T. Hannan, L.A. Cupples, and D.P Kiel. 2006. Colas, but not other carbonated beverages, are associated with low bone mineral density in older women: The Framingham Osteoporosis Study. *Am J Clin Nutr* 84(4):936-942.

Turner, R., R. Bauer, K. Woelkart, T. Hulsey, and J. Gangemi. 2005. An evaluation of Echinacea angustifolia in experimental rhinovirus infections. *New Eng J Med* 353(4):341-348.

USDA Pesticide Data Program. 2006. Annual summary calendar year 2005 [Online], p. 31. Available: www.ams.usda.gov/science/pdp/status.htm.

Van der Merwe, P., and E. Grobbelaar. 2005. Unintentional doping through the use of contaminated nutritional supplements. *S Afr Med J* 95(7):510-511.

van Loon L.J., R. Koopman, J.H. Stegen, A.J. Wagenmakers, H.A. Keizer, and W.H. Saris. 2003. Intramyocellular lipids form an important substrate source during moderate intensity exercise in endurance-trained males in a fasted state. *J Physiol* 553 (Pt. 2): 611-625.

Vander Wal, J.S., J.M. Marth, P. Khosla, C. Jen, and N.V. Dhurandhar. 2005. Short-term effect of eggs on satiety in overweight and obese subjects. *J Am Coll Nutr* 24(6):510-515.

Varner, L. 1995. Dual diagnosis: Patients with eating and substance-related disorders. *J Am Diet Assoc* 95(2):224-225.

Vega-Lopez, S., L.M. Ausman, J.L. Griffith, and A.H. Lichtenstein. 2007. Inter-individual reproducibility of glycemic index values for commercial white bread. *Diabetes Care* 30:1412-1417.

Vertanian, L., M. Schwartz, and K. Brownell. 2007. Effects of soft drink consumption on nutrition and health: A systematic review and meta-analysis. *Am J Public Health* 97:667-675.

Wagner, M., R. Keathley, and M. Bass. 2007. Developing a social norm intervention promotion campaign for student-athletes enrolled in a Division I-AA University. *Med Sci Sports Exerc* 39 (Suppl. no. 5): Abstract 1366.

Wallis, G., D. Rowlands, C. Shaw, R. Jentjens, and A. Jeukendrup. 2005. Oxidation of combined ingestion of maltodextrins and fructose during exercise. *Med Sci Sports Exerc* 37:426-432.

Wallis, G.A., S.E. Yeo, A.K. Blannin, and A.E Jeukendrup. 2007. Dose-response effects of ingested carbohydrate on exercise metabolism in women. *Med Sci Sports Exerc* 39(1):131-138.

Weaver, C. 2002. Adolescence: The period of dramatic bone growth. *Endocrine* 17:43-48.

Weaver, C.M., D. Teegarden, R.M. Lyle, et al. 2001. Impact of exercise on bone health and contraindication of oral contraceptive use in young women. *Med Sci Sports Exerc* 33:873-880.

Westerterp, K., G. Meijer, E. Janssen, W. Saris, and F. Ten Hoor. 1992. Long term effects of physical activity on energy balance and body composition. *Br J Med* 68(1):21-30.

Williams, P. 2007. Maintaining vigorous activity attenuates 7-year weight gain in 8340 runners. *Med Sci Sports Exerc* 39(5):801-809.

Wilmore, J., K. Wambsgans, M. Brenner, et al. 1992. Is there energy conservation in amenorrheic compared with eumenorrheic distance runners? *J Appl Physiol* 72(1):15-22.

Wing, R., and S. Phelan. 2005. Long-term weight loss maintenance. *Am J Clin Nutr* 82 (Suppl. no. 1): 222-225.

Wing, R.R., K.A. Matthews, L.H. Kuller, E.N. Meilahn, and P.L. Plantinga. 1991. Weight gain at the time of menopause. *Arch Intern Med* 151(1):97-102.

Winter, C., and S. Davis. 2006. Scientific status summary: Organic foods. *J Food Science* 71(9):R117.

Woo, R., J.S. Garrow, and F.X. Pi-Sunyer. 1982. Effect of exercise on spontaneous calorie intake in obesity. *Am J Clin Nutr* 36(3):470-477.

Woo, R., and F.X. Pi-Sunyer. 1985. Effect of increased physical activity on voluntary intake in lean women. *Metabolism* 34(9):836-841.

Woolsey, M. 2001. *Eating disorders: A clinical guide to counseling and treatment.* Chicago: American Dietetic Association.

World Cancer Research Fund and the American Institute for Cancer Research Expert Panel. 2007. Food, Nutrition, Physical Activity and the Prevention of Cancer; a Global Perspetive. www.dietandcancerreport.org

Wyatt, H.R., G.K. Grunwald, C.L. Mosca, M.L. Klem, R.R. Wing, and J.O. Hill. 2002. Long-term weight loss and breakfast in subjects in the National Weight Control Registry. *Obes Res* 10(2):78-82.

Wylie-Rosett, J., C.J. Segal-Isaacson, and A. Segal-Isaacson. 2004. Carbohydrates and increases in obesity: Does the type of carbohydrate make a difference? *Obes Res* 12 (Suppl. no. 2): 124-129.

Yoshioka, M., E. Doucet, S. St-Pierre, et al. 2001. Impact of high-intensity exercise on energy expenditure, lipid oxidation and body fatness. *Int J Obes Relat Metab Disord* 25(3):332-339.

Zachweija, J. 2002. Protein: Power or puffery? [Online]. Gatorade Sports Science Institute. Available: www.gssiweb.com

Zanker, C., and C. Cooke. 2004. Energy balance, bone turnover, and skeletal health in physically active individuals. *Med Sci Sports Exerc* 36(8):1372-1381.

Zarkadas, P., J. Carter, and E. Banister. 1994. Taper increases performance and aerobic power in triathletes. *Med Sci Sports Exerc* 26 (Suppl.): Abstract 194.

Zelasko, C. 1995. Exercise for weight loss: What are the facts? *J Am Diet Assoc* 95(12):1414-1417.

Zemel, M., W. Thompson, A. Milstead, K. Morris, and P. Campbell. 2004. Calcium and dairy acceleration of weight and fat loss during energy restriction in obese adults. *Obes Res* 12:582-590.

Zijp I., O. Korver, L. Tijburg. 2000. Effect of tea and other dietary factors on iron absorption. *Crit Rev Food Sci Nutr* 40(5):371-398.

APPENDIX C

Engineered Sports Fuels and Fluids

Athletes always ask me which brand of sports drink, gel, energy bar, protein bar or other commercial sports food is "the best." The answer is that the best product is the one that tastes best to *your* taste buds and settles well in *your* intestinal tract. Be sure to experiment with unfamiliar products during training, not during an important event.

While there is a time and place for many of these products, especially if you need fuel during intense exercise, these engineered products are more about convenience than necessity. They are neither magic nor better than natural foods. They are a commercial response to a marketing niche. The engineered sports food business is, indeed, a booming business!

As you look over this list, I invite you to appreciate the numerous categories of products, so you can see for yourself how enterprising businesses have developed a product for each market niche. Your job is to experiment with products during training to determine if they are worth the money, or if orange sections, bananas, water, defizzed cola, tea with honey, chocolate milk and other standard "sports foods" do as good a job at a lower price and with a better taste.

When making your choices, keep the following information in mind:

- Extra sodium is a good idea if you plan to exercise hard for more than two hours in the heat.
- Maltodextrins are often used for a sweetener because they are supposedly "longer lasting" than sucrose.
- Gels should always be tested during training. They can taste very sweet and are common contributors to diarrhea.
- Drinks labeled as recovery drinks offer a little protein along with the carbohydrate.

- Energy drinks offer concentrated sugar, often with added caffeine.

- Nutrition bars come in three basic types: energy-boosting preexercise snack bars, protein bars, and meal replacement bars. (You will also see diet or weight-loss bars in stores, but these are not listed here.)

- Energy bars should be eaten for extra energy, not as a meal replacement.

- Meal replacement bars offer some protein, vitamins and minerals, but they are better saved for emergency food than used as a standard meal replacement. They generally do not offer enough calories to replace an entire meal.

- Protein bars typically offer a blend of soy, whey, casein, and egg protein. They commonly offer 15 to 35 grams of protein. Because commercial-grade protein does not taste very good, these bars have strong flavors (such as chocolate mint) to mask the protein taste.

Sports Drinks

With Sodium
Gatorade, Edge Energy, Hydro-BOOM!, GU2O, Cytomax, Motor Tabs

Without Dye or Food Coloring
First Endurance EFS, Clif Shot Electrolyte Drink, Hammer Nutrition HEED, Recharge

Extra Sodium
Gatorade Endurance Formula, PowerBar Endurance, e-Fuel, First Endurance EFS, Clif Shot Electrolyte Drink, e load, Hydro Pro Cooler

Added Buffers
Cytomax, Perpetuem, Revenge Sport

Extra Carbohydrate
Carbo-Pro

Endurance Drinks
Perpetuem, Hammer Nutrition Sustained Energy, Edge Endless, Amino Vital

Maltodextrins as the Sweetener
Cytomax, Accelerade, PowerBar Endurance, HEED, GU2O

Added Protein
Amino Vital, Perpetuem, Accelerade, Revenge Pro

Recovery Drinks
Recoverite, Endurox R4, Ultragen

Added Extras
HEED (chromium, carnosine), Perpetuem (protein, fat, lactic acid buffer)

Fewer Calories For Dieters
PowerAde Option, Ultima Replenisher, Xxtra LowOz, Propel, nuun

For Women
Rain Sports Drink for Women (added calcium, folic acid, vitamin D)

Electrolytes
Endurolytes, nuun, e load Zone Caps

Gels
Gu, Carb-BOOM!, Clif Shot, Honey Stinger

Extra Sodium
PowerBar Gel, Crank Sports e-Gel, Cytomax Energy Gel

Added Protein
Accel Gel, Edge Endless, Hammer Gel

Added Caffeine

GU Espresso Love; Clif Shot Mocha, Cola, and Strawberry; Carb-BOOM! Chocolate Cherry; Hammer Gel Espresso; PowerBar Gel Double Latte, Tangerine, Chocolate, Green Apple, and Strawberry-Banana; Honey Stinger Ginsting and Strawberry

Added Extras

EAS Energy Gel (taurine), GU Energy Gel (histidine, ginger, chamomile)

Endurance Food

Jelly Belly Sport Beans (with sodium; kosher certified), Clif Shot Bloks (gummi candy in a block), Sharkies (organic fruit chew), SPIZ (liquid food), Revv Instant Energy (chocolate mint wafer)

Recovery Drinks

First Endurance E3, EAS Endurathon, Perpetuem, PowerBar Recovery Shake, Recoverite, Go Fast Energy Drink, Endurox R4, Gatorade Nutrition Shake, Hormel Health Labs Great Shake, GNC Pro Performance Distance, Clif Shot Recovery Drink, First Endurance Ultragen

Energy Drinks

Red Bull, Rock Star, Monster, Rebound*fx*, Full Throttle

Energy Bars

All Natural or Organic (No added vitamins or minerals)

Clif Bar, PeakBar, Perfect 10, Clif Nectar, Clif Mojo, LaraBar, Optimum, Trail Mix HoneyBar, Odwalla Bar, PowerBar Nut Naturals, Honey Stinger Bars, Kashi Bar, ReNew Life Organic Energy Bar, BoraBora Organic Bar, First Endurance

Granola-Type Bars

PowerBar Harvest, Nature Valley Granola Bar, Quaker Chewy Granola Bar, Nutri-Grain Bar

Women's Bars (Fewer calories; soy, calcium, iron, folic acid)

PowerBar Pria, Amino Vital Fit, Luna Bar, Balance Oasis

Low Carbohydrate Bars (40 percent carbohydrate calories)

Balance Bar, ZonePerfect

Kosher

Pure Fit Nutrition Bar, Lara Bar, ReNew Life Organic Energy Bar

Dairy-Free

Clif Nectar, Pure Fit, Perfect 10, LaraBar, Clif Builder's Bar

Soy-Based

Soyjoy

Fruit Only

Kalahari FruitTrekker Bar, Tropicana Fruitwise Strip

Gluten-Free

Perfect 10, Elev8Me, Hammer Bar, EnviroKidz Organic Crispy Rice Bar, Omega Smart Bar, ExtendBar, BumbleBar, ReNew Life Organic Energy Bar, Kalahari FruitTrekker Bar, Paleo-Bar

Wheat-Free (Not necessarily gluten-free)

Clif Nectar, Clif Builder's Bar, Odwalla Bar

Soy-Free

Carobar, Perfect-10, Clif Nectar, Vega Nutrition Bar, Organic Food Bar

Fructose-Free

JayBar, PaleoBar

Vegan

Pure Fit, LaraBar, Hammer Bar, Vega Whole Food Energy Bar, Clif Builder's Bar, Perfect 10, ReNew Life Organic Energy Bar

Bars With Caffeine

PeakBar Energy Plus

Vitamin and Protein-Pumped Candy Bars

Marathon Energy Bar, Detour Bar

Recovery Bar (4 to 1 Carbohydrate to Protein Ratio)

PowerBar Performance

Protein Bars

PowerBar ProteinPlus, EAS Myoplex Deluxe, High5 Protein Bar, Maximuscle Promax Meal, USN Pure Protein, Atkins Advantage, Tri-O-Plex, Clif Builder's Bar, Detour Bar, Honey Stinger Protein Bar, Special K Protein Meal Bar, AllGoode Organics, Boulder, GeniSoy, Spiru-Tein, Odwalla, Luna

Meal Replacement Bars

Kashi Go Lean Bar, Balance Satisfaction, MET-Rx Mr. Big, MET-Rx Big 100 Colossal

Meal Replacement Drinks

Carnation Instant Breakfast, Boost, Ensure, EAS Myoplex, MET-Rx RTD 40

Protein Powders

Hammer Soy, Hammer Whey, Bi-Pro Whey Protein Isolate, GNC Pro Performance 100% Whey Protein, CytoSport Muscle Milk

INDEX

Note: The italicized *f* and *t* following page numbers refer to figures and tables, respectively.

ABOUT THE AUTHOR

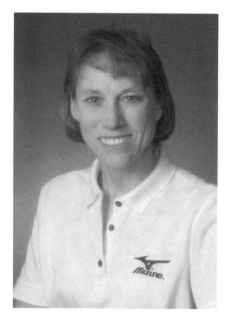

Nancy Clark, MS, RD, CSSD, renowned author and board-certified specialist in sports dietetics, is known for her ability to translate the science of nutrition for exercise and health into practical tips to enhance performance, manage weight, and resolve eating disorders. She has a private practice at Healthworks Fitness Center in Chestnut Hill, Massachusetts, where she offers nutrition consultations to both casual exercisers and competitive athletes. Her more renowned clients have included members of the Boston Red Sox, the Boston Celtics, and many collegiate, elite, and Olympic athletes from a variety of sports. She is also an advisory board member of Mizuno, Medical Wellness Association, and the Aerobics and Fitness Association of America.

An internationally known lecturer, Clark has given presentations to professional groups such as the American Dietetic Association (ADA) and the American College of Sports Medicine (ACSM), as well as team talks to athletes at Boston College and coaches with the Leukemia & Lymphoma Society's Team in Training national coaches certification program. She offers workshops nationally to health professionals with her sports nutrition workshop series. As a result of her renowned work, her photo and nutrition advice appeared on the back of the Wheaties box after the 2004 Summer Olympics.

Clark received her bachelor's degree in nutrition from Simmons College in Boston and her master's degree in nutrition from Boston University. She completed her internship in dietetics at Massachusetts General Hospital. She is a fellow of the American Dietetic Association, recipient of its Media Excellence Award, an active member of ADA's practice group of sports nutritionists (SCAN), and a recipient of that group's Honor Award. In addition, Clark is a fellow of the ACSM and a recipient of the Honor Award from ACSM's New England chapter. She is also the recipient of the 2007 Simmons College Distinguished Alumna Award.

Clark is the nutrition columnist for *New England Runner*, *Adventure Cycling*, and *American Fitness* and is a frequent contributor to sports and fitness publications such as *Shape* and *Runner's World*. Clark also writes a monthly nutrition column called "The Athlete's Kitchen," which appears regularly in over 100 sports publications and Web sites. She has authored *Nancy Clark's Food Guide for Marathoners: Tips for Everyday Champions* and *The Cyclist's Food Guide: Fueling for the Distance*.

Clark has competed at the 10K, half-marathon, and marathon distances. She has led many extended bike tours, including a Transamerica Trip and other tours through the Canadian and Colorado Rockies. She has trekked into the Himalayas and planned the high-altitude menu for a successful expedition. Her newest sport is rowing. She and her husband, son, and daughter live in the Boston area.

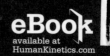